Late Effects of Treatment for Brain Tumors

Cancer Treatment and Research
Steven T. Rosen, M.D., *Series Editor*

Bashey, A., Ball, E.D. (eds): *Non-Myeloablative Allogeneic Transplantation.* 2002. ISBN 0-7923-7646-3.
Leong, S. P.L. (ed.): *Atlas of Selective Sentinel Lymphadenectomy for Melanoma, Breast Cancer and Colon Cancer.* 2002. ISBN 1-4020-7013-6.
Andersson, B., Murray D. (eds): *Clinically Relevant Resistance in Cancer Chemotherapy.* 2002. ISBN 1-4020-7200-7.
Beam, C. (ed.): *Biostatistical Applications in Cancer Research.* 2002. ISBN 1-4020-7226-0.
Brockstein, B., Masters, G. (eds): *Head and Neck Cancer.* 2003. ISBN 1-4020-7336-4.
Frank, D.A. (ed.): *Signal Transduction in Cancer.* 2003. ISBN 1-4020-7340-2.
Figlin, R. A. (ed.): *Kidney Cancer.* 2003. ISBN 1-4020-7457-3.
Kirsch, M.; Black, P. McL. (ed.): *Angiogenesis in Brain Tumors.* 2003. ISBN 1-4020-7704-1.
Keller, E.T., Chung, L.W.K. (eds): *The Biology of Skeletal Metastases.* 2004. ISBN 1-4020-7749-1.
Kumar, R. (ed.): *Molecular Targeting and Signal Transduction.* 2004. ISBN 1-4020-7822-6.
Verweij, J., Pinedo, H.M. (eds): *Targeting Treatment of Soft Tissue Sarcomas.* 2004. ISBN 1-4020-7808-0.
Finn, W.G., Peterson, L.C. (eds.): *Hematopathology in Oncology.* 2004. ISBN 1-4020-7919-2.
Farid, N. (ed.): *Molecular Basis of Thyroid Cancer.* 2004. ISBN 1-4020-8106-5.
Khleif, S. (ed.): *Tumor Immunology and Cancer Vaccines.* 2004. ISBN 1-4020-8119-7.
Balducci, L., Extermann, M. (eds): *Biological Basis of Geriatric Oncology.* 2004. ISBN
Abrey, L.E., Chamberlain, M.C., Engelhard, H.H. (eds): *Leptomeningeal Metastases.* 2005. ISBN 0-387-24198-1
Platanias, L.C. (ed.): *Cytokines and Cancer.* 2005. ISBN 0-387-24360-7.
Leong, S.P.L., Kitagawa, Y., Kitajima, M. (eds): *Selective Sentinel Lymphadenectomy for Human Solid Cancer.* 2005. ISBN 0-387-23603-1.
Small, Jr. W., Woloschak, G. (eds): *Radiation Toxicity: A Practical Guide.* 2005. ISBN 1-4020-8053-0.
Haefner, B., Dalgleish, A. (eds): *The Link Between Inflammation and Cancer.* 2006. ISBN 0-387-26282-2.
Leonard, J.P., Coleman, M. (eds): *Hodgkin's and Non-Hodgkin's Lymphoma.* 2006. ISBN 0-387-29345.
Leong, S.P.L. (ed): *Cancer Clinical Trials: Proactive Strategies.* 2006. ISBN 0-387-33224-3.
Meyers, C. (ed): *Aids-Associated Viral Oncogenesis.* 2007. ISBN 978-0-387-46804-4.
Ceelen, W.P. (ed): *Peritoneal Carcinomatosis: A Multidisciplinary Approach.* 2007. ISBN 978-0-387-48991-9.
Leong, S.P.L. (ed): *Cancer Metastasis and the Lymphovascular System: Basis for Rational Therapy.* 2007. ISBN 978-0-387-69218-0.
Raizer, J., Abrey, L.E. (eds): *Brain Metastases.* 2007. ISBN 978-0-387-69221-0.
Woodruff, T., Snyder, K.A. (eds): *Oncofertility.* 2007. ISBN 978-0-387-72292-4.
Angelos, P. (ed): *Ethical Issues in Cancer Patient Care, Second Edition.* 2008. ISBN 978-0-387-73638-9.
Ansell, S. (ed): *Rare Hematological Malignancies.* 2008. ISBN 978-0-387-73743-0.
Gradishar, W.J., Wood, W.C. (eds): *Advances in Breast Care Management, Second Edition.* 2008. 978-0-387-73160-5.
Blake, M., Kalra, M. (eds): *Imaging in Oncology.* 2008. ISBN 978-0-387-75586-1.
Bishop, M.R. (ed): *Hematopoietic Stem Cell Transplantation.* 2008. ISBN 978-0-387-78579-0.
Stockfleth, E., Ulrich, C. (eds): *Skin Cancer after Organ Transplantation.* 2008. ISBN 978-0-387-78573-8.
Fuqua, S.A.W. (ed): *Hormone Receptors in Breast Cancer,* 2008. ISBN: 978-0-387-09462-5.
Green, D., Kwaan H.C. (eds): *Coagulation in Cancer,* 2009. ISBN: 978-0-387-79961-2.
Stack, M.S., Fishman, D.A. (eds): *Ovarian Cancer, Second Edition,* 2009. ISBN: 978-0-387-98093-5.
Goldman, S., Turner, C.D. (eds): *Late Effects of Treatment for Brain Tumors,* 2009. ISBN: 978-0-387-77102-1.

Stewart Goldman · Christopher D. Turner

Editors

Late Effects of Treatment for Brain Tumors

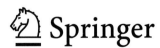 Springer

Editors

Stewart Goldman
Department of Pediatrics
Children's Memorial Hospital
Northwestern University
2300 Children's Plaza
Chicago IL 30614
USA
sgoldman@northwestern.edu

Christopher D. Turner
Department of Pediatric Oncology
Harvard Medical School
Dana-Farber Cancer Institute
44 Binney St.
Boston MA 02115
USA
christopher_turner@dfci.harvard.edu

ISSN 0927-3042
ISBN 978-0-387-77102-1   e-ISBN 978-0-387-77103-8
DOI 10.1007/b109924
Springer Dordrecht Heidelberg London New York

Library of Congress Control Number: 2008944167

Printed on acid-free paper

Springer is part of Springer Science+Business Media (www.springer.com)

Acknowledgments

We are forever indebted to our colleagues and friends for their perseverance and hard work in authoring this work.

We would like to thank and dedicate this book to our families, for their patience and encouragement as we completed this project. Thanks to Dee, Charlotte, Hannah and Kyle Goldman and Christen, Cameron and Kyle Turner. You are our inspiration and source of happiness.

To my father, Sol Goldman, who found such value, knowledge and compassion in books (SG) and to Ann and Joseph Turner who instilled a thirst for knowledge, a desire to heal, and modeled compassion and humility (CT).

We also would like to thank our patients, their families, and their communities for your courage and the lessons you teach us daily. We are honored that you allow us into your lives, may they be long and healthy.

Stewart Goldman & Christopher Turner

Contents

Part IV Additional Topics

Contributors

Vicki A. Anderson Australian Centre for Child Neuropsychology Studies, Murdoch Children's Research Institute and Department of Psychology, Royal Children's Hospital, Melbourne, VIC, Australia; Murdoch Children's Research Institute, Royal Children's Hospital, Melbourne, VIC, Australia; School of Behavioural Science, University of Melbourne, Melbourne, VIC, Australia

David M. Ashley, MD Children's Cancer Centre, Royal Children's Hospital, Melbourne, VIC, Australia; Murdoch Children's Research Institute, Royal Children's Hospital, Melbourne, VIC, Australia

Kanyalakshmi Ayyanar, MD Pediatric Hematology/Oncology, Kosair Children's Hospital, University of Louisville, Louisville, KY 40202, USA

Smita Bhatia, MD, MPH Division of Population Sciences, City of Hope National Medical Center, Duarte, CA, USA, sbhatia@coh.org

Melanie J. Bonner, PhD Departments of Psychiatry and Surgery, Preston Robert Tisch Brain Tumor Center, Duke University Medical Center, Durham, NC, USA; Department of Psychology and Neuroscience, Duke University, Durham, NC, USA, bonne002@mc.duke.edu

Daniel C. Bowers, MD Division of Pediatric Hematology-Oncology, University of Texas Southwestern Medical School, 5323 Harry Hines Blvd, Dallas, TX 75390-9063, USA, daniel.bowers@utsouthwestern.edu

Roberta D. Calhoun-Eagan, LCSW, ACSW, OSW-C Canandaigua VAMedical Center, 400 Fort Hill Avenue, Canandaigua, NY 14424, USA, roberta.calhoun-eagan@va.gov

Rowena Conroy Children's Cancer Centre, Royal Children's Hospital, Melbourne, VIC, Australia; Murdoch Children's Research Institute, Royal Children's Hospital, Melbourne, VIC, Australia

Karina Danner-Koptik, RN, MSN, APN, CPON Children's Memorial Medical Center, 2300 Children's Plaza, Box 30, Chicago, IL 60614-3394, USA

Elizabeth Dean-Clower, MD, MPH   Harvard Medical School, Boston, MA, USA; Leonard P. Zakim Center for Integrative Therapies, Dana-Farber Cancer Institute, Boston, MA, USA

B. Elizabeth Delasobera   Stanford University School of Medicine, Stanford, CA, USA

Cinzia R. De Luca   Children's Cancer Centre, Royal Children's Hospital, Melbourne, VIC, Australia; Australian Centre for Child Neuropsychology Studies, Murdoch Children's Research Institute and Department of Psychology, Royal Children's Hospital, Melbourne, VIC, Australia; School of Behavioural Science, University of Melbourne, Melbourne, VIC, Australia, cinzia.deluca@rch.org.au

Jörg Dietrich, MD, PhD   Department of Neurology, Brigham and Women's Hospital, 75 Francis Street, Boston, MA 02115, USA; Department of Neurology, Massachusetts General Hospital, 55 Fruit Street, Boston, MA 02114, USA, jdietrich1@partners.org

Kimberly J. Dilley, MD, MPH   Division of Hematology/Oncology/Transplant, Children's Memorial Hospital, Chicago, IL, USA; Northwestern University Feinberg School of Medicine, 2300 Children's Plaza, Box #30, Chicago, IL 60614, USA, kdilley@childrensmemorial.org

Arthur J. DiPatri Jr., MD   Department of Neurological Surgery, Northwestern University Feinberg School of Medicine, Chicago, IL, USA; Division of Pediatric Neurosurgery, Children's Memorial Hospital, Chicago, IL, USA, adipatri@childrensmemorial.org

Anne M. Doherty-Gilman, MPH   Leonard P. Zakim Center for Integrative Therapies, Dana-Farber Cancer Institute, Boston, MA, USA

María E. Echevarría, MD   San Jorge Children's Hospital, Division of Hematology/Oncology and Stem Cell Transplant, San Juan, PR, USA, mechevarria@sjcms.com

Jason R. Fangusaro, MD   Department of Pediatric Hematology/Oncology and Stem Cell Transplantation, Children's Memorial Hospital, 2300 Children's Plaza, Box #30, Chicago, IL, USA, jfangusaro@childrensmemorial.org

Paul Graham Fisher, MD, MHS   Departments of Neurology, Pediatrics, Neurosurgery, and Human Biology, Stanford University Medical Center, 875 Blake Wilbur Drive, Palo Alto, CA 94305-5826, USA, pfisher@stanford.edu

Stewart Goldman, MD   Children's Memorial Hospital, Northwestern University, Fienberg School of Medicine, 2300 Children's Plaza, Box #30, Chicago, IL 60614-3394, USA, sgoldman@childrensmemorial.org

Tress Goodwin   Stanford University, 875 Blake Wilbur Drive, Palo Alto, CA 94305-5826, USA, tgoodwin@stanford.edu

Dawn Grenier   National Brain Tumor Society, 124 Watertown Street, Suite 3H, Watertown, MA 02472-2500, USA, grenier@braintumor.org

Sarah Gupta, LICSW   National Brain Tumor Society, 124 Watertown Street, Suite 3H, Watertown, MA 02472-2500, USA, gupta@braintumor.org

A. Bebe Guill, MDiv   Duke Institute on Care at the End of Life, Duke Divinity School, Duke University Medical Center, Durham, NC 27710, USA, guill004@mc.duke.edu

Sridharan Gururangan MRCP (UK)   The Preston Robert Tisch Brain Tumor Center and the Departments of Pediatrics and Surgery, Duke University Medical Center, Durham, NC 27710, USA, gurur002@mc.duke.edu

David A. Jacobsohn, MD   Children's Memorial Medical Center, Chicago, IL, USA; Northwestern University's Feinberg School of Medicine, 2300 Children's Plaza, Box 30, Chicago, IL 60614, USA, djacobsohn@childrensmemorial.org

Santosh Kesari, MD, PhD   Department of Neurology, Brigham and Women's Hospital, 75 Francis Street, Boston, MA 02115, USA; Dana-Farber Cancer Institute, Center for Neuro-Oncology, 44 Binney Street, Boston, MA 02115, USA; Harvard Medical School, Boston, MA, USA, skesari@partners.org

Karen E. Kinahan, RN, MS, APRN,   Survivors Taking Action & Responsibility, Chicago, IL, USA; Robert H. Lurie Comprehensive Cancer Center of Northwestern University, Chicago, IL, USA, k-kinahan@northwestern.edu

Wendy Landier, RN, MSN, CPNP   Department of Population Sciences, Center for Cancer Survivorship, City of Hope National Medical Center, Duarte, CA, USA, wlandier@coh.org

Elizabeth Eaumann Littlejohn, MD   Department of Pediatrics, Section of Endocrinology, University of Chicago Hospital, Chicago, IL, USA, ebaumann@peds.bsd.uchicago.edu

Barbara Lockart, RN, MSN, CPNP   Division of Hematology/Oncology/ Transplant Children's Memorial Hospital, 2300 Children's Plaza, Box #30, Chicago, IL 60614, USA, blockart@childrensmemorial.org

Jay S. Loeffler, MD   Harvard Medical School, Boston, MA, USA; Department of Radiation Oncology, Massachusetts General Hospital, 100 Blossom St., Cox 3, Boston, MA 02114, USA, jloeffler@partners.org

Craig Lustig, MPA,   Children's Cause for Cancer Advocacy, 595 Second Street, Brooklyn, NY 11215-2601, USA

Maria McCarthy Children's Cancer Centre, Royal Children's Hospital, Melbourne, VIC, Australia; Murdoch Children's Research Institute, Royal Children's Hospital, Melbourne, VIC, Australia

Anna K. Meyer, MD Division of Pediatric Otolaryngology, Department of Otolaryngology-Head & Neck Surgery, University of California, San Francisco, CA, USA

Grace P. Monaco, JD Medical Care Management Corporation, The Candlelighters Childhood Cancer Foundation, Washington, DC, USA, gpmonaco@hughes.net

Michelle Monje, MD, PhD Department of Neurology, Brigham and Women's Hospital and Massachusetts General Hospital, 75 Francis Street, Boston, MA 02115, USA

Tracy Moore, LCSW Director of Social Work, North Shore University Hospital, 300 Community Drive, Manhassett, NY 11030, tmoore2@nshs.edu

Kenji Muro, MD Department of Neurological Surgery, Northwestern University Feinberg School of Medicine, Chicago, IL, USA; Division of Pediatric Neurosurgery, Children's Memorial Hospital, Chicago, IL, USA, kenji.muro@nmff.org

Sonia Partap, MD Stanford University, 875 Blake Wilbur Drive, Palo Alto, CA 94305-5826, USA, spartap@stanford.edu

Keith P. Pasichow Mount Sinai School of Medicine, New York, NY, USA

Martin Pham, BS Department of Neurological Surgery, Northwestern University Feinberg School of Medicine, Chicago, IL, USA; Division of Pediatric Neurosurgery, Children's Memorial Hospital, Chicago, IL, USA

David S. Rosenthal, MD Harvard Medical School, Boston, MA, USA; Leonard P. Zakim Center for Integrative Therapies, Dana-Farber Cancer Institute, 44 Binney Street, Boston, MA 02115, USA, drose@uhs.harvard.edu

Stephen A. Sands, PsyD, Herbert Irving Division of Child and Adolescent Oncology, Departments of Pediatrics and Psychiatry, Columbia University Medical Center, 161 Fort Washington Avenue, New York, NY 10032, USA, ss2341@columbia.edu

Susan Shaw, RN, MS, PNP Center for Children's Cancer and Blood Disorders, SUNY Upstate Medical University, Syracuse, NY, USA

Helen A. Shih, MD, MPH Harvard Medical School, Boston, MA, USA; Department of Radiation Oncology, Massachusetts General Hospital, 100 Blossom St., Cox 3, Boston, MA 02114, USA, hshih@partners.org

Gilbert Smith, JD Childhood Cancer Ombudsman Program, Burgess, VA, USA

Lisa G. Sorensen, PhD Children's Memorial Hospital, Chicago, IL, USA; Feinberg School of Medicine, Northwestern University, Chicago, IL, USA, lsorensen@chidrensmemorial.org

Nancy J. Tarbell, MD Harvard Medical School, Boston, MA, USA; Division of Pediatric Radiation Oncology, Massachusetts General Hospital, 55 Fruit Street, Bulfinch 370, Boston, MA 02114, USA, tarbell.nancy@mgh.harvard.edu

Christopher D. Turner, MD Harvard Medical School, Boston, MA, USA; Pediatric Neuro-Oncology Outcomes Research, Pediatric Representative, Leonard P. Zakim Center for Integrative Therapies, Dana-Farber Cancer Institute, 44 Binney Street, Boston, MA 02115, USA, christopher_turner@dfci.harvard.edu

Stacia Wagner, LSW Children's Brain Tumor Foundation, 274 Madison Avenue Suite 1004, New York, NY 10016, swagner@cbtf.org

Melody A. Watral, MSN, RN, CPNP, CPON Pediatric Neuro-Oncology, The Preston Robert Tisch Brain Tumor Center, Duke University Medical Center, Durham, NC, USA, watra001@mc.duke.edu

Joanna L. Weinstein, MD Division of Hematology, Oncology and Stem Cell Transplantation, Children's Memorial Hospital, Chicago, IL, USA

Patrick Y. Wen, MD Director of Neuro-Oncology, Packard Hospital, Center for Neuro-Oncology, Dana-Farber/Brigham and Women's Cancer Center, Boston, MA 02115, USA; Division of Neuro-Oncology, Department of Neurology, Brigham and Women's Hospital, Boston, MA 02115, USA, pwen@partners.org

Susan L. Weiner, PhD Children's Brain Tumor Foundation, 274 Madison Avenue, New York, NY 10016, USA, slweiner@childrenscause.org

Joanna L. Weinstein, MD Division of Hematology, Oncology and Stem Cell Transplantation, Children's Memorial Hospital, Chicago, IL, USA, jweinstein@childrensmemorial.org

Victoria W. Willard, MA Department of Psychology and Neuroscience, Duke University, Durham, NC, USA

Nancy M. Young, MD Section of Otology/Neurotology, Otolaryngology, Cochlear Implant Program and Audiology, Children's Memorial Medical Center, Chicago, IL 60614-3394, USA; Northwestern University's Feinberg School of Medicine, Children's Memorial Medical Center, 2300 Children's Plaza, Chicago, IL 60614-3394, USA

Frank A.J. Zelko, PhD Pediatric Neuropsychology, Children's Memorial Hospital, Chicago, IL, USA; Feinberg School of Medicine, Northwestern University, Chicago, IL, USA, fzelko@childrensmemorial.org

Part I
Overview of Brain Tumor Survivorship

Chapter 1
Introduction to Brain Tumor Survivorship and Historical Perspective

Stewart Goldman and Christopher D. Turner

Introduction

"Death precludes late effects." This attitude was our (and many others') first introduction to the issues of survivorship, and reflected the Oncologist's viewpoint of the late 1980s and early 1990s. Today, though neuro-oncologists are focused on increasing cure rates, we are increasingly aware that "the costs of the cure have a lifetime to be repaid" and, thus, our focus on late effects have taken on increased interest.

Background

The field of cancer survivorship is relatively new. Interest in cancer survivors and the late effects they experience has grown as the number of cancer survivors in the United States has tripled in the last 30 years to more than 11 million in 2005.[1] One should, therefore, not be surprised to learn that there has been a rapid increase in the number of publications on cancer late effects and survivorship issues within the last decade. A simple search of PubMed for the term "cancer survivorship" in the title or abstract reveals only 38 publications before the year 2000 and 186 publications since then [http://www.ncbi.nlm.nih.gov/pubmed/ accessed November 30, 2008] Many of the early publications on cancer survivors before 1990 dealt exclusively with a single type of cancer or a single late effect. In 1974, Meadows was one of the first to describe and advocate for a comprehensive approach to evaluate cancer survivors for treatment related late effects,[2] but the concept took time to catch on. Through the rest of the 1970s and 1980s there were relatively few broad publications of cancer

S. Goldman (✉)
Gus Foundation Chair Neuro-Oncology, Medical Director Neuro-Oncology,
Associate Professor of Pediatrics, Children's Memorial Hospital, Northwestern
University, Fienberg School of Medicine, Chicago, IL 60614-3394, USA
e-mail: sgoldman@childrensmemorial.org

S. Goldman, C.D. Turner (eds.), *Late Effects of Treatment for Brain Tumors*,
Cancer Treatment and Research 150, DOI 10.1007/b109924_1,
© Springer Science+Business Media, LLC 2009

survivorship issues across many disciplines that were published through the medical literature.[3-6] While the number of cancer survivors was growing during this period, their numbers were still relatively small when compared to the total number of patients diagnosed with cancer. The focus of oncologists and others that cared for cancer patients was justifiably focused on improving survival first, but by the end of the 1990s the five-year relative survival rate for all malignancies combined had increased to 64%.[7] It is notable to point out that beginning in the 1980s researchers began to focus attention on the central nervous system late effects associated with the treatment of childhood leukemia and brain tumors, and there were several important early studies reported.[8-16]

A second converging phenomenon was also occurring in the oncology community in the late 1980s and into the 1990s. Cancer survivors began to organize in greater numbers and the cancer survivorship advocacy community began to strengthen and grow. The National Coalition for Cancer Survivorship (NCCS), a broad reaching cancer advocacy coalition, was founded in 1986 and a more unified voice was being heard from survivors.[17] Instead of just being "happy to be alive" these groups brought increasing attention to the plethora of late effects experienced by the increasing number of cancer survivors.

The growing importance of these two trends, the increased number of survivors and a stronger, more unified cancer survivorship advocacy network, converged in 1996 when the National Cancer Institute (NCI) established an Office of Cancer Survivorship to focus research efforts on the short- and long-term consequences of cancer and its treatment.[18] Since then, there has been a rapid increase in grant support and publications on the late effects of cancer treatments.

Much of the early work in this field has focused on childhood cancer survivors, but in the last few years increased focus is being paid to survivors of adult malignancies. Unfortunately, survivors of CNS malignancies have been either excluded or underrepresented in many of the earlier late effect studies.

In the case of pediatric CNS tumor survivors, the concern was that their neurocognitive deficits would adversely affect the results and, in the case of adult CNS tumor survivors, the number of long-term survivors of malignant tumors was often not large enough to study. Recently, more attention has focused on CNS tumor survivors. The neurocognitive late effects of pediatric CNS tumor survivors due to the tumor or its treatment have been better described in recent publications.[19-21] There is also an ongoing effort to enrich a new cohort of the much-publicized Childhood Cancer Survivorship Study with survivors of CNS tumors, recognizing that this population was not adequately represented in the original cohort.

Research on survivors of adult CNS tumors has benefited from broader acceptance of the widening of the definition of cancer survivorship research to include patients from the time of diagnosis forward in examining the effects of treatment on an individual. Unfortunately, the percentage of adult CNS tumor survivors has not meaningfully changed, due in large part to limited advancement in the survival of those with high-grade gliomas.

As one proceeds through this book, it is important to recognize that cancer survivorship is a journey encompassing many phases, from recovery of the acute toxicities of therapy to the psychological adjustments of the survivor, their families, friends, teachers, coworkers and society. Survivors of brain tumors face the long-term late effects described in the subsequent chapters of this book, as well as challenges by a world not adequately prepared to adapt and accept this growing population.

Scope of this Book

The goal of this book is to present the current knowledge of late effects experienced by survivors of CNS malignancies for both children and adults in one comprehensive text.

The intended audience is physicians, nurses, psychologists and other health care professionals who care for CNS tumor survivors. We hope this book, together with our patients and their families, will be an aid for the future.

References

1. NCI. 2008. Estimated Number of Cancer Survivors in the United States from 1971 to 2005. Available at: http://cancercontrol.cancer.gov/ocs/prevalence/revalence.html. Accessed November 30, 2008.
2. Meadows AT, D'Angio GJ. Late effects of cancer treatment: methods and techniques for detection. *Semin Oncol.* 1974;1:87–90.
3. Hobbie WL. The role of the pediatric oncology nurse specialist in a follow-up clinic for long-term survivors of childhood cancer. *J Assoc Pediatr Oncol Nurses.* 1986;3:9–12, 24.
4. Welch-McCaffrey D, Hoffman B, Leigh SA, et al. Surviving adult cancers. Part 2: Psychosocial implications. *Ann Intern Med.* 1989;111:517–524.
5. Loescher LJ, Welch-McCaffrey D, Leigh SA, et al. Surviving adult cancers. Part 1: Physiologic effects. *Ann Intern Med.* 1989;111:411–432.
6. Hoffman B. Current issues of cancer survivorship. *Oncology.* (Williston Park) 1989;3:85–88; discussion 9–91, 4–5.
7. Ries LAG, Melbert D, Krapcho M, et al. (eds). *SEER Cancer Statistics Review, 1975–2005.* Bethesda, MD: National Cancer Institute. Available at: http://seer.cancer.gov/csr/1975_2005/, based on November 2007 SEER data submission, posted to the SEER web site, 2008.
8. Meadows AT, D'Angio GJ. Late effects of cancer treatment: methods and techniques for detection. *Semin Oncol.* 1974;1:87–90.
9. Hobbie WL. The role of the pediatric oncology nurse specialist in a follow-up clinic for long-term survivors of childhood cancer. *J Assoc Pediatr Oncol Nurses.* 1986;3:9–12, 24.
10. Danoff BF, Cowchock FS, Marquette C, et al. Assessment of the long-term effects of primary radiation therapy for brain tumors in children. *Cancer.* 1982;49:1580–86.
11. Duffner PK, Cohen ME, Thomas P. Late effects of treatment on the intelligence of children with posterior fossa tumors. *Cancer.* 1983;51:233–237.
12. Kun LE, Mulhern RK, Crisco JJ. Quality of life in children treated for brain tumors. Intellectual, emotional, and academic function. *J Neurosurg.* 1983;58:1–6.

13. Duffner PK, Cohen ME, Thomas PR, et al. The long-term effects of cranial irradiation on the central nervous system. *Cancer*. 1985;56:1841–1846.
14. Packer RJ, Meadows AT, Rorke LB, et al. Long-term sequelae of cancer treatment on the central nervous system in childhood. *Med Pediatr Oncol*. 1987;15:241–253.
15. Mulhern RK, Kovnar EH, Kun LE, et al. Psychologic and neurologic function following treatment for childhood temporal lobe astrocytoma. *J Child Neurol*. 1988;3:47–52.
16. Packer RJ, Sutton LN, Atkins TE, et al. A prospective study of cognitive function in children receiving whole-brain radiotherapy and chemotherapy: 2-year results. *J Neurosurg*. 1989;70:707–713.
17. NCCS (National Coalition for Cancer Survivorship) 1996. Imperatives for Quality Cancer Care: Access, Advocacy, Action, and Accountability. Clark EJ, Stovall EL, Leigh S, Siu AL, Austin DK, Rowland JH. Silver Spring, MD:NCCS.
18. Committee on Cancer Survivorship: Improving Care and Quality of Life. From cancer patient to cancer survivor: lost in transition. In: Hewit M, Greenfield S, Stovall E. eds. *National Cancer Policy Board*. Washington, DC: The National Academies Press; 2005: 28–30.
19. Moore BD, 3rd. Neurocognitive outcomes in survivors of childhood cancer. *J Pediatr Psychol*. 2005;30:51–63.
20. Mulhern RK, Merchant TE, Gajjar A, et al. Late neurocognitive sequelae in survivors of brain tumours in childhood. *Lancet Oncol*. 2004;5:399–408.
21. Packer RJ, Mehta M. Neurocognitive sequelae of cancer treatment. *Neurology*. 2002;59:8–10.

Chapter 2
Late Effects of Neurosurgery

Arthur J. DiPatri, Jr., Martin Pham, and Kenji Muro

Introduction

For most diagnoses in neuro-oncology, surgery plays a key role in the multi-disciplinary patient management strategy. While the goals of surgery will vary between specific cases, most procedures are performed with the intention to procure tissue to establish the histological diagnosis, to alleviate mass effect on the surrounding structures, and to achieve maximal cytoreduction in anticipation of subsequent adjuvant therapy. Since many patients will go on to require other treatments such as chemotherapy and radiation therapy, the long-term effects of the surgery itself can be difficult to determine. In this chapter, we will provide a historical perspective on the specialty of neurosurgery and discuss the evolution of techniques and noteworthy innovations that have contributed to a reduction in morbidity and mortality and, ultimately, in an improvement in the incidence and severity of late effects. Since the neurological, cognitive and endocrinological late effects of treatment are discussed elsewhere in this text, we will limit our discussion to the late effects related to the surgical treatment of central nervous system tumors.

Historical Perspectives and Technical Innovations

The field of neurological surgery had its origins near the end of the 19th century in England. Up until that time, little progress had been made since the Middle Ages and most attempts at surgery on the central nervous system were doomed to failure. Without concurrent advances in the fields of antisepsis and anesthesia and perhaps, more importantly, the development of the concepts of cerebral localization, the establishment of neurosurgery as a separate surgical discipline

A.J. DiPatri (✉)
Department of Neurological Surgery, Northwestern University Feinberg
School of Medicine, Division of Pediatric Neurosurgery,
Children's Memorial Hospital, Chicago, IL, USA
e-mail: adipatri@childrensmemorial.org

S. Goldman, C.D. Turner (eds.), *Late Effects of Treatment for Brain Tumors*,   7
Cancer Treatment and Research 150, DOI 10.1007/b109924_2,
© Springer Science+Business Media, LLC 2009

would not have been possible. During this era, general surgeons who had a special interest in the nervous system performed most of the surgery on the brain. Oftentimes, these cases were undertaken under a neurologist's direction and misdiagnosis was common. Due to the high risk associated with these procedures, surgery on the brain and spinal cord was usually considered only as a last resort and reserved for only the most moribund of patients.

William Macewen, a Scottish surgeon, is credited with being the first surgeon to use localizing signs to guide surgery for lesions within the brain.[1] By 1879 he had successfully treated disorders such as abscesses and cysts[2] whereas prior to that time most surgery on the head was restricted to the management of trauma. In the last part of the 19th century, Victor Horsley, an English neurosurgeon, began to persuade his medical colleagues that more could be achieved in the treatment of gliomas and epilepsy, particularly with earlier diagnosis.[3] Other leading European surgeons would also make important contributions to the field. During the early part of the 20th century, Harvey Cushing pioneered various techniques that would become instrumental in establishing neurosurgery as a distinct surgical specialty and for that he is commonly regarded as the father of American neurosurgery. In 1901, with Cushing just embarking on his neurosurgical career, morbidity was excessive and mortality rates varied between 30–50% for brain tumor surgery.[4] While many of Cushing's original contributions to neurosurgery were in the area of brain tumor surgery he also added to our understanding of vasomotor physiology, the control of intracranial hemorrhage, and to our knowledge of and treatment of elevated intracranial pressure. Notably, by 1910 his reported mortality rate for brain tumor surgery had decreased to only 13%.[5]

Closely related to the development of improved neurosurgical techniques were advances in the related fields of anatomy, physiology and pathology. Much of what was and would soon be accomplished by pioneering neurosurgeons would not have occurred were it not for simultaneous improvements in the field of anesthesia. From the first successfully administered anesthetics near the end of the 19th century through the first few decades of their use, the primary goal of the anesthetist was to see to it that the patient survived the operation.[2] Improvements in the delivery of volatile agents, the development of local anesthetics, the increased utilization of endotracheal intubation and the development of modern inhalational anesthetics enabled the anesthetist to not only increase the safety of the procedure, but also to provide optimal conditions for neurosurgical procedures.[2] Today, the neuroanesthesiologist plays an important role in reducing the morbidity and mortality associated with surgery of the central nervous system and the surgical management of brain lesions. The selection of specific anesthetic agents and techniques is tailored to facilitate surgical exposure, optimize the balance between cerebral blood flow and metabolism, preserve cerebral autoregulation, and allow for rapid emergence from anesthesia to provide for rapid intraoperative or post-operative neurological assessment.[6] Neuroanesthetic techniques also facilitate specialized neurosurgical procedures, like awake craniotomy with cortical mapping, as well as other types of neurosurgical procedures that require intraoperative electrophysiological mapping or monitoring.

The development of neuroimaging techniques would improve the surgeon's ability to precisely localize intracranial lesions, and continued progress in the field has been instrumental in advancing the field of neurosurgery. While radiographs could detect the presence of calcified lesions or areas of erosion of the skull, they only indirectly inferred the presence of a lesion. With the introduction of pneumoencephalography by Walter Dandy in 1918,[7] direct views of the ventricular system could be obtained, but the presence of a lesion within the brain parenchyma still had to be inferred. With the introduction of cerebral angiography in 1927[8] and its ability to accurately define the cerebral vasculature, details about brain surface anatomy could now be deduced. These techniques would continue to be the primary neuroimaging modalities until the introduction of computed tomography (CT) in the 1970s.[9] CT surpassed all other types of brain imaging by providing real-time images of intracranial structures. The location of an intracranial lesion would no longer have to be inferred from indirect information, and CT had the added benefit of being more comfortable for the patient. With the introduction of magnetic resonance imaging (MRI) into clinical practice in the early 1980s, MRI would soon become the premier imaging method by providing precise structural information.

The development of frame-based stereotactic surgery gave the neurological surgeon the ability to precisely target subcortical structures for the treatment of movement disorders, pain disorders and epilepsy, as well as perform abscess drainage, tumor biopsies and resections.[10–12] While considered by many to be the gold standard for the three-dimensional localization of an intracranial target or lesion, there are certain disadvantages of having a stereotactic frame in place. First, frame application may need to be performed under general anesthesia and may be technically difficult in children with thin skulls. Lesions in the posterior fossa can be difficult to target and in some cases the frame itself may restrict access to some areas of the surgical field. Additionally, since changing the stereotactic target during surgery can be cumbersome, only a limited number of end points can be targeted during any one surgical setting.[13] An alternative technique, frameless stereotactic neuronavigation, was later developed to obviate the need for a head-mounted frame. Stereotactic workstations translate cross-sectional CT or MRI data into stereotactic coordinates, and an optical tracking system is utilized to determine the position of a selected instrument tip in relation to the patient's three-dimensionally defined anatomy. These frameless systems provide the surgeon with more flexibility during various types of cranial and spinal neurosurgery.[14,15] Regardless of the type of system utilized, stereotactic-guided biopsies and stereotactic resections are commonly performed, particularly for deep-seated lesions or for lesions situated in eloquent or hazardous areas of the brain.

One of the guiding principles of surgical neuro-oncology is to minimize injury to adjacent structures whenever possible, and the use of stereotactic techniques has made this increasingly possible. The development of both frame-based and frameless stereotactic systems have allowed neurosurgeons to precisely localize the targeted lesion, design an incision and plan a trajectory or a surgical corridor before any incision is made.[16] While it is generally accepted that the application of image guidance techniques can often minimize the degree of invasiveness of a particular procedure, the routine use of neuronavigation in cytoreductive surgery has not been corroborated with significant improvements in patient outcome.[17] One prospective randomized controlled trial performed by Willems and colleagues demonstrated that, for a specific population of patients containing a single intracerebral contrast-enhancing tumor, there was no beneficial effect on radicality of resection, postoperative course, or survival in the acute postoperative setting when neuronavigation was used.[18] This suggests that while neuronavigation may increase the surgeon's confidence, there may not be a rationale for its routine use when it has not already been deemed advantageous because of either the size or location of the lesion or the surgeon's experience.[13]

Although preoperative imaging is important to determine the anatomical location and the degree of invasivity of a particular tumor, the use of real-time intraoperative imaging is also crucial for a variety of reasons.[19] Intraoperative imaging allows the surgeon to monitor the extent of tumor resection and adapt to brain shift as a result of cerebrospinal fluid (CSF) leakage or surgical retraction. Complications such as ischemia and hemorrhage can also be detected early.[20,21] Intraoperative sonography has the advantage over CT and MRI in that it produces true real-time images; when enhanced via sonographic, magnetic, and optical tracking methods, a tool of choice can also be used to navigate a surgical trajectory.[22] Sonographic images, however, are often difficult to interpret because lesions cannot be easily distinguished echogenically from healthy brain tissue. Blood products in the surgical field can also cause misinterpretation.[21] Both intraoperative CT and MRI can provide updates to data sets for frame-based and frameless stereotaxy, and mobile CT scanners have been developed for both the operating room and critical care areas.[23] In contrast to CT, however, intraoperative MRI provides excellent soft tissue delineation for discriminating between healthy and pathologic tissue in the interests of detecting tumor margins. Although this technology is expensive, high resolution and near real-time image acquisition avoids using ionizing radiation and is currently considered the best method for interactive image-guided neurosurgery.[20,24] The neurological surgeon can avoid critical brain structures while navigating the surgical field with greater accuracy.[25] Several studies have shown that patients benefit from the additional information provided by intraoperative MRI, but its exact role still needs to be determined as well as whether or not the cost of the technology is justified.[21,26–30]

One of the goals in treating brain tumors is to avoid causing an iatrogenic neurologic injury to eloquent brain regions, and advanced imaging techniques are helping to determine the anatomic location of these important structures. Functional MRI (fMRI) is a noninvasive technique that can identify functionally important areas of the brain involved in language, motor, and memory function. With this information a preoperative plan can be developed to minimize injury and maximize the extent of resection.[31,32] Data from the fMRI exam can be fused to the preoperative stereotactic reference images to further increase the safety of surgery, particularly when it comes to deciding upon an approach and the choice of a surgical corridor for tumor resection. There are limitations in that while fMRI can provide information as to which areas of the brain are involved in a certain task, this technology cannot distinguish if that area is essential for that task.[19] Another technique used for neurophysiologic monitoring during surgical resection is direct bipolar electrocortical stimulation (ECS).[33,34] This technology is more invasive and demanding of the patient and on the operating team to conduct and, therefore, is utilized only in specific situations. For motor cortex mapping, ECS can be performed while the patient is under general anesthesia without muscle relaxation; low frequency cortical stimulation causes contralateral muscle contractions that can be detected by electrophysiological monitoring techniques.[33,35] The use of monopolar ECS to measure muscle action potentials instead of movement can also be used in the primary motor cortex, and this method has been shown to decrease the risk of intraoperative seizure. Monopolar ECS, however, is not as sensitive as bipolar ECS for mapping motor function in the premotor frontal cortex.[36] Language mapping necessitates an "awake craniotomy" so that the patient can perform certain tasks such as counting or naming.[37] Once these eloquent brain regions have been identified they can be excluded from the area of planned resection to minimize the risk of injury to important language functions. A surgical series reviewed by Haglund and colleagues found that 87% of patients who presented without preoperative language deficits had no permanent postoperative language deficits following awake craniotomy for language mapping; for the subgroup of patients whose resection margins were more than 1 cm away from vital language areas, patients retained normal language function by the end of the first postoperative week. All patients were followed for at least one year and no improvement at the one-year follow-up was considered a permanent deficit.[38]

Another important innovation that would revolutionize the field of neurosurgery was the introduction of the operating microscope. In 1957, Theodore Kurze became the first neurosurgeon to use a microscope in an operating room[39] and, despite initial resistance to its use, the technology would gradually gain acceptance. The operating microscope provided stereoscopic magnification and illumination which, when used in conjunction with specially designed microsurgical instrumentation, opened new surgical corridors to the surgeon.[40] Proponents of radical surgery would now argue that resections could be performed with much less risk to vital structures and ultimately the patient. Surgical exposures that were previously considered dangerous or unattainable were now possible and skull base approaches such as the transsphenoidal, transpetrosal, translabyrinthine, and transclival approaches became more widely utilized, and microsurgical techniques have enabled neurosurgeons to safely and effectively remove basal, cerebellopontine angle (CPA), intraventricular, and intramedullary tumors.[41] A surgical series review by Symon and Rosenstein found that use of the operating microscope in the surgical management of suprasellar meningiomas appeared to lower mortality rates and improve overall outcome in patients.[42] Facial nerve preservation during vestibular schwannoma removal was also found to be much more feasible[43,] and the operating microscope also reduced the incidence of nerve and vessel injury during skull base tumor removal.[44]

While many advances within the field of neurosurgery have been achieved through the development and adoption of new technologies or techniques, certain medical innovations also deserve mention. Prior to 1950, patients who underwent radical surgery for craniopharyngioma would often suffer cardiovascular collapse or hyperthermic crises and die within hours or days of their surgery.[45] This changed in 1952 after Ingraham[46] reported his successful use of ACTH and cortisone in the treatment of patients harboring these tumors. Since it was now possible to support patients through the difficult postoperative period, radical surgery was now seen as possible and the pessimism that was associated with the treatment of craniopharyngioma began to fade, albeit temporarily. In another review of a series of craniopharyngioma patients, Tytus described the postoperative course of patients who received cortisone as "impressively benign"[47] and he hypothesized that the drug minimized post-operative edema in the hypothalamic area. While his hypothesis was never proven, peritumoral cerebral edema had been long recognized as a significant problem in neurosurgery. Extracellular vasogenic edema is the most common type of cerebral edema associated with brain tumors and it often contributes to increased intracranial pressure and neurologic dysfunction.[48,49] In what some have described as one of the greatest translational contributions in the history of neurosurgery,[50] Joseph Galicich, Lyle French and James Melby described their use of dexamethasone for the treatment and prevention of peritumoral cerebral edema.[51] In early 1960, the authors administered high doses of dex-amethasone to all patients with brain tumors undergoing craniotomy and their results suggest a reduction in the amount of cerebral edema. Their observations revolutionized neurosurgical practice and are responsible for reducing the morbidity and improving outcomes in uncountable neurosurgical patients.[52,53]

Late Effects of Neurosurgery

Intracranial tumors account for nearly 30% of all childhood cancers diagnosed in the United States[54] and an estimated 3,750 new primary malignant and nonmalignant central nervous system tumors were predicted in children in the United States in 2007.[55] The survival of children with these tumors is influenced by many factors including histology, location, size and the intrinsic behavior of the neoplasm. Advances in early diagnosis, advanced imaging techniques, surgical techniques and postoperative critical care have all contributed to considerable improvements in the prognosis for children with CNS tumors over the last few decades but, in general, children with CNS malignancies do not share the same favorable prognosis as children with most other common pediatric malignancies.[56] With increased survival rates has come the recognition of late effects of both the disease itself and its treatment, and a wide range of complications have been identified.

Neurocognitive late effects and abnormalities of growth and endocrine function are the most common complications seen in long-term pediatric brain tumor survivors[57–61] and can result from any of the major modalities used in their treatment. Since the management of CNS tumors frequently involves a combination of surgery, craniospinal irradiation and chemotherapy, separating the effects of the various treatments remains enigmatic. While a considerable body of knowledge has developed describing the late effects of chemotherapy and craniospinal radiation,[62,63] little is known about the isolated effects of surgical resection.

Even in patients with benign tumors who undergo only surgical resection, disentangling the cause of sequelae that may be related to the intrinsic properties of the tumor itself from those related to surgery is difficult. Prior to treatment, brain tumors can interfere with normal function through various mechanisms. Tumors can exert mass effect, and displace and potentially damage adjacent structures, interfere with the normal circulation of cerebrospinal fluid leading to hydrocephalus, cause an increase in intracranial pressure and infiltrate normal intracranial structures, to name a few. Neurosurgical procedures by their very nature are invasive and can have both positive and negative effects. There is little doubt that the alleviation of mass effect and the restoration of the normal CSF pathways are beneficial, but any intrinsic tumor that does not present to a pial surface will require some degree of dissection through cortex, and the underlying white matter and sequelae that may ensue are directly related to the size and location of the surgical corridor.

Craniospinal irradiation has been associated with the highest risk of significant cognitive morbidity, but increasing evidence has shown that patients with certain types of damage to the cerebellum may exhibit cognitive disabilities that are similar to those seen in patients with damage to the cerebral cortex.[64] The postoperative syndrome of cerebellar mutism usually manifests 1–2 days after posterior fossa surgery and can be seen in up to 25% of patients following resection of medulloblastoma, and less commonly with other tumors.[65,66] The syndrome consists of mutism, emotional lability ataxia and profound axial hypotonia.[67] The mutism is transient with recovery occurring in nearly all patients, but speech rarely normalizes and permanent cognitive and behavioral problems can occur.[65,67] The pathogenesis of this disorder is still debated and is likely multifactorial. Injury to the cerebellar vermis during the surgical approach to the fourth ventricle, retraction on the vermis and injury to the dentato-thalamo-cortical pathways have all been implicated as possible mechanisms. Other possible etiologies include direct invasion of the brain stem by tumor,[67] postoperative ischemia and edema that may develop as a result of surgery in afferent supranuclear pathways.[68]

The development of focal neurological deficits following the surgical resection of brain tumors is a well-recognized complication that, in most cases, is dependent on the location of the tumor. Local or regional injuries may occur when normal or surrounding tissue is removed or damaged during a surgical resection, and retraction may also disrupt adjacent nerve fiber tracts leading to further white matter injury. Depending on the area of brain involved, focal neurological deficits or seizures may occur. In a population-based study from Denmark on patients who underwent surgery alone for their brain tumor, only 31% were free of neurological deficits at long-term follow-up.[69] Ataxia is the most commonly occurring deficit observed after posterior fossa surgery, and while most occurrences are mild and resolve shortly after surgery, some patients can exhibit severe cerebellar dysfunction that may persist. Facial nerve palsy, oculomotor abnormalities, swallowing dysfunction, vocal cord paralysis and motor disturbances occur less frequently.[69–72] Focal neurological deficits and seizures are known complications in patients undergoing surgery for hemispheric tumors. In most cases the morbidity associated with the procedure is evident immediately after surgery and most minor deficits improve within months. Seizures can occur at any time after surgical resection of hemispheric tumors, with the incidence of postoperative seizures varying between 15[73] and 70%.[74] The results of several surgical series suggest that complete tumor resection and short duration of seizures prior to resective surgery increases the likelihood of a seizure-free outcome.[75–77]

Certain types of tumors occur more frequently in adult patients and the common complications associated with these tumors deserve mention. Meningiomas are the second most common primary intracranial tumor, accounting for 13–26% of all primary intracranial tumors; 90% of meningiomas are histologically benign.[78] Although the use of fractionated radiotherapy and stereotactic radiosurgery is increasing for those tumors that are surgically inaccessible or recurrent and either atypical or anaplastic, surgery remains the primary treatment of choice with complete surgical resection resulting in cure of the disease.[79,80] Meningiomas, therefore, represent a unique opportunity to study the morbidities that may result from neurosurgical care. Depending on the location of the tumor, total excision of the lesion and its dural attachment is the primary surgical goal; however, partial excision is preferable when total removal of the lesion is associated with an unacceptable risk of neurologic deficit.[81] Tumors located in the cerebral convexities, olfactory groove, lateral sphenoid wing, anterior falx, and anterior third of the superior sagittal sinus are more surgically accessible than tumors in the medial sphenoid wing, posterior falx, posterior two-thirds of the superior sagittal sinus, cavernous sinus, optic nerve sheath, and petroclival region. The most critical factor in determining postoperative morbidity is location.[78–81]

For complete tumor excision of meningiomas involving the supratentorial convexities, Kinjo and colleagues reported no operative mortalities or postoperative neurologic deficits in a study of 37 patients who underwent Simpson grade zero removal of their lesions, which constitutes removal of an additional dural margin of about 2 cm around the tumor. Nineteen of these patients had a follow-up period of more than five years.[82] Similarly, Tuna and colleagues reported that in a study of 93 patients with meningiomas, of which 14 patients harbored very large meningiomas (>6 cm) of the cerebral convexities, total resection was performed in 12 patients and 11 were free from postoperative major neurological deficit. There was one postoperative death due to pulmonary embolus. Two patients in this study underwent subtotal resection due to tumor involvement of the middle cerebral artery, and their preoperative deficits did not fully recover postoperatively. The mean follow-up period was 4 ± 0.6 years.[83]

Several studies have been performed to demonstrate the efficacy of total removal of meningiomas occupying the olfactory groove. Tuna and colleagues reported no postoperative major neurological deficit in 14 patients who underwent total resection of very large (>6 cm) olfactory groove meningiomas. The mean follow-up period was 4.2 ± 0.5 years.[84] In a surgical case series of 81 patients, Spektor and colleagues found no instances of operative mortality and no new permanent focal neurologic deficit beside anosmia. The mean follow-up period was 5.9 years.[85] Another surgical series review by Bassiouni and colleagues found that of 56 patients who underwent total resection of their olfactory groove meningiomas, there was olfactory function deterioration in 15, visual deterioration in one, mental function deterioration in two, and postoperative deaths in three patients due to rebleeding, pneumonia, and pulmonary embolism. The mean follow-up period in this series was 5.6 years.[86]

Vestibular schwannomas, also known as acoustic neuromas, are benign intracranial tumors that originate from the vestibular portion of the eighth cranial nerve, and are the most common tumor that presents at the CPA.[87] As with meningiomas, they have been shown to be completely resectable and, therefore, represent an opportunity to study morbidities that may result from neurosurgical treatment. The natural history of symptomatic vestibular schwannomas is the onset of hearing loss or other auditory complaints such as tinnitus, ipsilateral facial paresthesias due to compression of the trigeminal nerve, compression of the brain stem with possible contralateral hemiparesis, obstruction of the CSF pathways leading to hydrocephalus, and, rarely, facial nerve weakness. The most common morbidity associated with treatment of vestibular schwannomas is injury to the cochlear and facial nerves.[88]

Using a retrosigmoid endoscopic approach, Kabil and Shahinian reported postoperative hearing deterioration in 40 of 101 patients in their surgical series review.[89] In a retrospective analysis of 20 patients under the age of 21 performed by Mirzayan and colleagues, hearing could not be preserved in 55% of cases. Although the facial nerve was anatomically preserved in all patients, one patient had postoperative facial nerve palsy that did not show signs of reinnervation after 12 months of follow-up. A hypoglossal-facial anastomosis for reanimation was performed in that case.[90] Roehm and Gantz conducted a retrospective review of 216 patients that were 65 years of age and older with vestibular schwannomas. Of 108 patients who underwent surgical resection of their lesions, 30 had postoperative facial paralysis that did not recover over a mean follow-up period of 2.95 years. Three of these patients, however, had less than six months' follow-up, so paralysis may not reflect their true functional outcome. Eleven of 15 patients with initial useful hearing who underwent middle fossa approaches lost useful hearing postoperatively.[91] Gormley and colleagues stratified the functional outcomes of 179 patients based on tumor size (small <2 cm, medium 2–3.9 cm, large >4 cm). Mean follow-up time in this series was 5.8 years. In patients with functional preoperative hearing defined as Gardner-Robertson Class I or II, hearing could not be preserved in 22 (52%) of 42 patients with small tumors, 18 (75%) of 24 patients with medium tumors, and three (100%) of three patients with large tumors. For patients with excellent preoperative facial nerve function defined as House-Brackmann Grade I or II, excellent facial nerve function could not be fully preserved in three (4%) of 67 patients with small tumors, 21 (26%) of 80 patients with medium tumors, and 16 (62%) of 26 patients with large tumors. One patient sustained a lasting cerebellar and brain stem injury in this study.[92] Other studies have reported similar results for preservation of excellent facial nerve function in small tumors (96–97% preservation of House-Brackmann Grade I or II) as well as hearing preservation (34–59% preservation).[87,92–98]

Non-functioning pituitary macroadenomas are benign lesions that can cause visual field defects, decreased visual acuity, and pituitary insufficiency due to mass effect.[99] As with meningiomas and vestibular schwannomas, surgical treatment of these benign tumors offers an opportunity to study the late effects that may result from these surgeries.

Zhang and colleagues reported that in a series of 187 patients with non-functioning pituitary adenomas with suprasellar extensions, transphenoidal microsurgery caused no postoperative deterioration in either visual field defects or visual acuity (mean follow-up of 3.8 years). Twenty-eight patients had postoperative diabetes insipidus that resolved after 1–6 weeks of symptomatic therapy.[100] In a study of 109 consecutive patients treated with transphenoidal microsurgery, Dekkers and colleagues reported postoperative transient diabetes insipidus in 28% of cases, visual field deterioration in three patients, and one perioperative mortality due to subarachnoid bleeding two days after surgery.[101] Of 10 patients with giant non-functioning pituitary adenomas who underwent a combined transsphenoidal and pterional craniotomy approach, Alleyne and colleagues reported no instances of worsening of vision or postoperative hypopituitarism that did not already exist preoperatively.[102] In determining if quality of life (QOL) was affected, Nielson and colleagues conducted a retrospective analysis on 192 patients who underwent surgery for their non-functioning pituitary macroadenomas. Postoperatively, 51 (27%) patients had panhypopituitarism, and nine (5%) of patients had permanent diabetes insipidus (median follow-up of 12 years, range 5–20). Of 139 patients who were still alive at the time of the study, 109 responded to the QOL questionnaires. Perceived quality of life was based on a Danish version of Short Form (SF-36) and Major Depression Inventory (MDI-10) questionnaires, and was meant to assess physical, mental, social, and general health aspects. Overall, QOL of these patients was not different than those of the control background population when matched for age and sex, including those patients with postoperative hypopituitarism. When compared to controls, patients reported better physical functioning, less bodily pain, and a better overall physical component score (p<0.05). All other areas of the SF-36 questionnaire (physical role, general health, vitality, social functioning, emotional role, mental health, and mental component score) showed no statistically significant difference between patients and population controls.[103] In contrast, both Dekkers and Johnson reported an overall significant decrease in perceived QOL in their studies of 99 and 51 patients treated successfully for their non-functioning pituitary macroadenomas when compared with the normal population, respectively.[104,105]

Conclusion

Considerable progress has been made in the field of neurosurgery and the related disciplines during the past century. Our knowledge of the natural history of oncologic diseases, combined with a greater understanding of anatomy and neurophysiology has increased surgeon confidence in and around eloquent locations of the brain. Neurosurgeons, neuro-oncologists and radiation oncologists have all contributed to improving the survival rates for most central nervous system tumors, but the risk of cognitive, neurological and endocrinological impairment remains high amongst survivors. While the biology of a tumor will ultimately determine the prognosis of the patient, aggressive treatment strategies also contribute to the morbidity faced by these patients. Whether or not new surgical techniques or innovative technologies will improve survival and outcomes in these patients remains to be determined and a multi-institutional, prospective collection of outcome data will be needed to draw more definitive conclusions.

References

1. Lyons AE. The Crucible Years 1880 to 1900: Macewen to Cushing. In: Greenblatt SH, Dagi TF, Epstein MH, eds. *A History of Neurosurgery*. Park Ridge: American Association of Neurological Surgeons; 1997:153–166.
2. Kiss I. From Anesthesia for Neurosurgery to Neuroanesthesia. A Historical Note. *Acta Neurochir* (Wien). 2000;142:1391–1395.
3. Horsley V. On the technique of operations of the central nervous system. *Br Med J*. 1906;2:411–423.
4. Greenblatt SH. Harvey Cushing's paradigmatic contribution to neurosurgery and the evolution of his thoughts about specialization. *Bull Hist Med*. 2003;77(4):789–822.
5. Jay V. The Legacy of Harvey Cushing. Archive Pathol Lab Med 2001;125(12):1539–1541.
6. Engelhard K, Werner C. Inhalational or intravenous anesthetics for craniotomies? Pro inhalational. *Curr Opin Anaesthesiol*. 2006;19(5):504–508.

7. Dandy WE. Ventriculography following the injection of air into the cerebral ventricles. *Ann Surg*. 1918;68:5–11.

8. Moniz E. L'encephalographie arterielle. Son importance dans la localisaztion des tumeurs cerebrales. *Rev Neurol* (Paris). 1927;34:72–90.

9. Ommaya A. Computed axial tomography of the head: the EMI scanner – a new device for direct examination of the brain "in vivo". *Surg Neurol*. 1973;1:217–222.

10. Gildenberg PL. Computerized tomography and stereotactic surgery. In: Spiegel EA, ed. *Guided Brain Operations*. Karger: Basel, 1982:24–34.

11. Gildenberg PL, Franklin PO. Survey of CT-guided stereotactic surgery. *Appl Neurophysiol*. 1985;48:477–480.

12. Lunsford LD, Deutsch M, Yoder V. Stereotactic interstitial brachytherapy: Current concepts and concerns in 20 patients. *Appl Neurophysiol*. 1985;48:117–120.

13. Willems PWA, van der Sprenkel JW, Tulleken CA, et al. Neuronavigation and surgery of intracerebral tumors. *J Neurol*. 2006;253(9):1123–1136.

14. Germano IM, Villalobos H, Silvers A, et al. Clinical use of the optical digitizer for intracranial neuronavigation. Neurosurgery 1999;45:261–269.

15. Gumprecht HK, Widenka DC, Lumenta CB. BrainLab VectorVision Neuronavigation System: technology and clinical experiences in 131 cases. *Neurosurgery*. 1999;44:97–104.

16. Spetzger U, Laborde G, Gilsbach JM. Frameless neuronavigation in modern neurosurgery. *Minim Invasive Neurosurg*. 1995;38(4):163–166.

17. Ostertag CB and Warnke PC. Neuronavigation computer-assisted neurosurgery. *Nervenartz*. 1999;70(6):517–521.

18. Willems PWA, Taphoorn MJB, Burger H, et al. Effectiveness of neuronavigation in resecting solitary intracerebral contract-enhancing tumors: a randomized controlled trial. *J Neurosurg*. 2006;104:360–368.

19. Jacobs AH, Kracht LW, Gossmann A, et al. Imaging in neurooncology. *NeuroRx*. 2005;2(2):333–347.

20. Zakhary R, Keles GE, Berger MS. Intraoperative imaging techniques in the treatment of brain tumors. *Curr Opin Oncol*. 1999;11(3):152–156.

21. Fenchel S, Boll DT, Lewin JS. Intraoperative MR imaging. *Magn Reson Imaging Clin N Am*. 2003;11(3):431–447.

22. Comeau RM, Fenster A, Peters TM. Intraoperative US in interactive image-guided neurosurgery. *Radiographics*. 1998;18:1019–1027.

23. Butler WE, Piaggio CM, Constantinou C, et al. A mobile computed tomographic scanner with intraoperative and intensive care unit applications. *Neurosurgery*. 1998;42:1304–1310.

24. Mittal S, Black PM. Intraoperative magnetic resonance imaging in neurosurgery: the Brigham concept. *Acta Neurochir Suppl*. 2006;98:77–86.

25. Jolesz FA, Talos IF, Schwartz RB. Intraoperative magnetic resonance imaging and magnetic resonance imaging-guided therapy for brain tumors. *Neuroimaging Clin N Am*. 2002;12(4):665–683.

26. Keles GE. Intracranial neuronavigation with intraoperative magnetic resonance imaging. *Curr Opin Neurol*. 2004;17(4):497–500.

27. Seifert V. Intraoperative MRI in neurosurgery: technical overkill or the future of brain surgery? *Neurol India*. 2003;51(3):329–332.

28. Black PM, Moriarty T, Alexander E III, Stieg et al. Development and implementation of intraoperative magnetic resonance imaging and its neurosurgical applications. *Neurosurgery*. 1997;41:831–845.

29. Tronnier VM, Wirtz CR, Knauth M, et al. Intraoperative diagnostic and interventional magnetic resonance imaging in neurosurgery. *Neurosurgery*. 1997;40:891–902.

30. Wirtz CR, Bonsanto MM, Knauth M, et al. Intraoperative magnetic resonance imaging to update interactive navigation in neurosurgery: method and preliminary experience. *Comput Aided Surg*. 1997;2:172–179.

31. Tharin S, Golby A. Functional brain mapping and its applications to neurosurgery. *Neurosurgery*. 2007;60(4 Suppl 2):185–201.
32. Taylor MD, Bernstein M. Surgical Management. In: Schiff D, O'Neill BP, eds. *Principles of Neuro-Oncology*. New York: McGraw-Hill; 2005:121–142.
33. Ojemann G, Ojemann J, Lettich E, et al. Cortical language localization in left, dominant hemisphere. An electrical stimulation mapping investigation in 117 patients. *J Neurosurg*. 1989;71:316–326.
34. Penfield W. The cerebral cortex and consciousness. In: Penfield W, ed. *The Harvey Lectures*. Baltimore: Williams & Wilkins Co.; 1937:35–69.
35. Berger MS, Kincaid J, Ojemann GA, et al. Brain mapping techniques to maximize resection, safety, and seizure control in children with brain tumors. *Neurosurgery*. 1989;25:786–792.
36. Kombos T, Suess O, Kern BC, et al. Comparison between monopolar and bipolar electrical stimulation of the motor cortex. *Acta Neurochir*. (Wien) 1999;141(12):1295–1301.
37. Meyer FB, Bates LM, Goerss SJ, et al. Awake craniotomy for aggressive resection of primary gliomas located in eloquent brain. *Mayo Clin Proc*. 2001;76:677–687.
38. Haglund MM, Berger MS, Shamseldin M, et al. Cortical localization of temporal lobe language sites in patients with gliomas. *Neurosurgery*. 1994;34:567–576.
39. Kriss TC, Kriss VM. History of the operating microscope: from magnifying glass to microneurosurgery. *Neurosurgery*. 1998;42(4):899–907.
40. Hernesniemi J, Niemela M, Karatas A, et al. Some collected principles of microneurosurgery: simple and fast, while preserving normal anatomy. *Surg Neurol*. 2005;64(3):195–200.
41. Yasargil, MG. Intracranial microsurgery. *Proc R Soc Med*. 1972;65(1):15–16.
42. Symon L, Rosenstein J. Surgical management of suprasellar meningioma. Part 1: The influence of tumor size, duration of symptoms, and microsurgery on surgical outcome in 101 consecutive cases. *J Neurosurg*. 1984;61(4):633–641.
43. Samii M. Facial nerve grafting in acoustic neurinoma. *Clin Plast Surg*. 1984;11(1):221–5.
44. Pan JW, Zhan RY, Tong Y, et al. Treatment of skull base communicating tumor with endoscope-assisted microneurosurgery and diode laser. *Chin Med J*. (Engl). 2007;120(4):342–344.
45. DiPatri, AJ Jr., Prabhu V. A history of the treatment of craniopharyngioma. *Childs Nerv Syst*. 2005;21(8–9):606–621.
46. Ingraham FD, Matson DD, McLaurin RL. Cortisone and ACTH as an adjunct to the surgery of craniopharyngiomas. *N Eng J Med*. 1952;246:568–571.
47. Tytus JS, Seltzer HS, Kahn EA. Cortisone as an aid in the surgical treatment of craniopharyngiomas. *J Neurosurg*. 1955;12:555–564.
48. Kaal C, Vecht CJ. The management of brain edema in brain tumors. *Curr Opin Oncol*. 2004;16(6):593–600.
49. Thapar K, Taylor MD, Laws ER, et al. Brain edema, increased intracranial pressure, and vascular effects of human brain tumors. In: Kaye AH, Laws ER, eds. *Brain Tumors. An Encyclopedic Approach*. London: Churchill Livingstone; 2001:189–216.
50. McClelland S, Long DM. Genesis of the use of corticosteroids in the treatment and prevention of brain edema. *Neurosurgery*. 2008;62(4):965–968.
51. Galicich JH, French LA, Melby JC. Use of dexamethasone in treatment of cerebral edema associated with brain tumors. *J Lancet*. 1961;81:46–53.
52. Gutin PH. Corticosteroid therapy in patients with brain tumors. *Natl Cancer Inst Monogr*. 1977;46:151–166.
53. Koehler PJ. Use of corticosteroids in neuro-oncology. *Anticancer Drugs*. 1995;6(1):19–33.
54. Wingo PA, Tong T, Bolden S. Cancer Statistics. *CA Cancer J Clin* 1995;45:8–30.
55. Central Brain Tumor Registry of the United States data, 2000–2004. Chicago, Illinois. CBTRUS. Available at: http://www.cbtrus.org. Released April 2007.
56. Gurney JG, Smith MA, Bunin GR. CNS and miscellaneous intracranial and intraspinal neoplasms. In: Ries LAG, Smith MA, Gurney JG, et al., eds. *Cancer Incidence and*

Survival Among Children and Adolescents: Unites States SEER program 1975–1995. NIH Pub. No. 99-4649. Bethesda, MD 1999.

57. Anderson NE. Late complications in childhood central nervous system tumor survivors. *Curr Opin Neurol.* 2003;16:677–683.

58. Briere, ME, Scott JG, McNall-Knapp RY, et al. Cognitive outcome in pediatric brain tumor survivors: delayed attention deficit at long-term follow-up. *Pediatr Blood Cancer.* 2008;50:337–340.

59. Reimers SR, Ehrenfels S, Mortensen EL, et al. Cognitive deficits in long-term survivors of childhood brain tumors: identification of predictive factors. *Med Pediatr Oncol.* 2003;40:26–34.

60. Packer RJ, Gurney JG, Punkyo JA, et al. Long-term neurologic and neurosensory sequelae in adult survivors of a childhood brain tumor: childhood cancer survivor study. *J Clin Oncol.* 2003;21(17):3255–3261.

61. Muirhead SE, Hsu E, Grimard L, et al. Endocrine complications of pediatric brain tumors: case series and literature review. *Pediatr Neurol.* 2002;27(3):165–170.

62. Mulhern RK, Merchant TE, Gajjar A, et al. Late Neurocognitive sequelae in survivors of brain tumors in children. *Lancet Oncol.* 2004;5(7):399–408.

63. Moore III BD. Neurocognitive outcomes in survivors of childhood cancer. *J Ped Psych.* 2005;30(1)51–63.

64. Cantelmi D, Schweizer TA, Cusimano MD. Role of cerebellum in the Neurocognitive sequelae of treatment of tumors of the posterior fossa: an update. *Lancet Oncol.* 2008;9:569–576.

65. Wells EM, Walsh KS, Khademian ZP, et al. The cerebellar mutism syndrome and is relation to cerebellar cognitive function and the cerebellar cognitive affective disorder. *Dev Disabil Res Rev.* 2008;14(3):221–228.

66. Levison L, Cronin-Golomb A, Schmahmann JD. Neuropsychological consequences of cerebellar tumour resection in children: cerebellar cognitive affective syndrome in children. *Brain.* 2000;123:1041–1050.

67. Robertson PL, Muraszko KM, Holmes EJ, et al. Incidence and severity of postoperative cerebellar mutism syndrome in children with medulloblastoma: A prospective study by the Children's Oncology Group. *J Neurosurg* (6 Suppl Pediatrics). 2006;105:444–451.

68. Wisoff JH, Epstein FJ. Pseudobulbar palsy after posterior fossa operation in children. *Neurosurgery.* 1984;15:707–709.

69. Sonderkaer S, Schmiegelow M, Carstensen H, et al. Long-term outcome of childhood brain tumors treated by surgery only. *J Clin Oncol.* 2003;21(7):1347–1351.

70. Pencalet P, Maixner W, Sainte-Rose C, et al. Benign cerebellar astrocytomas in children. *J Neurosurg.* 1999;90:265–273.

71. Merchant TE, Fouladi M. Ependymoma: new therapeutic approaches including radiation and chemotherapy. *J Neurooncol.* 2005;75(3):287–299.

72. Cochrane DD, Gustavson B, Poskitt KP, et al. The surgical and natural morbidity of aggressive resection for posterior fossa tumors in childhood. *Pediatr Neurosurg.* 1994;20:19–29.

73. Pollack IF, Claasen D, al-Shboul Q, et al. Low-grade gliomas of the cerebral hemispheres in children: an analysis of 71 cases. *J Neurosurg.* 1995;82:536–547.

74. Hildebrand J, Lecaille C, Perennes J, et al. Epileptic seizures during follow-up of patients treated for primary brain tumors. *Neurology* 2005;65:212–215.

75. Ianelli A, Guzzetta F, Battaglia D, et al. Surgical treatment of temporal tumors associated with epilepsy in children. *Pediatr Neurosurg.* 2000;32:248–254.

76. Khajavi K, Comair YG, Wyllie E, et al. Surgical management of pediatric tumor-associated epilepsy. *J Child Neurol.* 1999;14:15–25.

77. Packer RJ, Sutton LN, Patel KM, et al. Seizure control following tumor surgery for cortical low-grade gliomas. *J Neurosurg.* 1994;80:998–1003.

78. Loius DN, Scheithauer BW, Budka H, et al. Meningiomas. In: Kleihues P, Caenee WK, eds. *Pathology and Genetics of Tumours of the Nervous System: World Health Organization Classification of Tumours.* Lyon: IARC Press; 2000:176–184.

79. Whittle IR, Smith C, Navoo P, et al. Meningiomas. *Lancet.* 2004;363(9420):1535–1543.
80. Taylor MD, Bernstein M. Primary Meningeal Neoplasms. In: Schiff D, O'Neill BP, eds. *Principles of Neuro-Oncology.* New York: McGraw-Hill; 2005:369–379.
81. Drummond KJ, Zhu JJ, Black PM. Meningiomas: updating basic science, management, and outcome. *Neurologist.* 2004;10(3):113–130.
82. Kinjo T, al-Mefty O, Kanaan I. Grade zero removal of supratentorial convexity meningiomas. *Neurosurgery.* 1993;33(3):394–399.
83. Tuna M, Gocer AI, Gezercan Y, et al. Huge meningiomas: a review of 93 cases. *Skull Base Surg.* 1999;9(3):227–238.
84. Spektor S, Valarezo J, Fliss DM, et al. Olfactory groove meningiomas from neurosurgical and ear, nose, and throat perspectives: approaches, techniques, and outcomes. *Neurosurgery.* 2005;57(4 Suppl):268–280.
85. Bassiouni H, Asgari S, Stolke D. Olfactory groove meningiomas: functional outcome in a series treated microsurgically. *Acta Neurochir* (Wien). 2007;149(2):109–121.
86. Bennett M, Haynes DS. Surgical approaches in the removal of vestibular schwannomas. *Otolaryngol Clin North Am.* 2007;40(3):589–609.
87. Samii M, Matthies C. Management of 1000 vestibular schwannomas (acoustic neuromas): hearing function in 1000 tumor resections. *Neurosurgery.* 1997;40(2):248–260.
88. Kabil MS, Shahinian HK. A series of 112 fully endoscopic resections of vestibular schwannomas. *Minim Invasive Neurosurg.* 2006;49(6):362–368.
89. Mirzayan MJ, Gerganov VM, Ludemann W, et al. Management of vestibular schwannomas in young patients-comparison of clinical features and outcome with adult patients. *Childs Nerv Syst.* 2007;23(8):891–895.
90. Roehm PC, Gantz BJ. Management of acoustic neuromas in patients 65 years or older. *Otol Neurotol.* 2007;28(5):708–714.
91. Gormley WB, Sekhar LN, Wright Dc, et al. Acoustic neuromas: results of current surgical management. *Neurosurgery.* 1997;41(1):50–58.
92. Ojemann RG. Management of acoustic neuromas (vestibular schwannomas): Honored guest presentation. *Clin Neurosurg.* 1993;40:498–535.
93. Ojemann RG, Martuza RL. Acoustic neuromas. In: Youmans JR, ed. *Neurological Surgery.* Philadelphia: W.B. Saunders Co.; 1990:3316–3350.
94. Ebersold MJ, Harner SG, Beatty CW, et al. Current results of the retrosigmoid approach to acoustic neurinoma. *J Neurosurg.* 1992;76:901–909.
95. Gardner G, Robertson JH. Hearing preservation in unilateral acoustic neuroma surgery. *Ann Otol Rhinol Laryngol.* 1988;97:55–66.
96. Nadol JB, Chiong CM, Ojemann RG, et al. Preservation of hearing and facial nerve function in resection of acoustic neuroma. *Laryngoscope.* 1992;102:1153–1158.
97. Tatagiba M, Samii M, Matthies C, et al. The significance for postoperative hearing of preserving the labyrinth in acoustic neurinoma surgery. *J Neurosurg* 1992;77:677–684.
98. Shelton C, Brackmann DE, House WF, et al. Middle fossa acoustic tumor surgery: Results in 106 cases. *Laryngoscope.* 1989;99:405–408.
99. Dekkers OM, Biermasz NR, Pereira AM, et al. Mortality in patients treated for Cushing's disease is increased, compared with patients treated for nonfunctioning pituitary macroadenoma. *J Clin Endocrinol Metab.* 2007;92(3):976–981.
100. Zhang X, Fei Z, Zhang J, et al. Management of nonfunctioning pituitary adenomas with suprasellar extensions by transsphenoidal microsurgery. *Surg Neurol.* 1999;52(4):380–385.
101. Dekkers OM, Pereira AM, Roelfsema F, et al. Observation alone after transsphenoidal surgery for nonfunctioning pituitary macroadenoma. *J Clin Endocrinol Metab.* 2006;91(5):1796–801.
102. Alleyne CH, Barrow DL, Oyesiku NM. Combined transsphenoidal and pterional craniotomy approach to giant pituitary tumors. *Surg Neurol.* 2002;57(6):380–390.
103. Nielsen EH, Lindholm J, Laurberg P, et al. Nonfunctioning pituitary adenoma: incidence, causes of death and quality of life in relation to pituitary function. *Pituitary.* 2007;10(1):67–73.

104. Dekkers OM, van der Klaauw AA, et al. Quality of life is decreased after treatment for nonfunctioning pituitary macroadenoma. *J Clin Endocrinol Metab.* 2006;91(9):3364–3369.
105. Johnson MD, Woodburn CJ, Vance ML. Quality of life in patients with a pituitary adenoma. *Pituitary.* 2003;6(2):81–87.

Chapter 3
Late Effects of CNS Radiation Therapy

Helen A. Shih, Jay S. Loeffler, and Nancy J. Tarbell

Introduction

Radiation therapy is used as a primary or adjuvant treatment modality for many types of newly diagosed and recurrent/progressive brain tumors. For over 50 years, standard radiotherapy has utilized photons; that is, high energy X-rays, as the therapeutic source. Energy delivered to targeted tissues causes cell injury, growth arrest, and cell death. DNA damage is believed to be the principle biological event leading to cell death, but a variety of molecular changes and damage are known to occur to nucleic acids and proteins which may also contribute to the mechanism of tumor killing by radiation therapy. The fields of diagnostic radiology and therapeutic radiation therapy have had several technological advancements in recent years. Introduction and advancements in computed tomography (CT) and magnetic resonance imaging (MRI) have greatly impacted the methods of disease detection and subsequent targeting for radiation therapy planning and delivery. Technical innovations have led to greater precision of radiation delivery to targeted sites while minimizing exposure to normal tissues. The clinical application of proton radiation has expanded in recent decades with growing recognition of its unique and favorable physical characteristics. Choice of radiation modality depends upon multiple patient, disease, and anatomical factors. Despite the multiple clinical advancements in radiation therapy, there are inherent risks. As long-term survival of patients with brain tumors improves, the late effects of radiation therapy become increasingly salient to understand, minimize, and manage.

H.A. Shih (✉)
Assistant Professor of Radiation Oncology, Harvard Medical School, Department of Radiation Oncology, Massachusetts General Hospital, 100 Blossom St., Cox 3, Boston, MA, 02114, USA
e-mail: hshih@partners.org

S. Goldman, C.D. Turner (eds.), *Late Effects of Treatment for Brain Tumors*, Cancer Treatment and Research 150, DOI 10.1007/b109924_3, © Springer Science+Business Media, LLC 2009

Modalities of Radiation Therapy

Conventional Radiation Therapy of the pre-Three-Dimensional Planning Era

Until the turn of the 21st century, the majority of therapeutic radiation therapy plans were designed by clinical measurements alone, or with the assistance of fluoroscopy. The use of more advanced imaging data, primarily by CT, became increasingly widespread throughout the 1990s and has significantly improved the clinician's ability to deliver conformal radiation therapy such that excess radiation to surrounding normal tissues could be limited. Prior to this, the volume of the radiation treatment target was much larger so as to more securely encompass the full extent of the disease. This contributed to a higher risk of radiation-related adverse effects. The techniques of radiation delivery were also less sophisticated, leading to both an increased volume of surrounding normal tissues irradiated and an increased dose to these areas. The majority of external beam radiation therapy is delivered by machines called linear accelerators that generate megavoltage (MV) photon and electron beams. Most therapeutic radiation is delivered with 4–25 MV beams. This is in comparison to lower energy machinery such as the Van de Graaff generator and cobalt-60 machines which provided energies of 1–2 MV in the clinic. The result of using these lower energies was increased heterogeneity of delivered radiation such that adverse effects from radiation were much more common. Much of the long-term reported radiation toxicities today are a result of these older treatment modalities, and current morbidity risks with newer technology are often estimated to be significantly less, with true rates yet to be realized.

Photon Versus Proton Radiation Therapy

Photons are a form of electromagnetic energy. They carry no mass or charge. They are bundles of energy that pass easily through matter and are partially absorbed by the materials that they pass through. Protons are the nucleus of hydrogen atoms and are isolated from stripping of the orbital electron from hydrogen. They carry both mass and a positive charge. They travel a finite length in tissues and deliver a disproportional amount of their energy in the last few millimeters of their track. With regard to radiation therapy, proton and photon radiation share similar biological effects. Protons offer the distinct benefit of depositing less excess radiation to surrounding nontarget tissues. Due to the complexity and expense of building and maintaining such facilities, there are limited clinical proton treatment facilities in the United States. However, this number is growing as the clinical benefit in minimizing adverse effects of excess radiation exposure is increasingly realized.

3-D Conformal Radiation Therapy (3D-CRT)

Standard photon-based radiation therapy is delivered by machines called linear accelerators. Linear accelerators can be adapted to deliver radiation in a variety of methods. 3-D conformal radiation therapy (3D-CRT) is the most widely available form of radiation planning. It utilizes CT and/or MRI scans with physician-specified areas of treatment target and of neighboring normal tissues with varying radiation sensitivity. Both types of areas are defined on each slice of the CT scan, creating three-dimensional volumes for targeting or avoidance. A combination of multiple radiation treatment beams is used. An intersection of beams defines the target region of high radiation dose. The surrounding tissue receives a lower radiation dose that is hopefully below clinically significant thresholds.

Intensity Modulated Radiation Therapy (IMRT)

Intensity modulated radiation therapy (IMRT) is a form of image-based radiation planning. It is delivered with a linear accelerator that is adapted with the capability of delivering a more variable radiation dose to each point within the target. The net result is a more highly conformal treatment to the target and comparatively much lower doses delivered to adjacent tissues. IMRT allows for improved radiation dose sparing to radiation-sensitive tissues that may be in proximity to the treatment site. A common example is avoiding a high dose to the optic chiasm or brain stem for an adjacent frontotemporal lobe tumor. The downside of delivering this highly conformal therapy is an increased integral dose and more inhomogeneity of dose.

Stereotactic Radiosurgery (SRS)

Stereotactic radiosurgery (SRS) can be delivered by linear accelerator, Gamma Knife (GK, Elekta, Stockholm, Sweden), or cyclotron (protons). Other new modalities of SRS delivery are actively being developed, but incorporate the basic principles of one of these methods. It refers to high radiation dose delivery in one setting. Because the target is typically small in volume and because such high doses delivered in one setting can be extremely harmful to normal tissues, great care must be taken to ensure accuracy of setup. SRS is most useful when the target/normal tissue interface is clear and the target volume is quasi-spherical.

SRS was first implemented in clinical practice by the Gamma Knife system in the late 1960s. It was developed to treat intracranial targets. GK utilizes cobalt-60, a radioactive isotope that emits photons as its radiation source. In its most common design, 201 sources of ^{60}Co are distributed in a hemisphere around the patient's head, thereby distributing the integral normal tissue exposure while creating a high dose target where all the radiation beams intersect. The dose gradient between high and low doses is very narrow such that small targets can be treated to high doses, yet are juxtaposed to radiation-sensitive structures that will receive a negligible dose. The dose heterogeneity between the edge of the treatment target and its center is typically a 50% dose gradient. This can be either very useful or sometimes harmful, depending upon the tissue being irradiated. GK is the most widely published radiosurgical methodology.

Linear accelerators have been adapted to deliver stereotactic radiosurgical treatments intracranially.[1] To reduce the dose to tissues between skin surface and target, linear accelerator-based SRS typically employ moving arcs around a central axis that creates a spherical or elliptoid treatment volume. Arcs refer to the radiation source of the linear accelerator moving in an arc around the patient during radiation delivery; that is, while the radiation beam is on. The irradiated tissues span between the entrance site on skin that is constantly changing and the fixed central axis, the target. The created irradiated volume is the shape of a paper fan. Multiple arcs are typically used to deliver the daily treatment. A high dose is delivered to the rotational center and a low dose is delivered elsewhere. Because higher accuracy is often required for small targets, a more sophisticated method of immobilizing the patient, as compared to normal fractionated radiation therapy, is used. Radiation delivered by linear accelerator-based SRS is more homogeneous in dose as compared to GK. This is helpful to avoid *hot spots* when irradiated targets that include radiation-sensitive normal tissues, such as a diffuse disease process that includes normal brain tissue. Linear accelerator-based SRS is used most commonly for treatment targets in the brain; however, in recent years, the concept has been applied to extracranial sites as well.[2]

Proton radiation can be delivered in a single fraction as proton stereotactic radiosurgery. Again, strong emphasis is placed on accuracy of setup. The dose delivered is often more favorable in terms of conformality to target and sparing of normal tissue irradiation. This advantage becomes greater with larger or irregularly shaped targets. Despite the inherent superiority of proton treatment plans as compared to photon-based systems, scarce resources limit its widespread use.

Stereotactic Radiotherapy (SRT)

Stereotactic radiotherapy (SRT) is a form of fractionated SRS. Treatment volumes are generally small, thus making them amenable to arc therapy. It utilizes a CT-based radiation treatment planning system similar to SRS. An important difference is the method of immobilization. Instead of the SRS frame that typically involves invasive pins fixed to the head, SRT most commonly uses a dental mold attached to a stereotactic frame. A customized occipital head mold is used to improve the reproducibility of the setup. For edentulous patients, customized head molds of both the occiput and frontal cranium can be created as an alternate form of immobilization. These setups can easily be replicated daily with no discomfort to the patient. The radiation planning is virtually identical to that of SRS. The difference is that small doses are delivered over several treatments with SRT, rather than in one large dose as in SRS. Arcs are applied when possible to dilute the integral dose to the normal tissues, but fixed fields can also be used if the target size is larger than can be ideally applied with arcs. This is a clinical judgment determined by the radiation oncologist. Fixed field SRT is very similar to 3D-CRT, but the immobilization with the stereotactic frame lends greater precision in setup and, thus, superior conformal treatment delivery. Fractionation schedules for SRT used for targets within the brain often require 20–30 treatments delivered over 4–6 weeks.

Brachytherapy

Brachytherapy uses implantable radioactive substances shaped into pellets, strands, or, more rarely, liquids to deliver highly conformal radiation therapy. The dose gradient is extremely high due to the low energy of most isotopes used. This translates to high doses delivered to tissues abutting the radioactive source and negligible doses at only a few millimeters away. The most common permanent isotope implant is iodine-125. Phosphorus-32 has been used for cystic lesion instillations such as recurrent craniopharyngiomas or recurrent pituitary adenomas. The use of most brachytherapy has largely fallen out of favor because of the technological advancements of SRS, SRT and IMRT that offer comparatively high conformal methods of treating small targets in the brain. Dose distributions in brachytherapy are often poorly reconstructed and typically only calculated from posttreatment imaging.[3] Brachytherapy has the additional disadvantage of exposing personnel to the radioactive source during the implantation procedure. It can be costly in preparation and has potential limitations in timing, both with regard to availability from manufacturers and factoring for its radioactive decay. Potential late effects of brachytherapy are similar to those of other radiation treatments.

Complexity in Understanding Late Effects of Radiation Therapy

Treatment successes must be balanced with potential adverse effects of therapies. One of the difficulties in shaping the role of radiation therapy in the treatment of brain tumors is the limited understanding of radiation late effects in the CNS. Radiobiological models have been proposed to describe late effects, but none come close to recognizing all contributory variables. Factors of radiation treatment that contribute to the risks of normal tissue injury include consideration of size of treatment volume, specific tissues being irradiated, fraction size, time between treatment fractions, total dose, and overall length of radiation treatment course. Clinical practice has evolved over the years such that current long-term clinical data may not reflect late effect risks of modern treatments. In particular, improved imaging, conformal planning, and treatment methods have resulted in a significant reduction of normal CNS tissue volumes irradiated and dose delivered such that reported risks of radiation therapy are likely an overestimation of current risks of treatment.[4–5]

Additional factors that may either confound understanding or compound the effects of radiation include comorbidities of the patient (e.g., diabetes, collagen vascular diseases, neurofibromatosis), patient's age, previous radiation or other treatment history, concurrent therapies, and potential future systemic therapies (e.g., chemotherapy-associated recall effect). The disease process itself is an important source of functional compromise.[6–8] In fact, one study has shown that in a group of glioma patients that all had some baseline neurocognitive impairment, those patients with low-grade gliomas improved neurocognitively following radiation treatment at a posttreatment interval mean of 2.6 months, whereas patients with high-grade gliomas remained largely unchanged or dropped slightly in performance at a mean of 2.9 months.[9] More intuitively, neurofibromatosis type II is an example of a complex disease in which radiation therapy may increase the susceptibility of radiation-induced morbidity such as hearing loss in the setting of treatment of vestibular schwannomas.[10] Those patients at a younger age at time of irradiation may have a markedly increased risk of potential morbidities, such as in the case of endocrinopathies following cranial irradiation.[11] The potential late effects of radiation will be discussed briefly here and elaborated in more detail in other chapters.

Radiation-Related Adverse Effects

Technological advancements in radiation therapy have led to an improved delivery of therapeutic radiation while achieving steep dose gradients at target edges, thereby reducing unnecessary irradiation of juxtaposed normal tissues. While the increased treatment conformality is expected to translate into a decrease of radiation-related toxicity, these unwanted treatment adverse effects are not entirely eliminated.

Neurocognitive Effects

Irradiation of the brain in children clearly increases the risk of neurocognitive decline.[12] Increased susceptibility is seen with younger ages and in females. A greater decline in IQ is also associated with those children beginning with higher baseline function. Neurocognitive deficits have been reported with doses as little as 18 Gy given to the brain along with concurrent chemotherapy.[13] Conversely, other investigators have found no decrement in IQ or memory as compared to age expected means among 61 patients with a history of cranial irradiation to 18 Gy for a similar indication of high-risk ALL.[14] Instead, comprehensive neuropsychiatric testing revealed a reduced ability to complete complex figure drawings and an age-related verbal deficit in children irradiated at less than 36 months. Hyperfractionation in this population has not been shown to improve cognitive function; patients treated with either conventional or hyperfractionated irradiation schedules demonstrated equivalent normal cognitive function.[15] At higher doses, there seems to be a dose dependency as suggested by a single institutional experience that craniospinal irradiation at 23.4 Gy has less neuropsychological sequelae than at 36 Gy.[16] Understanding the components of cognitive function that are affected by therapy will also enable better intervention in survivors. In a series of 16 patients with craniopharyngiomas treated with surgery and conformal postoperative radiation therapy, overall cognitive function was found to be equivalent to age-specific norms, but memory was found to be worse in both language and visuospatial function.[17] Whether this decrement is a result of radiation therapy, surgery, or the primary tumor is difficult to decipher, but it enables clinicians to better address sources of quality of life issues. Some studies suggest early radiation effects may be largely attention deficits, offering an opportunity to intervene in these children to limit secondary neurocognitive decline.[18,19] From behavioral and social outcomes studies conducted on 2,927 children treated through the Childhood Cancer Survivor Study, there was a 1.4 to 1.7 times higher incidence of depression, anxiety, antisocialism, or attention deficit as compared to paired unaffected siblings.[19] If these effects are a result of stresses inherent to having a diagnosis of cancer and undergoing therapy, it is plausible that psychotherapeutic intervention with or without pharmacotherapy may be able to temporize these late effects.

While the fear for neurocognitive injury following radiation therapy for brain tumors is of great concern for many adult patients, the existing data characterizing this radiation effect in adults is poor. This is a multifactorial result reflecting the difficulty to capture an effect that is slow in evolution, with variable rates of progression to varying degrees of deficit, and overlying a frequent baseline of disease-related neurocognitive compromise. Clinically, a subtle effect that is easily missed on insufficiently sensitive tests may have significant life altering effects on affected individuals. Animal studies show whole-brain irradiation results in decreased cognitive function that correlates with histological changes such as demyelination; however, these studies invariably use hypofractionated courses such as 25 Gy in a single fraction, which would never be considered in clinical use.[20] Clinical studies report radiation-related neurocognitive deficits using end points of short-term memory loss, inattentiveness, slowness of executive function, changes in judgment, and decreased insight. However, most studies are retrospective and single armed such that treatment and tumor effects cannot be differentiated.[18,21,22] Treatment details such as total dose and irradiated brain volume are largely a reflection of primary disease which may be the primary cause for any neurocognitive decline, rather than the radiation.[21] Yet other studies suggest that neurocognitive changes are truly multifactorial with the primary disease as the primary source of symptoms and both irradiation and systemic therapies as additional causes of cognitive sequelae.[6] While personal experiences of clinicians suggest that neurocognitive effects are prevalent, formal clinical evaluations to characterize them are still in need.

Hypopituitarism

The loss of one or more hormonal functions of the hypothalamic-pituitary axis is a common adverse effect of cranial radiation therapy in both pediatric and adult populations. Children are particularly sensitive to pituitary or hypothalamic irradiation.

In one series of 87 children treated with or without radiation, the most common unique radiation sequelae was endocrine deficiency, which was seen in 88% if irradiated patients, but 0% in patients who received only surgery as an intervention.[7] Other pediatric series show similar rates of endocrine dysfunction following cranial irradiation, particularly when targeting the parasellar region.[23] Risk of endocrine dysfunction also appears to increase when chemotherapy is a component of treatment in addition to radiation.[24] Hormonal deficiencies resulting from cranial irradiation often impact children more than adults because of the radiation-sensitivity of the growth hormone axis.[25] In adults, this often has no clinical significance. Unless corrected, this will cause a compromise in growth and development in prepubertal children.[26]

Among adults, endocrine dysfunction can occur insidiously, developing over months to years and often undiagnosed. Given our ability to correct for most pituitary deficiencies, patients should be counseled on the importance of regular endocrine evaluation if their radiation therapy will involve the parasellar or hypothalamic regions. Hypopituitarism develops slowly over months to years and is documented at 20–50% at five years among patients receiving direct irradiation to the pituitary.[27–30] Minniti et al.[27] report long-term results of 47 patients with GH-secreting tumors and otherwise normal pituitary function prior to irradiation. New hypopituitarism developed following standard fractionated 45–50 Gy at a rate of 57% at five years, 78% at 10 years, and 85% at 15 years, distributed over gonadal, thyroid, and cortisol insufficiency. Similar rates of hypopituitarism develop with either radiosurgery or fractionated therapy.[28] Retrospective data suggests that radiation-induced hypopituitarism is both dose-related and site-related in that irradiation of the pituitary stalk or hypothalamus increases the risk for endocrine deficits.[25,29,31] Feigl et al.[29] report that the dose difference of 7.7 Gy ± 3.7 Gy versus 5.5 ± 3 Gy to the infundibulum among 92 patients treated with GK for pituitary adenomas was statistically different and correlative to pituitary dysfunction at five years. A moderate dose of 50 Gy to the hypothalamus has also been shown to be predictive of pituitary insufficiency.[25] Awareness of the effects of hypothalamic and stalk irradiation should be weighed and minimized during radiation planning. Where irradiation is unavoidable, neuroendocrine surveillance is important because deficiencies are usually correctable with pharmacotherapy.

Visual Pathway Injury

Although uncommon, radiation-induced vision injury or blindness has a devastating impact on the quality of life of patients. Following a review of 1,621 patients from 35 studies of patients with pituitary adenomas treated with radiosurgery, Sheehan et al.[32] found 16 cases of vision injury with dose to the optic pathways ranging between 0.7–12 Gy. Most retrospective analyses attempting to determine the threshold of single fraction radiation tolerance to the optic system determine 8–10 Gy as the maximal tolerance, with 8 Gy considered as a safe threshold and 10 Gy associated with rare occurrences of optic neuropathy.[33-34] Leber et al.[34] studied 50 patients who underwent GK for benign tumors not limited to pituitary adenomas and found no cases of visual impairment among 31 patients whose optic system received less than 10 Gy, 26.7% rate of injury among 22 patients treated between doses of 10 to less than 15 Gy, and 77.8% risk at doses of ≥ 15 Gy among 13 patients. However, case reports of optic nerve or chiasm injury at lower doses support the importance of minimizing unnecessary doses and the volume of tissue exposed to radiation. Fractionated radiation is associated with a substantially lower risk of optic pathway injury with an estimate of 1.5% at 20 years in one large series of 411 patients, and no visual complications were often detected in smaller series.[28,35] The critical dose threshold for visual pathway injury appears to be at 50 Gy when fractionated.[36] Although fractionation can reduce radiation side effects, the historical use of substantially larger treatment volumes may account for the treatment-related vision impairment reported in some series.[36] Retrospective studies on retinal tolerance have reaffirmed that both total dose and daily dose are important factors in determining risk. Parsons et al.[37] found that, at doses of less than 1.9 Gy per day, the risk for retinal injury is far less at retinal doses of 45–55 Gy at 44%, compared to 67% for fractional doses above 1.9 Gy. In regard to optic nerve tolerance to radiation at doses ≥ 60 Gy, optic neuropathy developed in 11% of patients with fractionation of <19.9 Gy, compared to 47% for ≥ 1.9 Gy daily treatments.[38] Based upon these and similar experiences, most radiation oncologists regard 8 Gy to be the tolerance dose to the optic nerve for single fraction treatment, and 50–54 Gy as the dose tolerance for standard (1.8–2 Gy) fractionations. Preexisting comorbidities or compromised nerve function prior to irradiation may decrease these dose tolerances.

Other Cranial Nerve Deficits

Hearing can be affected by radiation. In studies within the pediatric population, there is a dose-dependent risk of ototoxicity correlating with fractionated radiation doses above 32 Gy.[39] A series of 33 adults treated for primary brain tumors with irradiation including the entire temporal bone and hearing apparatus on one side was evaluated after 6–25.6 years from completion of cranial irradiation.[40] Approximately one-third of patients (10/33) in this cohort developed sensorineural hearing loss, consistent with findings in the head and neck malignancy literature.[41,42] In one series, dose dependency for hearing loss was found with no hearing loss associated with a standard fractionated radiation dose of less than 54 Gy.[41] Increasing age and the use of concurrent chemotherapy were also associated with a higher risk for hearing loss.[42] In this report of 325 head and neck cancer patients treated with radiation, sensorineural hearing loss was experienced in 15.1% of patients and associated with doses to the cochlea exceeding 60.5 Gy.

Many other smaller series report few if any cases of cranial neuropathies with single fraction doses as high as 30 Gy to segments of nerves traversing through the cavernous sinus, indicating the high resiliency of these nerves.[34] Tischler et al.[33] report eight cases of cranial neuropathies, two of which occurred on the background of prior high-dose irradiation; all others occurred at doses > 18 Gy, and at least three cases had symptoms that were either temporary or intermittent. The history of prior irradiation and comorbidities such as baseline cranial nerve injury, diabetes mellitus, and vascular disease likely define an inherently higher risk population for nerve injury. Fractionation is an important means of decreasing this risk when there is a concern about a high dose being delivered to nerves that are unavoidably in the treatment field.

Brain Injury and Necrosis

Brain necrosis is seen most commonly with large conventional radiation fields.[4] The use of modern conformal techniques that greatly reduce radiation exposure to nontarget tissues should reduce some of the previously experienced brain necrosis. Conversely, concurrent chemotherapy with cranial irradiation in high-grade gliomas has been increasingly used, and data from phase III trials have shown this combination to yield a survival benefit.[43] However, long-term toxicity of combined modality therapy, such as a potential increase in tissue necrosis, has yet to be defined. Although uncommon, brain parenchyma injury is also seen with modern radiosurgical techniques for pituitary adenomas with 13 cases reported among 35 series reviewed by Sheehan and colleagues.[32] Prior irradiation appears to be a strong risk factor for radiation-induced brain necrosis in the sense that a high cumulative dose will eventually exceed normal tissue tolerance.[44] Risk of brain necrosis is also a function of the volume of tissue irradiated, with a lower risk associated with smaller treatment volumes as is the current trend with more conformal radiation therapy techniques.

Secondary Tumors

Radiation-induced malignancies are rare, but devastating when they occur. Secondary tumors are a recognized risk in patients treated for brain tumors. It is unclear whether the 1–3% long-term risk is a result of longer follow-up of a continuous increasing risk with time or if there is an inherently higher susceptibility for second tumors in the pediatric population.[45–47] In an analysis of the SEER database between 1973 and 1998, there were 2,056 patients with at least a five-year survival and there continued to be an increased risk of second malignancy after controlling for radiation therapy, suggesting that systemic therapies contribute to the risk.[11] In a review of outcomes from St. Jude Children's Research Hospital of 1,612 patients with acute lymphocytic leukemia, a 20-year cumulative incidence of brain tumors was 1.39% for all patients and 1.6% for those children treated with cranial irradiation.[45] There was a correlation of increased risk with increasing doses. For groups receiving ≤20 Gy, 21–30 Gy, and > 30 Gy, second tumor risks were 1.03%, 1.65%, and 3.23%, respectively. Similarly, long-term follow-up of 1,597 high-risk acute lymphoblastic leukemia (ALL) children treated on a Dana-Farber Cancer Institute Consortium protocol reported a total of 13 second malignancies.[47] Median time to occurrence was 6.7 years and the cumulative incidence for a second malignancy as a first follow-up event was 2.7%. Only 61% (8 of 13) of these second malignancies occurred within the radiation treatment field, again suggestive of risk factors other than radiation exposure as contributing to the secondary malignancy risk.

Long-term follow-up of pediatric cranial irradiation has shown a late effect correlation with gliomas and meningiomas that occur at a median time of nine and 17 years after irradiation, respectively.[48] Odds ratios with radiation exposure as compared to age, sex, and diagnosis-matched controls were 6.98 for gliomas and 9.94 for meningiomas with risk that correlated with dose in a fairly linear relationship. Tsang et al.[49] report on long-term follow-up of 305 patients with pituitary adenomas that were treated with radiation and found a rate of radiation-induced gliomas of 1.7% at 10 years and 2.7% at 15 years. Similarly, Brada and colleagues[35] reported on long-term results of 411 patients with pituitary adenomas and had a 20-year rate of radiation-induced tumors of 1.9%. Radiation treatments in the first study were delivered between 1972–1986, and in the second study between 1962–1986, both using older technical methods that treated substantially larger volumes of tissue than modern day techniques of visualization, localization, and radiation delivery. Because the risk of radiation-induced tumors requires long-term follow-up of ideally 10 or more years, there currently is insufficient data to accurately describe the risk with modern radiotherapy.

Survivors of irradiation prior to the 1990s will largely continue to harbor the risks of the older treatment methods, thus continued close surveillance is important to optimal management in those individuals who do develop second tumors. Most common types of radiation-induced tumors include meningiomas, high-grade gliomas, and sarcomas.[35,50] Poor prognosis is expected with malignant histologies. Radiation-induced malignancies are particularly concerning in the setting of treating patients with benign tumors who often have an otherwise normal life expectancy. Although current patients can be advised that the risk is expectedly much lower than those quoted from historical reports, long-term survivors of older methods of radiotherapy should thus be all the more closely observed. Additional discussion on radiation-induced malignancies can be found in the Secondary Cancer Chapterin this book.

Vascular Stenosis – Internal Carotid Artery Stenosis

Radiation is a well-recognized risk factor for vascular stenosis when irradiation occurs in childhood.[51] Moyamoya is a vascular response to irradiation that characteristically occurs in the pediatric population.[11] Analysis of a series of 20 pediatric patients who experienced intracranial hemorrhage after cranial irradiation found that poor clinical outcome correlated with hemorrhages located in the brain stem.[52] No other predictors of outcome were otherwise established among factors assessed, including radiation dose, type of malignancy, systemic therapy, time interval to bleed, or patient factors.

In adults, the risk of late-occurring cerebral vascular accident (CVA) appears real, but small. In a recent report from the Childhood Cancer Survivor Study of 4,828 leukemia survivors and 1,871 brain tumor patients, 37 and 63 cases of CVA were subsequently documented with the greatest risks occurring among children receiving doses of 50 Gy or higher.[51] In contrast, vascular stenosis following radiation therapy for pituitary adenomas, a tumor of the adult population, is a very uncommon event reported in few numbers.[53–55] In one long-term series of 331 patients treated with fractionated radiation for pituitary adenomas, the investigators reported five-, 10-, and 20-year risks for a cerebrovascular accident of 4%, 11%, and 21%, respectively.[53] This approximate 1%/year rate of stroke was equivalent to a relative risk of 4.1 as compared to the normal population. Concerns of this study are the lack of other substantial data to support these findings and the lack of detail of the study population, including no information about the types of strokes, possible inherent risk factors of patients, details of radiation, or locations of strokes. Whereas there may be small evidence consistent with radiation-related carotid stenosis, this risk currently appears to be minimal at a clinically significant level. As with all other tissues not intended for irradiation, treatment-related risks are best avoided by minimizing any unnecessary irradiation of neighboring tissues when possible.

Radiation-Associated Cavernous Malformations

Uncommonly, young patients can develop de novo cavernous malformations following exposure to therapeutic irradiation. The mean latency period to development is about nine years following radiation (45–60 Gy). These lesions tend to bleed at the same risk as cavernous malformations not associated with radiation exposure (1% per year) and should be resected if symptoms, most commonly seizures, develop. It is important to recognize this phenomena since these cavernomas can be mistaken for recurrent tumor or brain necrosis.[56] The occurrence of intracranial hemorrhage has also been seen in the pediatric population following cranial irradiation, but with predisposing risk factors found in a series of 20 patients.[52]

Radiation-Induced Alopecia

Frequently overlooked as a minor cosmetic side effect to cranial radiation therapy, hair loss can have devastating consequences to the quality of life of patients. Whereas most clinicians recognize that hair loss is a by-product of cranial irradiation that may or may not be permanent, few investigators have studied this carefully. Lawenda et al.[57] found that permanent alopecia correlated with radiation dose to hair follicles with a 50% risk for permanent moderate to complete alopecia with a fractionated follicular dose of 43 Gy. Modifications in radiation techniques, such as selection of energy used and scalp blocks, can vary the risk of permanent alopecia. The use of IMRT, in addition to increased conformality of high doses to targets, is also able to achieve lower doses to the scalp such that there can be both lower risks of alopecia and increase the probability of hair regrowth in areas where alopecia does occur.

Unique Concerns of Radiation Therapy in the Pediatric Population

Myelination and neurological maturation continues through the first few years of life. Radiation has been shown to have devastating effects on stunting development of the neurological system. Neurological deficits in children with brain tumors are common, whether or not radiation therapy is used, but the compounded insults to the immature nervous system can take a significant toll on later quality of life. Overall, rates reported of radiation-associated late complications from irradiation of the CNS in children range from 41% to 75% and appear to be higher when irradiation occurs at a younger age.[23,58] An evaluation of 342 adults with histories of childhood tumors showed a correlation between unfavorable adult quality of life and history of radiation therapy, but whether this reflects poor outcomes inherent to more aggressive tumors that are treated with radiation versus purely effects of radiation therapy remains unclear.[59] Accurate prospective data that is sensitive in analysis and reflective of modern therapy and techniques is lacking.

General trends in pediatric brain tumor protocols have attempted to delay the use of radiation therapy at young ages to allow for maximal time for neurological maturation. In addition, there is a trend to use lower doses of radiation when possible and to substitute chemotherapy for reduction in radiation dose. In long-term evaluation of 618 high-risk ALL children treated on one of two Dana-Farber Cancer Institute Consortium protocols, there was no negative effect of cranial irradiation on either height or weight.[60] Total dose delivered to these patients was 18 Gy at 1.8 Gy daily or 0.9 Gy twice daily separated by at least six hours, and was limited to the cranium in all cases. With slightly higher doses of 20–24 Gy to either the cranium or full craniospinal irradiation, there is blunting of growth that has been well-recognized.[61,62] Whereas effects of radiation are variable with dose dependency, this is in contrast to clear risk factors of young age and chemotherapy.[60] Depending upon the tumor type, advancements in radiation therapy such as improved imaging with MRI-CT fusion and increasingly conformal techniques, such as stereotactic radiotherapy or proton radiotherapy, allow for reasonably high local control of disease while minimizing normal brain radiation exposure.[63,64] These steps are promising towards developing efficacious therapies with reduced treatment toxicities.

Radiographic End Points

The use of MRI to characterize late radiation changes is relatively new. Most patients show white matter changes postcranial irradiation.[65] Preliminary data suggests a positive correlation between patients with neurocognitive deterioration and detectable MRI changes.[66,67] Changes include decreased perfusion in high injury regions, radiographic necrosis, both white and gray matter lesions, blood-brain barrier disruption, and hemosiderin deposits.[67,68] Calcifications and asymptomatic foci of hemorrhages also appear to be associated with cranial irradiation.[69] How closely or predictive MRI changes are to clinical manifestations is not known, but in one small series of 21 patients treated with craniospinal irradiation, 50% of cases had radiographic changes while no patients had developed neurological symptoms at a median follow-up of 14 years.[70]

Importance of Posttreatment Care

Following completion of radiation therapy, close surveillance is imperative. In addition to monitoring disease response to therapy and consideration for salvage as needed, it is important to screen for potential treatment-related adverse effects. Potential late effects generally arise insidiously over months to many years. Many late effects are treatable, thereby improving a patient's quality of life. Symptomatic edema is often responsive to a limited course of steroids. Hypopituitarism is a common effect of radiation therapy when the hypothalamus or pituitary are irradiated, occurring in about one-third of patients within five years from radiation treatment and with continued gradual rise in rate with time. These deficits can generally be restored with symptomatic improved well-being.

Future Directions

As retrospective long-term data on the late effects of radiation therapy becomes increasingly available, it will be important to compare these results with the difference in radiotherapy delivered today. The advancements of better imaging and in increasingly conformal radiation delivery have markedly reduced the volume of normal CNS tissue irradiated and this will surely have an impact on future risks of late effects.

Understanding radiation biology, both in terms of normal tissue and tumor radiosensitivity, is important to optimizing treatment schedules. Some preliminary data suggests hyperfractionation of craniospinal irradiation in medulloblastoma cases may significantly decrease the risk for long-term hypothyroidism; however, conducting these trials comes with risks of uncertain effects on disease control.[71]

The significance of ever improving and new MRI techniques has yet to be fully realized. If changes detected on MRI are found to be predictive of future clinical sequelae, this may be a means of identifying high-risk patients to intervene upon prophylactically.

Another area of new investigation will be to understand the molecular events following CNS irradiation. If CNS exposure to radiation cannot be entirely eliminated, another direction to investigate is pharmacotherapies that may selectively protect normal tissue or selectively potentate radiation effect in tumor cells and perhaps thus offer a means of intelligent targeted treatment delivery.

References

1. Kooy HM, Nedzi LA, Loeffler JS, et al. Treatment planning for stereotactic radiosurgery of intra-cranial lesions. *Int J Radiat Oncol Biol Phys.* 1991;21:683–693.
2. Kavanagh BD, McGarry RC, Timmerman RD. Extracranial radiosurgery (stereotactic body radiation therapy) for oligometastases. *Semin Radiat Oncol.* 2006;16:77–84.
3. Viola A, Major T, Julow J. Comparison of (125)I stereotactic brachytherapy and LINAC radiosurgery modalities based on physical dose distribution and radiobiological efficacy. *Radiat Res.* 2006;165:695–702.
4. Bhansali A, Banerjee AK, Chanda A, et al. Radiation-induced brain disorders in patients with pituitary tumors. *Australas Radiol.* 2004;48:339–346.

5. Gregor A, Cull A, Traynor E, et al. Neuropsychometric evaluation of long-term survivors of adult brain tumours: relationship with tumour and treatment parameters. *Radiother Oncol.* 1996;41:55–59.

6. Klein M, Heimans JJ, Aaronson NK, et al. Effect of radiotherapy and other treatment-related factors on mid-term to long-term cognitive sequelae in low-grade gliomas: a comparative study. *Lancet.* 2002;360:1361–1368.

7. Benesch M, Lackner H, Sovinz P, et al. Late sequela after treatment of childhood low-grade gliomas: a retrospective analysis of 69 long-term survivors treated between 1983 and 2003. *J Neurooncol.* 2006;78:199–205.

8. Stuschke M, Eberhardt W, Pöttgen C, et al. Prophylactic cranial irradiation in locally advanced non-small-cell lung cancer after multimodality treatment: long-term follow-up and investigations of late neuropsychologic effects. *J Clin Oncol.* 1999;17:2700–2709.

9. Costello A, Shallice T, Gullan R, et al. The early effects of radiotherapy on intellectual and cognitive functioning in patients with frontal brain tumours: the use of a new neuropsychological methodology. *J Neurooncol.* 2004;67:351–359.

10. Combs SE, Volk S, Schulz-Ertner D, et al. Management of acoustic neuromas with fractionated stereotactic radiotherapy (FSRT): long-term results in 106 patients treated in a single institution. *Int J Radiat Oncol Biol Phys.* 2005;63:75–81.

11. Kortmann RD, Timmerman B, Taylor RE, et al. Current and future strategies in radiotherapy of childhood low-grade glioma of the brain. Part II: Treatment-related late toxicity. *Strahlenther Onkol.* 2003;179:585–597.

12. Ris MD, Packer R, Goldwein J, et al. Intellectual outcome after reduced-dose radiation therapy plus adjuvant chemotherapy for medulloblastoma: a Children's Cancer Group study. *J Clin Oncol.* 2001;19:3470–3476.

13. Langer T, Martus P, Ottensmeier H, et al. CNS late-effects after ALL therapy in childhood. Part III: neuropsychological performance in long-term survivors of childhood ALL: impairments of concentration, attention, and memory. *Med Pediatr Oncol.* 2002;38:320–328.

14. Waber DP, Shapiro BL, Carpentieri SC, et al. Excellent therapeutic efficacy and minimal late neurotoxicity in children treated with 18 Gray of cranial radiation therapy for high-risk acute lymphoblastic leukemia: a 7-year follow-up study of the Dana-Farber Cancer Institute Consortium Protocol 87-01. *Cancer.* 2001;92:15–22.

15. Waber DP, Silverman LB, Catania L, et al. Outcomes of a randomized trial of hyperfractionated cranial radiation therapy for treatment of high-risk acute lymphoblastic leukemia: therapeutic efficacy and neurotoxicity. *J Clin Oncol.* 2004;22:2701–2707.

16. Mulhern RK, Kepner JL, Thomas PR, et al. Neuropsychologic functioning of survivors of childhood medulloblastoma randomized to receive conventional or reduced-dose craniospinal irradiation: a pediatroc Oncology Group study. *J Clin Oncol.* 1998;16:1723–1728.

17. Carpentieri SC, Waber DP, Scott RM, et al. Memory deficits among children with craniopharyngiomas. *Neurosurgery.* 2001;49:1053–1058.

18. Kiehna EN, Mulhern RK, Li C, et al. Changes in attentional performance of children and young adults with localized primary brain tumors after conformal radiation therapy. *J Clin Oncol.* 2006;24:5283–5290.

19. Schultz KA, Ness KK, Whitton J, et al. Behavioral and social outcomes in adolescent survivors of childhood cancer: a report from the Childhood Cancer Survivor Study. *J Clin Oncol.* 2007;25:3649–3656.

20. Akiyama K, Tanaka R, Sato M, et al. Cognitive dysfunction and histological findings in adult rats one year after whole brain irradiation. *Neurol Med Chir (Tokyo).* 2001;41:590–598.

21. Moretti R, Torre P, Antonello RM, et al. Neuropsychological evaluation of late-onset post-radiotherapy encephalopathy: a comparison with vascular dementia. *J Neurol Sci.* 2005;229–230:195–200.

22. Surma-aho O, Niemelä M, Vilkki J, et al. Adverse long-term effects of brain radiotherapy in adult low-grade glioma patients. *Neurology*. 2001;56:1285–1290.
23. Heikens J, Michiels EM, Behrendt H, et al. Long-term neuro-endocrine sequelae after treatment for childhood medulloblastoma. *Eur J Cancer*. 1998;34:1592–1597.
24. Livesey EA, Hindmarsh PC, Brook CG, et al. Endocrine disorders following treatment of childhood brain tumours. *Br J Cancer*. 1990;61:622–625.
25. Pai HH, Thornton A, Katznelson L, et al. Hypothalamic/pituitary function following high-dose conformal radiotherapy to the base of skull: demonstration of a dose-effect relationship using dose-volume histogram analysis. *Int J Radiat Oncol Biol Phys*. 2001;49:1079–1092.
26. Oberfield SE, Allen JC, Pollack J, et al. Long-term endocrine sequelae after treatment of medulloblastoma: prospective study of growth and thyroid function. *J Pediatr*. 1986;108:219–223.
27. Minniti G, Jaffrain-Rea M-L, Osti M, et al. The long-term efficacy of conventional radiotherapy in patients with GH-secreting pituitary adenomas. *Clin Endocrinol*. 2005;62:210–216.
28. Mitsumori M, Shrieve DC, Alexander E III, et al. Initial clinical results of linac-based stereotactic radiosurgery and stereotactic radiotherapy for pituitary adenomas. *Int J Radiat Oncol Biol Phys*. 1998;42:573–580.
29. Feigl GC, Bonelli CM, Berghold A, et al. Effects of gamma knife radiosurgery of pituitary adenomas on pituitary function. *J Neurosurg*. 2002; 97 (Suppl 5):415–421.
30. Zierhut D, Flentje M, Adolph J, et al. Eternal radiotherapy of pituitary adenomas. *Int J Radiat Oncol Biol Phys*. 1995;33:307–314.
31. Vladyka V, Liscak R, Novotny J, et al. Radiation tolerance of functioning pituitary tissue in gamma knife surgery for pituitary adenomas. *Neurosurgery*. 2003;52:309–317.
32. Sheehan JP, Niranjan A, Sheehan JM, et al. Stereotactic radiosurgery for pituitary adenomas: an intermediate review of its safety, efficacy, and role in the neurosurgical treatment armamentarium. *J Neurosurg*. 2005;102:678–691.
33. Tischler RB, Loeffler JS, Lunsford LD, et al. Tolerance of cranial nerves of the cavernous sinus to radiosurgery. *Int J Radiat Oncol Biol Phys*. 1993;27:215–221.
34. Leber KA, Berglöff J, Pendl G. Dose-response tolerance of the visual pathways and cranial nerves of the cavernous sinus to stereotactic radiosurgery. *J Neurosurg*. 1998;88:43–50.
35. Brada M, Rajan B, Traish D, et al. The long-term efficacy of conservative surgery and radiotherapy in the control of pituitary adenomas. *Clin Endocrinol*. 1993;38:571–578.
36. Movsas B, Movsas TZ, Steinberg SM, et al. Long-term visual changes following pituitary irradiation. *Int J Radiat Oncol Biol Phys*. 1995;33:599–605.
37. Parsons JT, Bova FJ, Fitzgerald CR, et al. Radiation retinopathy after external-beam irradiation: analysis of time-dose factors. *Int J Radiat Oncol Biol Phys*. 1994;30:765–773.
38. Parsons JT, Bova FJ, Fitzgerald CR, et al. Radiation optic neuropathy after megavoltage external-beam irradiation: analysis of time-dose factors. *Int J Radiat Oncol Biol Phys*. 1994;30:755–763.
39. Merchant TE, Gould CJ, Xiong X, et al. Early neuro-otologic effects of three-dimensional irradiation in children with primary brain tumors. *Int J Radiat Oncol Biol Phys*. 2004;58:1194–1207.
40. Johannesen TB, Rasmussen K, Winther FO, et al. Late radiation effects of hearing, vestibular function, and taste in brain tumor patients. *Int J Radiat Oncol Biol Phys*. 2002;53:86–90.
41. Raaijmakers E, Engelen AM. Is sensorineural hearing loss a possible side effect of nasopharyngeal and parotid irradiation? A systematic review of the literature. *Radiother Oncol*. 2002;65:1–7.
42. Bhandare N, Antonelli JP, Morris CG, et al. Ototoxicity after radiotherapy for head and neck tumors. *Int J Radiat Oncol Biol Phys*. 2007;67:469–479.

43. Stupp R, Mason WP, van den Bent MJ, et al. Radiotherapy plus concomitant and adjuvant temozolomide for gliobalstoma. *N Engl J Med*. 2005;352:987–996.

44. Mayer R, Sminia P. Reirradiation tolerance of the human brain. *Int J Radiat Oncol Biol Phys*. 2008;70:1350–1360.

45. Peterson KM, Shao C, McCarter R, et al. An analysis of SEER data of increasing risk of secondary malignant neoplasms among long-term survivors of childhood brain tumors. *Pediatr Blood Cancer*. 2006;47:83–88.

46. Walter AW, Hancock ML, Pui CH, et al. Secondary brain tumors in children treated for acute lymphoblastic leukemia at St Jude Children's Research Hospital. *J Clin Oncol*. 1998;16:3761–3767.

47. Dalton VMK, Gelber RD, Li F, et al. Second malignancies in patients treated for childhood acute lymphoblastic leukemia. *J Clin Oncol*. 1998;16:2848–2853.

48. Neglia JP, Robison LL, Stovall M, et al. New primary neoplasms of the central nervous system in survivors of childhood cancer: a report from the Childhood Cancer Survivor Study. *J Natl Cancer Inst*. 2006;98:1528–1537.

49. Tsang RW, Laperriere NJ, Simpson WJ, et al. Glioma arising after radiation therapy for pituitary adenoma. *Cancer*. 1993;72:2227–2233.

50. Bembo SA, Pasmantier R, Davis RP, et al. Osteogenic sarcoma of the sella after radiation treatment of a pituitary adenoma. *Endocr Pract*. 2004;10:335–338.

51. Bowers DC, Liu Y, Leisenring W, et al. Late-occurring stroke among long-term survivors of childhood leukemia and brain tumors: a report from the Childhood Cancer Survivor Study. *J Clin Oncol*. 2006;24:5277–5282.

52. Poussaint TY, Siffert J, Barnes PD, et al. Hemorrhagic vasculopathy following the treatment of CNS neoplasia in childhood: diagnosis and followup. *Am J Neuroradiol*. 1995;16:693–699.

53. Brada M, Burchell L, Ashley S, et al. The incidence of cerebrovascular accidents in patients with pituitary adenoma. *Int J Radiat Oncol Biol Phys*. 1999;45:693–698.

54. Pollock BE, Nippoldt TB, Stafford SL, et al. Results of stereotactic radiosurgery in patients with hormone-producing pituitary adenomas: factors associated with endocrine normalization. *J Neurosurg*. 2002;97:525–530.

55. Lim YJ, Leem W, Park JT, et al. Cerebral infarction with ICA occlusion after gamma knife radiosurgery for pituitary adenoma: a case report. *Stereotact Funct Neurosurg*. 1999;72:132–129.

56. Nimjee SM, Powers CJ, Bulsara KR. Review of the literature on de novo formation of cavernous malformations of the central nervous system after radiation therapy *Neurosurg Focus*. 2006;21:1–6.

57. Lawenda BD, Gagne HM, Gierga DP, et al. Permanent alopecia after cranial irradiation: dose-response relationship. *Int J Radiat Oncol Biol Phys*. 2004;60:879–887.

58. Chapman CA, Waber DP, Bernstein JH, et al. Neurobehavioral and neurologic outcome in long-term survivors of posterior fossa brain tumors: role of age and perioperative factors. *J Child Neurol*. 1995;10:209–212.

59. Mostow EN, Byrne J, Connelly RR, et al. Quality of life in long-term survivors of CNS tumors of childhood and adolescence. *J Clin Oncol*. 1991;9:592–599.

60. Dalton VK, Rue M, Silverman LB, et al. Height and weight in children treated for acute lymphoblastic leukemia: relationship to CNS treatment. *J Clin Oncol*. 2003;21:2953–2960.

61. Chow EJ, Friedman DL, Yasui Y, et al. Decreased adult height in survivors of childhood acute lymphoblastic leukemia: a report from the Childhood Cancer Survivor Study. *J Pediatr*. 2007;150:370–375.

62. Schriock EA, Schell MJ, Carter M, et al. Abnormal growth pattern and adult short stature in 115 long-term survivors of childhood leukemia. *J Clin Oncol*. 1991;9:400–405.

63. Marcus KJ, Goumnerova L, Billett AL, et al. Stereotactic radiotherapy for localized low-grade gliomas in children: final results of a prospective trial. *Int J Radiat Oncol Biol Phys*. 2005;61:374–379.

64. Yock TI, Tarbell NJ. Technology insight: proton beam radiotherapy for treatment in pediatric brain tumors. *Nat Clin Pract Oncol.* 2004;1:97–103.
65. Johannesen TB, Lien HH, Hole KH, et al. Radiological and clinical assessment of long-term brain tumour survivors after radiotherapy. *Radiother Oncol.* 2003;69:169–176.
66. Cheung M, Chan AS, Law SC, et al. Cognitive function of patients with nasopharyngeal carcinoma with and without temporal lobe radionecrosis. *Arch Neurol.* 2000;57:1347–1352.
67. Chan YL, Leung SF, King AD, et al. Late radiation injury to the temporal lobes: morphologic evaluation at MR imaging. *Radiology.* 1999;213:800–807.
68. Chan YL, Yeung DK, Leung SF, et al. Dynamic susceptibility contrast-enhanced perfusion MR imaging in late radiation-induced injury of the brain. *Acta Neurochir Suppl.* 2005;95:173–175.
69. Paakko E, Talvensaari K, Pyhtinen J, et al. Late cranial MRI after cranial irradiation in survivors of childhood cancer. *Neuroradiology.* 1994;36:652–655.
70. Russo C, Fischbein N, Grant E, et al. Late radiation injury following hyperfractionated craniospinal radiotherapy for primitive neuroectodermal tumor. *Int J Radiat Oncol Biol Phys.* 1999;44:85–90.
71. Ricardi U, Corrias A, Einaudi S, et al. Thyroid dysfunction as a late effect in childhood medulloblastoma: a comparison of hyperfractionated versus conventionally fractionated craniospinal radiotherapy. *Int J Radiat Oncol Biol Phys.* 2001;50:1287–1294.

Chapter 4
Late Effects of Chemotherapy

Sridharan Gururangan

Introduction

While surgery and radiotherapy have long been established as treatment modalities of patients with brain tumors, the usefulness of chemotherapy is being increasingly recognized as an important therapeutic strategy, especially in young children, with the view of delaying radiotherapy or avoiding this modality altogether. Combination chemotherapy in standard and myeloablative doses is now regularly utilized to treat pediatric and adult brain tumors including low-grade gliomas, central primitive neuroectodermal tumors (PNET), ependymomas, germ cell tumors, and malignant gliomas. Traditionally, the types of chemotherapeutic agents used in patients with brain tumors have included microtubule disrupting drugs (e.g., vincristine) and alkylating agents including platinum analogs (cisplatin and carboplatin), nitrosoureas (e.g., carmustine, lomustine), cyclophosphamide, and ifosfamide, and more recently temozolomide (Temodar™, Schering Plough Corporation, Kenilworth, NJ). Inhibitors of Topoisomerase I and II (camptothecins, etoposide) have also been used either as single agents or in combination with alkylating drugs.[1] While the use of chemotherapy has most certainly improved outcomes in patients with CNS tumors, both acute and chronic toxicities from these drugs compromise their therapeutic intent and limits their effectiveness. Also, chronic organ damage due to chemotherapy results in significant impairment in quality of life of long-term survivors and impairs their ability to lead a productive existence. It is therefore mandatory for health care providers to have a proper understanding of these side effects in the long-term follow-up of brain tumor survivors. Table 4.1 lists the most common chemotherapeutic drugs used in the treatment of patients with brain tumors, common acute and chronic side effects, and a suggested plan

S. Gururangan (✉)
Director, and the Pediatric Clinical Services, Associate Professor of Pediatrics and Surgery, The Preston Robert Tisch Brain Tumor Center departments of Pediatrics and Surgery, Duke University Medical Center, Durham, NC 27710, USA
e-mail: gurur002@mc.duke.edu

S. Goldman, C.D. Turner (eds.), *Late Effects of Treatment for Brain Tumors*,
Cancer Treatment and Research 150, DOI 10.1007/b109924_4,
© Springer Science+Business Media, LLC 2009

Table 4.1 Common chemotherapeutic agents used in patients with brain tumors, related acute and chronic side effects, screening and diagnostic tests, and management plan

Agent	Acute side effects	Chronic side effects	Screening and diagnostic tests	Management and intervention
Nitrosoureas (BCNU, CCNU)	Thrombophlebitis (carmustine) Delayed bone marrow suppression	Renal failure Pulmonary fibrosis Hypogonadism	Urine analysis, serum BUN, creatinine annually Chest X-ray, PFTs including DLCO once a year Serum testosterone/estradiol, FSH/LH	Low salt and protein diet, dialysis, renal transplant Pulmonary evaluation, steroid therapy, avoidance of infections, flu vaccines annually Referral to fertility clinic Sex hormone replacement
Cisplatin	Acute renal failure Myelosuppression (not severe) Nausea and vomiting Hypokalemia Hypomagnesemia Hypocalcemia	Sensorineural hearing loss Chronic renal failure Peripheral neuropathy Hypomagnesemia Hypogonadism Secondary leukemia (moderate risk)	Pure tone audiometry, DPOAE, BAER Serum BUN/ creatinine, Cr^{51} EDTA clearance Neurologic examinations, nerve conduction studies Serum Mg^{++} levels CBC with diff annually	Preferential seating in class, avoid noise exposure and ototoxic agents, hearing aids Mg^{++} supplementation
Carboplatin	Allergic reactions Myelosuppression (severe) Nausea and vomiting (mild)	Same as cisplatin but only at high doses	As above	-
Cyclophosphamide	Nausea and vomiting Alopecia Myelosuppression (severe) Hemorrhagic cystitis Cardiac necrosis (high doses only) Syndrome of inappropriate ADH secretion (SIADH)	Pulmonary fibrosis Hypogonadism Bladder fibrosis possibly leading to bladder cancers Secondary MDS / leukemia	Chest X-ray, PFTs including DL_{CO} Serum testosterone/estradiol, FSH/LH, serum inhibin A and B CBC with diff q annually	Pulmonary evaluation, steroid therapy, avoidance of infections, flu vaccines annually Referral to fertility clinic Sex hormone replacement

Table 4.1 (continued)

Agent	Acute side effects	Chronic side effects	Screening and diagnostic tests	Management and intervention
Ifosfamide	Nausea and vomiting Alopecia Myelosuppression (severe) Hemorrhagic cystitis Acute encephalopathy Renal tubular acidosis Hyperphosphaturia Glycosuria Hypokalemia Renal failure (rare)	Hypophosphatemic rickets Renal tubular acidosis Hypokalemia Chronic renal failure Bladder fibrosis possibly leading to bladder cancers Hypogonadism Secondary MDS/leukemia	blood pressure, height, weight, hemoglobin/hematocrit, urinalysis, creatinine, annually Serum testosterone/estradiol, FSH/LH, serum inhibin A and B annually	Low salt and protein diet, dialysis, renal transplant Electrolyte and phosphorus supplements Counseling regarding bladder cancer
Temozolomide	Myelosuppression Fatigue Constipation	Not known	NA	NA
Procarbazine	Myelosuppression Nausea and vomiting Drowsiness, depression, agitation, and paresthesias Hypersensitivity reactions Hypertension when given with tricyclic antidepressants or sympathomimetics	Hypogonadism Secondary leukemia Leucoencephalopathy (following intra-arterial therapy)	Serum testosterone/estradiol, FSH/LH, serum inhibin A and B CBC with diff q annually	Referral to fertility clinic Sex hormone replacement

Table 4.1 (continued)

Agent	Acute side effects	Chronic side effects	Screening and diagnostic tests	Management and intervention
Busulfan	Myelosuppression (acute and delayed) Seizures (high doses) Addisonian syndrome	Pulmonary fibrosis Hypogonadism Secondary leukemia	Chest X-ray, PFTs including DL_{CO} Serum testosterone/estradiol, FSH/LH, serum inhibin A and B CBC with diff q annually	Pulmonary evaluation, steroid therapy, avoidance of infections, flu vaccines annually Referral to fertility clinic Sex hormone replacement
Vincristine	Alopecia (mild) Myelosuppression (mild) Jaw pain Ptosis Foot drop Myalgias Abdominal pain Constipation Loss of deep tendon reflexes Hepatic dysfunction Seizures SIADH	Peripheral neuropathy	Neurologic examination Nerve conduction studies	AFO braces for foot drop Orthopedic evaluation for ankle stabilization Analgesics for neuropathic pain
Etoposide	Alopecia Myelosuppression Mucositis Liver dysfunction Allergic reactions	Secondary leukemia	CBC with differential q annually	Appropriate management of secondary leukemia

of assessment of organ function in a long-term follow-up clinic. The following discussion will be limited to some of the common long-term side effects of chemotherapy. It must be kept in mind that in most instances, there is additional damage to these organs from exposure to non-chemotherapeutic treatments including irradiation and supportive care measures (e.g., antibiotics, diuretics, steroids etc.,), and environmental factors (e.g., the influence of noise exposure in children with hearing loss from cisplatin).

Late Effects of Chemotherapy

Sensorineural Hearing Loss

Chemotherapy-induced sensorineural hearing loss (SNHL) in patients with brain tumors is invariably due to exposure to platinum analogs mostly cisplatin (CDDP), and less so from carboplatin or oxaliplatin. The platinum group of agents has been in use since the early 1970s and has been the mainstay of therapy in most childhood brain tumors, including embryonal tumors like medulloblastoma, ependymoma, and germ cell tumors.[2,3] Despite its effectiveness, the use of CDDP is limited by its tendency to cause hearing loss and renal damage.[4–8] The mechanism of the toxicity of CDDP on the inner ear has been extensively studied and reported in the literature and recently reviewed by Rybak et al.[9] Preclinical toxicity studies in guinea pigs and gerbils have demonstrated that the ototoxic effects of CDDP are due to cochlear damage, particularly the organ of Corti (specifically the outer hair cells), spiral ganglion, and the lateral wall (stria vascularis and the lateral ligament). Microscopic examination in these animals following CDDP exposure shows that cells of the Type I spiral ganglion undergo detachment of myelin sheaths.[9] Examination of the stria vascularis demonstrates edema, bulging, rupture, and cytoplasmic depletion of organelles.[9] TUNEL staining reveals apoptosis in all three areas of the cochlea. Platinum DNA adducts were identified in outer hair cells, spiral ganglion, and stria vascularis, suggesting that these were indeed the targets for the drug. Experimental studies on the biochemical basis for CDDP-induced ototoxicity indicate that reactive oxygen species (ROS, including hydroxide, hydrogen peroxide, and lipid peroxides) might be the cause of cellular destruction in the cochlea. Such reactive radicals are generated due to CDDP mediated depletion of antioxidants including direct binding of the agent to active sulfhydryl groups of antioxidant enzymes, depletion of copper and selenium (active components of enzymes superoxide dismutase and glutathione peroxidase), direct inhibition of antioxidant enzymes by the ROS, depletion of glutathione and its cofactor NADPH, and induction of NOX-3 (an isoform of NADPH oxidase) that results in an accumulation of free oxygen radicals.[9] Accumulation of ROS in the cochlea results in calcium influx into the cells triggering cellular apoptosis.[11] Cisplatin has also been shown to directly affect the potassium channels in the stria vascularis resulting in K^+ efflux from the cells and impaired generation of endocochlear potential within this structure following transmission of sound signals into the cochlea.[9]

Clinical hearing loss following CDDP treatment can be graded according to severity as described by Brock et al.[10] This system grades hearing loss based on pure tone thresholds from grade 0 (no hearing loss), grade 1 (minimal hearing loss, ≥ 40 dB at or >8000 Hz), grade 2 (moderate hearing loss, ≥ 40 dB at or >4000 Hz), and grade 3 or 4 (severe hearing loss, ≥ 40 dB at or >1000 Hz). This grading system helps to recognize high-frequency hearing loss and is more useful in assessing ototoxicity from CDDP compared to other grading systems including the NCI common toxicity criteria of adverse events (CTCAE).[6] The incidence of hearing loss in children receiving CDDP for various solid tumors varies between 35–50% in most published studies.[4-6,8] However, most children suffer from high-frequency hearing loss (i.e., Brock grade I) and $\leq 15\%$ of children have severe hearing impairment that affects the speech frequencies requiring hearing aids. Ototoxicity from CDDP is typically asymptomatic although patients can complain of tinnitus. The effect on hearing can be seen as soon as 2–3 weeks from the last dose of treatment. As one would expect, several risk factors have been established that can predict severe hearing loss following CDDP therapy. The two most important risk factors for CDDP-induced ototoxicity include age and cumulative exposure to the drug. Patients younger than five years of age have a higher risk of developing SNHL for a given cumulative dose of CDDP as compared to older children.[6,7] In a study published from the Children's Hospital of Philadelphia, Li et al. evaluated hearing impairment in 153 children who had received CDDP containing regimens for various solid tumors (excluding those who had received cranial irradiation).[6] Among patients who developed moderate to severe hearing loss, 69% were less than five years of age as compared to only 5% who were older than 15 years at the time of treatment (Fig. 4.1).[6] For a given cumulative dose, younger children develop more hearing loss than older patients. For example, a three-year-old infant who receives four cycles of CDDP will have a 15 dB higher hearing loss compared to a 13-year-old child who receives the same treatment.[7] This difference increases to 30 dB after seven courses.[7] Identifying hearing loss in this patient population is particularly important since such defective hearing will impair speech development.[8] Similarly, Li et al. have shown that a cumulative dose of CDDP (as compared to magnitude of individual doses) has a significant impact on the incidence and degree of hearing loss (Fig. 4.1).[6] Only 13% of children developed Brock Grade 2 or worse hearing loss when the cumulative dose was $100-300$ mg/m^2; that increased to 22% with doses of $700-1130$ mg/m^2.[6] In a study from St. Jude Children's Hospital, Schell et al. showed that hearing loss from CDDP follows a triphasic pattern.[9] In most cases, the hearing threshold remains at baseline levels for typically 3–4 courses, after which a minimal shift occurs; this increases with further treatment past a substantial level (at least 50 dB) and then plateaus despite continuing exposure to the drug.[7] In patients with brain tumors, the addition of cranial irradiation

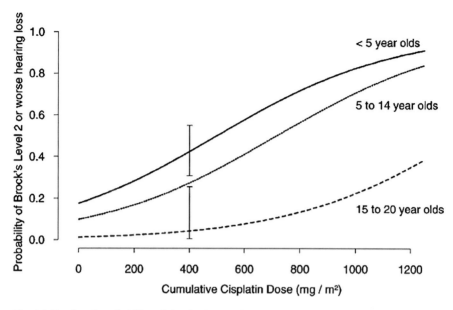

Fig. 4.1 Predicted probability of developing moderate to severe losses as a function of age at treatment and the total cumulative dosage of cisplatin. The 95% confidence intervals (CIs) for the predicted risk probability at the overall median dose, 400 mg/m2, are also identified. At 400 mg/m2, the younger group would have a significantly higher risk than the older group in developing moderate to severe loss

and/or posterior fossa radiotherapy compounds the risk of worsening ototoxicity due to CDDP. Irradiation of the cochlear apparatus adds an additional 25–30 dB to the hearing loss caused by CDDP alone.[7] While one report in children with brain tumors suggested that cranial irradiation given post-CDDP does not worsen hearing loss, the follow-up period in this study was relatively short to accurately estimate the delayed effect of this modality on hearing.[4] Hearing loss from CDDP can also be aggravated from the concurrent use of other ototoxic drugs including aminoglycosides, genetic conditions that predispose to hearing loss, and chronic noise exposure before or after CDDP therapy.[11–14] In contrast to CDDP, carboplatin in conventional doses typically causes only mild ototoxicity.[15] However, when used in myeloablative doses, it can cause severe hearing impairment especially in patients who have had prior insults related to CDDP exposure, cranial irradiation, or exposure to other ototoxic drugs.[12]

Sensorineural hearing loss from CDDP is usually permanent with very little improvement following cessation of therapy.[7] However, the benefits of the drug in sustained tumor control outweighs this risk, especially since patients can be fitted with suitable hearing aids to overcome this deficit. However, there has been a concerted effort in identifying strategies to minimize hearing loss in patients who receive CDDP with or without cranial irradiation. Obtaining a baseline pure tone audiogram (PTA) prior to starting therapy and prior to each cycle of CDDP will enable the clinician to screen for hearing impairment prior to and during therapy. Younger children who cannot cooperate well for PTA should have their hearing measured by behavioral audiometry, distortion product otoacoustic emission (DPOAE), or brain stem auditory evoked responses (BAER).[16] Most contemporary protocols that use CDDP containing regimens have specific dose modification guidelines to offset further damage; a 50% dose reduction is recommended for Brock Grade 2 hearing loss and, for those with more severe damage, the drug is withheld altogether. **Such dose reductions should be carefully weighed against the risk of losing tumor control from decreasing CDDP exposure**. Newer radiotherapy techniques including 3-D conformal radiotherapy, intensity modulated radiotherapy (IMRT), or proton therapy are effective in avoiding or minimizing radiation exposure to the cochlear apparatus and, thus, the compounding risk from this modality. In addition, otoprotective drugs including amifostine and sodium thiosulfate are being tested in the clinic in patients receiving CDDP for various malignancies to ameliorate hearing loss, renal damage, and peripheral neuropathy.[17] Amifostine (Ethyol, WR-2721; Medimmune, Gaithersburg, MD) is a phosphorylated thiol that is converted to its active metabolite WR-1065 that is then dephosphorylated by membrane-bound alkaline phosphatase (ALK). The selectivity of amifostine for normal tissue as compared to tumor is based on the higher expression of ALK in normal versus tumor tissue. The active metabolite scavenges ROS within the cells and thus prevents damage. Although FDA-approved for certain indications including prevention of chemotherapy-induced renal dysfunction, myelosupression, and radiation-induced xerostomia and mucositis, the role of amifostine in preventing chemotherapy-induced toxicities including hearing impairment remains unclear.[17] The drug is associated with significant toxicities including hypotension, hypersensitivity reactions, and hypocalcemia.[17] Two recent pediatric studies of the use of amifostine as an otoprotectant in children with solid tumors receiving CDDP-containing regimens have not shown any measurable benefit.[18,19] However, in a recent large prospective study of children with newly diagnosed average risk medulloblastoma who received upfront radiotherapy, followed by four cycles of dose intensive CDDP, cyclophosphamide, and vincristine plus stem cell rescue, the use of two doses of intravenous amifostine (600 mg/m^2 given 5 minutes prior to and 3 hours post start of a 6-hour CDDP infusion) resulted in a more than 20% reduction in severe hearing loss as compared to a control group of patients who were treated on the same study, but did not receive amifostine (Amar Gajjar MD; Memphis, TN, personal communication 2007). Similarly, sodium thiosulfate (STS) is being utilized as an otoprotectant in patients with brain tumors who receive high-dose intra-arterial carboplatin following blood-brain barrier disruption with some preliminary evidence of efficacy.[20,21]

Peripheral Neuropathy

Peripheral nerves are made up of sensory, motor, and autonomic nerve fibers and can be small (unmyelinated, made up of microtubules, and sense pain and temperature) or large (myelinated and made up of neurofilaments – the framework of axons – and control muscles, position, and vibration).[22] The nerve fibers terminate at the level of skin and muscle distally, and proximally extend to the dorsal root ganglion where the cell body is present with further transmission via the spinal cord via the dorsal column (large fibers) and spinothalamic tract (small fibers).[22] Peripheral neuropathy can be defined as injury, inflammation, or degeneration of peripheral nerve fibers and is one of the important and frequently underestimated long-term side effects of chemotherapy in patients with brain tumors.[22] Agents typically associated with this debilitating side effect are the vinca alkaloids and platinum drugs, including CDDP and oxaliplatin. The anti-inflammatory/antiangiogenic drug thalidomide (Thalomid®, Celgene Corporation, USA) that is used in patients with brain tumors either alone or in combination with chemotherapy, is another drug that can cause significant peripheral nerve damage.

In general, the incidence of polyneuropathy due to chemotherapeutic drugs is not clearly known in children, but is found in about 20% of adults with cancer.[22] The neuropathy is temporally related to drug administration (except in the case of CDDP), is related to the dose of the drug, depends on the drug crossing the blood-nerve barrier, occurs in a stocking glove distribution (typically first in fingertips and toes) and progresses medially towards the trunk, affecting one fiber type more than the other.

Although most vinca alkaloids (vincristine, vinblastine, or vindesine) can cause neuropathic symptoms, vincristine is unique in its tendency to cause polyneuropathy and is perhaps its only long-term toxicity. This microtubule inhibiting agent classically causes early loss of deep tendon reflexes (mediated by unmyelinated small nerve fibers) and a symmetrical sensory impairment and paresthesias in the distal extremities. **Nerve damage is dependent on dose and duration of treatment. Those who receive more than 6 mg/m^2 of vincristine (or a cumulative dose of 15–20 mg) begin to experience neuropathic symptoms.**[22,23] Patients frequently complain of limb, back, and abdominal pain following treatment. Paresthesias of the hands and feet can occur in up to 67% of patients who receive vincristine. About 30–40% of patients develop a motor neuropathy manifested as foot or wrist drop. Cranial nerves are particularly affected and can present as ptosis, vocal cord paralysis (causing stridor), diplopia, and facial palsy. Rarely optic atrophy or sensorineural hearing loss has been reported.[22,24] Vincristine also affects the autonomic nervous system that is most frequently manifested as constipation. When used in high doses or in the presence of hepatic dysfunction, it is possible to observe orthostatic hypotension, cardiac autonomic dysfunction, or urinary retention.[22,24] Patients at risk of severe neuropathy from vincristine include elderly patients, those with preexisting conditions that already predispose them to peripheral nerve damage (e.g., diabetes mellitus) or inherited neuropathies like

Charcot-Marie-Tooth disease, who receive high individual doses of the drug (more than 2 mg/m^2), or have hepatic dysfunction.[22,24]

The neuropathic symptoms following vincristine usually resolve after discontinuation of the drug in over two-thirds of patients. However, in some cases, patients experience intractable symptoms for years following cessation of therapy.[22,24] It is, therefore, prudent to minimize the duration of the drug's administration, decrease the drug's dose, or discontinue treatment at the earliest sign of motor or severe sensory neuropathy. Concurrent administration of specific agents to ameliorate the effects of the drug including pyridoxine, vitamin B-12, glutamic acid, folinic acid, or a mixture of gangliosides have not shown to be of benefit. In the author's experience, patients with long-standing polyneuropathy associated with intractable pain or paresthesias might benefit from drugs like gabapentin (Neurontin^{TM}, Pfizer pharmaceuticals, New York, NY) or Amitryptiline (Elavil$^®$, Astra Zeneca, USA) in controlling symptoms.

Unlike vincristine, the polyneuropathy associated with CDDP affects large fibers and causes a sensory neuropathy characterized by loss of sense of position and vibration. Some patients even complain of a lightning like sensation that starts in the neck and travels down the arms and legs following flexion of the neck – the *Lhermitte's sign*. Neuropathologic studies have shown that there is aggregation of microfilaments and swelling/loss of axons. **Cisplatin associated neuropathy occurs in 50–70% of patients following a cumulative dose of ≥ 300 mg/m^2, especially in bleomycin-containing regimens either at the end of therapy or even 2–3 months following completion of treatment.**[22,24] Recovery occurs in about 60% of patients, but in some it can be a chronic and debilitating side effect.[22,24] No specific antidote has been conclusively shown to protect patients from the neuropathic effects of CDDP.

Thalidomide (Thalomid$^®$, Celgene Corporation, USA) is an oral anti-inflammatory/antiangiogenic drug that is being used for several inflammatory conditions (Systemic lupus erythematosus, Behcet's disease), hematologic malignancies (multiple myeloma), and for malignant glioma.[25,26] The main side effects associated with this drug are sedation, constipation, and peripheral neuropathy.[25,26] Thalidomide typically produces a sensorimotor neuropathy and affects mostly nonmyelinated nerve fibers.[22,26] Thalidomide-induced peripheral neuropathy is dependent on the duration of exposure rather than the cumulative dose or dose intensity.[26] In one study of 75 adults who received thalidomide for multiple myeloma, over 75% of patients developed clinical neuropathy by 12 months of treatment.[26] Reversibility of neuropathy following discontinuation of the drug is not clearly known since most patients did not receive formal evaluations after stopping therapy.

Renal Dysfunction

The kidneys are susceptible to toxic effects of chemotherapy due to high blood flow through this organ and its role, in conjunction with the liver, in drug elimination. Chemotherapy-induced renal dysfunction can be caused by damage to the renal structures or vasculature, hemolytic–uremic syndrome, or prerenal perfusion deficits.[27] **The drugs that typically cause renal injury in patients with brain tumors include platinum analogs, ifosfamide, and nitrosoureas.**[27] In general terms, the extent of renal damage from most chemotherapeutic agents is related to age at diagnosis, cumulative exposure to the drug, prior renal dysfunction related to disease or nephrectomy, and exposure to other nephrotoxic agents including radiotherapy, aminoglycoside antibiotics, and loop diuretics (e.g., furosemide).

Cisplatin (CDDP). CDDP is the chemotherapeutic drug that is most likely to cause renal damage in patients with brain tumors due to its frequency of use in this patient population and its selective accumulation in the liver and kidneys.[28] Nephrotoxicity is a dose limiting side effect of CDDP and is clearly dependent on dose intensity (higher dose per course) and cumulative dose exposure. The mechanism of CDDP-mediated damage has been extensively studied and reported in the literature.[28] It is interesting to note that although CDDP typically targets rapidly dividing tumor cells, its toxic effect on the kidneys is mediated by damage to the nondividing proximal tubular cells (PTC) by a process distinct from formation of platinum-DNA adducts.[28] Cisplatin combines with extracellular glutathione (GSH) and is then cleaved to a CDDP-cysteine-glycine or CDDP-cysteine conjugate by the enzyme gamma glutamyl transpeptidase (GGT). These conjugates are highly reactive thiols that cause apoptosis of the cell either via mitochondrial apoptotic pathways (caspase c) or through tumor necrosis factor (TNF) and Fas receptor.[28] Such proximal tubular damage results in K^+, Na^+, Mg^{++}, and water loss through the kidneys.[29] Through an auto feedback mechanism between PTC and the glomerulus, Na^+ and water loss triggers increased renovascular resistance, decreased glomerular blood flow [and, hence, glomerular filtration rate (GFR)], and a rise in serum creatinine as early as two or three days after CDDP administration.[29] In the clinic, CDDP nephrotoxicity can be ameliorated by the use of pre- and post-hydration with normal saline, mannitol, or furosemide-induced diuresis.[29] Although a decrease in GFR as measured by Cr^{51} EDTA clearance following CDDP (about 8–10% per course) has been reported in children with solid tumors receiving CDDP containing chemotherapy regimens along with acute electrolyte disturbances, frank renal failure requiring dialysis is distinctively uncommon in such patients unless there has been a drug overdose.[28] Decrease in renal dysfunction and electrolyte abnormalities usually occur following a cumulative dose of 300–500 mg/m^2 and can be exacerbated by the use of other nephrotoxins, including drugs like ifosfamide and aminoglycoside antibiotics.[8,30]

Monitoring renal function during CDDP therapy is very important and is best achieved by measuring GFR using Cr^{51} EDTA clearance at baseline and prior to each or every other course. In this context, it should be emphasized that monitoring blood urea nitrogen (BUN), serum creatinine, or 24-hour urine creatinine clearance as surrogate markers of renal function can be misleading since these tests, although specific, are not sensitive enough to detect decline until significant renal function has been lost.[31] In addition, they are dependent on hydration (BUN), nutritional status and muscle mass of the patient (serum creatinine), and proper urine collection (24-hour urine creatinine clearance).[31] Unlike CDDP-induced ototoxicity, Brock et al. have observed that nephrotoxicity due to this drug is at least partially reversible over several years following cessation of therapy.[32]

Carboplatin. Carboplatin, on the other hand, is not nephrotoxic in conventional doses (500–600 mg/m^2/course) when given with pre- and post-hydration, possibly due to its poor retention in renal tubules.[29] However, prior renal dysfunction (from CDDP or other causes) and higher doses of drug (as in high-dose chemotherapy settings) can cause renal dysfunction.

Amifostine has been utilized to decrease the nephrotoxicity from platinum analogs and has been shown to be useful in protecting the kidneys from the toxic effects of CDDP.[17,33] However, dose reduction or switching to carboplatin might be a cheaper and more effective strategy to protect from further damage.[33]

Nitrosoureas. Carmustine (BCNU) and lomustine (CCNU) and other chlorethylnitrosoureas have been used with good results in patients with brain tumors, including low-grade gliomas, medulloblastoma, and malignant gliomas.[34] While the main dose limiting toxicities with this drug group is delayed myelosuppression and pulmonary fibrosis, delayed renal damage has been observed in almost all patients who receive cumulative doses of $\geq 1,400$ mg/m^2 of BCNU for malignant glioma.[35] In most patients, damage is insidious and becomes evident several months following discontinuation of therapy due to storage of these extremely lipid soluble drugs in adipose tissue and slow release into systemic circulation even after cessation of therapy.[35] Renal dysfunction manifests as azotemia, raised serum creatinine levels, and proteinuria. None of these patients show any acute renal impairment during treatment.[35] Renal biopsies in such patients reveal glomerulosclerosis, tubular atrophy, and focal interstitial fibrosis.[37] Renal damage from nitrosoureas is not reversible and no specific chemoprotectant is available. **Nephrotoxicity can be prevented by not giving treatment beyond a cumulative dose of 600 mg/m^2.**

Ifosfamide. Ifosfamide, an oxazophosphorine analog similar to cyclophosphamide, is used to treat sarcomas and intracranial germ cell tumors.[30,36] Nephrotoxicity due to this agent has been well characterized and includes renal tubular damage and decreased glomerular function.[27,30] The exact mechanism of nephrotoxicity due to this drug is unknown, but could be related to some of the reactive metabolites generated by drug activation in the liver.[27] Clinical manifestations of renal toxicity are predominantly from PTC damage and can be subtle in about 90% of patients with only subclinical glycosuria.[30] In about 30% of children receiving ifosfamide, PTC dysfunction is more pronounced with hypokalemia, glycosuria, aminoaciduria, renal tubular acidosis (due to loss of urinary HCO_3^-), proteinuria phosphaturia, and hypophosphatemic rickets, that is collectively termed renal Fanconi's syndrome.[32]

Rarely, distal tubular dysfunction can occur with impairment of urinary acidification and concentration (nephrogenic diabetes insipidus).[30] Glomerular impairment as evidenced by rising serum creatinine and decreasing GFR usually follows tubular damage and is sometimes the only feature of renal toxicity in adolescents.[30] Glomerular disease rarely results in chronic renal failure requiring hemodialysis. Ifosfamide-induced renal toxicity typically occurs in patients following cumulative doses above 45 gm/m^2, age < 5 years, and especially following prior or concomitant CDDP exposure.[30] **It is important to note that nephrotoxicity from ifosfamide cannot be prevented by mesna rescue.**[27] While stopping the drug usually results in some reversal of renal function, renal abnormalities can persistent up to 10 years post-exposure.[30] Such patients will continue to need management of abnormal bone growth due to rickets, supplementation to correct electrolyte imbalances, especially phosphate and bicarbonate, and occasionally vitamin D$_3$ treatment for osteomalacia.[30]

Pulmonary Fibrosis

The drugs that have become the mainstay of therapy for patients with brain tumors have also been associated with pulmonary damage, including pulmonary fibrosis (restrictive lung disease, RLD).[37,38] Such patients are also increasingly prone to recurrent pneumonia and worsening of reactive airway disease.[39] Drugs that have a predilection for causing pulmonary disease include nitrosoureas, cyclophosphamide, bleomycin, busulfan, and methotrexate.[38] Craniospinal irradiation further contributes to this RLD.[37]

Nitrosoureas, including BCNU and CCNU, have been known to cause pulmonary damage since the 1970s.[40] The cause for this lung injury due to these agents is unknown although it is possibly related to free radical mediated damage of the alveolar epithelium and associated endothelial cells.[40] **Pulmonary toxicity usually occurs in about 50–70 % of patients who receive nitrosoureas at a young age and a cumulative dose that reaches 1,500 mg/m^2 over a span of two years.**[40] The use of craniospinal irradiation and other alkylating agents, including cyclophosphamide, can exacerbate this damage.[40] The symptoms start insidiously 3–6 years following cessation of therapy and usually consist of cough, dyspnea, fever, and weight loss.[38,41] The radiologic pattern is one of fibrosis, especially involving the upper lobes. Pneumothorax is another characteristic complication of the BCNU lung.[38,41] Pulmonary changes are rarely reversible even with the use of corticosteroids. Most patients eventually die of respiratory failure. Pulmonary function tests, including diffusion capacity of carbon monoxide (DL$_{CO}$), should be routinely monitored during treatment with nitrosoureas, and every effort should be made to keep the cumulative drug exposure to < 500–600 mg/m^2. Patients who have received nitrosoureas should be monitored for pulmonary symptoms, exercise intolerance, and unexplained fatigue. Decline in DL$_{CO}$ has been shown to predate radiologic appearance of lung damage.[38] The other listed chemotherapeutic agents cause symptoms and radiologic signs that are fairly similar to that of BCNU lung, with some exceptions.

Bleomycin causes lung damage after a cumulative dose of 450 I.U. Computed tomography of the chest is more sensitive in detecting lung injury from bleomycin than plain X-rays.[38] Like BCNU, bleomycin toxicity is exacerbated by older age, coexisting respiratory diseases, craniospinal irradiation, and high inhaled oxygen concentrations, and is rarely reversible.[38] Occasionally, the radiologic picture of bleomycin pulmonary toxicity can appear as huge nodules mimicking lung metastases.[38] A hypersensitivity pneumonitis with eosinophilia has been associated with bleomycin that is responsive to drug withdrawal and corticosteroid therapy.[38]

Busulfan is used mostly in combination with melphelan as a preparative regimen prior to auto or allogenic bone marrow transplant. The incidence of lung damage from this drug varies from 6%–43% and can be insidious in onset with a clinical picture similar to other agents that cause pulmonary toxicity.[38]

Cyclophosphamide-induced pulmonary toxicity is frequently underestimated, but can cause pulmonary damage in two forms: an early onset pneumonitis that occurs 1–6 months following exposure and responds to drug withdrawal, and a late onset pulmonary fibrosis that is irreversible.[38]

Methotrexate. Chronic exposure to *Methotrexate* can cause pneumonitis that is preceded by cough, dyspnea, and fever.[38] The chest X-ray reveals a diffuse interstitial infiltrate associated with pleural effusions and hilar adenopathy.[38,42] About one-third of patients demonstrate granulomas on lung biopsy. Methotrexate lung is rarely fatal and responds to drug withdrawal.

Infertility

Gonadal dysfunction due to chemotherapy for malignancies has been described for more than 60 years following the first reports of azoospermia in patients receiving nitrogen mustard in 1948.[43] In fact, chemotherapy can interfere with the structure and function of the reproductive organs and have profound or lasting effects on the reproductive system.[43] These effects are related to the age and pubertal status of the patients along with the particular class, dosage, and combination of antineoplastic agents used to treat brain tumors.[43]

The testes in males consist of the seminiferous tubules and interstitial cells of Leydig (secrete testosterone), along with supporting and vascular tissue for nourishment of the spermatozoa. The tubules are lined by stratified epithelium and consist of spermatogenic cells and Sertoli cells (maintain the blood-testes barrier and regulate release of spermatozoa from the germinal cells). The spermatogonia (germinal cells), spermatocytes, spermatids, and mature spermatozoa reside within this tubule. It takes 64–90 days for the initial cycling of the spermatogonia to the final release of spermatazoa. Cytotoxic chemotherapy can affect any of these different stages of sperm production and support structures. Alkylating agents including platinum analogs, nitrosoureas, busulfan, cyclophosphamide, chlorambucil, procarbazine, and temozolomide used in brain tumor therapy affect the germinal cells, early to late spermatogonia, and spermatocytes. The degree of gonadal damage is based on the intensity of each dose, cumulative doses, and duration of treatment; patients who receive higher doses per course and treated for a prolonged duration have a higher incidence of azoospermia.[43] The use of combination alkylator therapy worsens this toxicity on testicular function. Leydig cells can also be damaged in up to 30% of patients receiving alkylating agents, although overt testosterone deficiency is rare.[43] On the other hand, antimetabolite therapy (e.g., methotrexate) has only a minimal effect on gonadal function. Clinical manifestations of chemotherapy-induced testicular damage, irrespective of the agent used, include testicular atrophy, severe oligo or azoospermia, and infertility. In the presence of a normal hypothalamic-pituitary (HP) axis, follicular stimulating hormone (FSH) and lutenizing hormone (LH) levels are high due to negative feedback inhibition. In addition, the levels of inhibin A and B (hormones secreted by sertoli cells and germinal epithelium) are low and suggest damage to the seminiferous tubules. In patients who receive cranial irradiation of >35 Gy to the HP axis as part of brain tumor control, hypogonadism is accentuated by a marked decrease in FSH and LH levels. Testicular biopsy reveals atrophied tubules, germinal aplasia, and peritubular fibrosis. Sertoli cells remain in the background since they are more resistant to the effects of chemotherapy. In a population study from Denmark, Schmiegelow et al. followed the gonadal function of 30 male children (<15 years of age at diagnosis) with brain tumors for at least 18 years following either radiotherapy (RT, involving the hypothalamic–pituitary axis) or RT + chemotherapy.[44] While both groups had evidence of secondary hypogonadism, patients who received RT +chemo had significantly higher levels of FSH and LH, and lower inhibin B levels suggesting gonadal damage.[44] In addition, there was a significant inverse correlation between basal FSH and inhibin B levels and testicular volume.[44] Recovery of gonadal function following completion of therapy can be unpredictable for each patient, but is probably related to age at treatment, type of drug, total dose administered, and duration of time off therapy.[43] Prepubertal testes are probably more resistant to the toxic effects of moderate doses of alkylator chemotherapy, but germinal epithelial injury will occur even in this group at higher doses, especially in the context of malnutrition.[43] **Similarly, patients who receive myeloablative doses of any alkylator therapy, cumulative doses of >11 gm/m^2 of cyclophosphamide, or total body irradiation for allogenic bone marrow transplant are not expected to recover gonadal function.**[43]

In females, the process of oogenesis begins in intrauterine life during which germ cells increase in number and then begin to divide by meiosis to reduce the diploid number of chromosomes to half. At the time of birth, the oocytes are in the long prophase of the first meiotic division and remain in this state until the formation of mature follicle before ovulation. The primary oocyte covered by granulose cells is called a primordial follicle and develops during gestation. About 2 million such follicles can be present in the postnatal ovary, which decreases by atresia to 500,000 by menarche and 25,000 by 38 years. About

15 years later, the number of follicles falls below a threshold level, triggering menopause. Following menarche, during the cyclical process of ovulation, the primary oocyte completes its meiotic division, and becomes a secondary oocyte and is surrounded by proliferating granulosa cells and follicular fluid (graafian follicle). Only about 300–400 oocytes mature and ovulate to this stage during the entire lifespan of a woman. Similar to males, the alkylating agents cause destruction of ovarian follicles in a dose-dependent fashion, decrease the number of maturing follicles, and cause premature menopause. **The histological hallmark of alkylator toxicity on the ovary is follicular destruction and ovarian fibrosis.**[43] Clinically, this is manifested as amenorrhea, a decrease in serum estradiol, and a rise in FSH/LH levels. Lack of estrogens results in vaginal dryness and dyspareunia. Menopausal symptoms such as "hot flashes" occur frequently. The ovarian reserve in such patients can be reliably determined using a transvaginal ultrasonogram (TVU) early in the menstrual cycle (day 2–5) to measure ovarian volume and count the number of antral follicles.[45] The onset and recovery of amenorrhea following alkylator therapy is dependent on the age of the patient and duration of therapy.[43] Women age 40 years or older develop amenorrhea after lower cumulative doses of treatment and within a short interval (1–2 months) after starting therapy.[43] The risk of permanent amenorrhea is worse with combination alkylator therapy, especially in older women given myeloablative doses of treatment. While it is possible that the prepubertal ovary is more resistant to alkylator therapy, in one study of 13 prepubertal girls with brain tumors treated with nitrosoureas or procarbazine, nine showed evidence of primary ovarian failure and only three had normal pubertal development and menarche.[46] In a recent population-based study of ovarian function in 100 women who were childhood cancer survivors treated with RT and alkylator-based chemotherapy, the volume of the ovary and the number of antral follicles as measured by TVU were significantly reduced in patients who either had ovarian failure (on hormone replacement therapy) or had diminished ovarian reserve due to gonadal damage for chemo/radiotherapy, as compared to a group of controls with normal ovarian function.[45]

Studies have shown that the risk of infertility associated with chemotherapy is of paramount importance in the patient's and parents' minds, and treating oncologists should discuss fertility issues with all patients of childbearing age and to parents of prepubertal children who are imminently starting chemotherapy.[47] Sperm banking is a viable option for adolescent boys and men before starting any therapy; however, guidelines for successful sperm banking suggest that the sperm count must be 20×10^6/ml and the post-thaw motility has to be $>40\%$.[43] In some patients, the quality of the sperm can be suboptimal even prior to starting any treatment due to their underlying malignancies.[43,47] While semen is usually obtained by masturbation, it is also possible to obtain sperm by penile vibration and electro-ejaculation under general anesthesia.[44] While sperm banking is an effective method of preserving fertility, insurance companies do not routinely reimburse the cost of storage.[47] It has also been observed that few men return to the banks to retrieve their sperm for use.[47] The use of lutenizing hormone releasing hormone (LH-RH) agonists plus testosterone to protect spermatogonia following chemotherapy has not been successful and the failure of this preventative treatment is probably related to the intensity of chemotherapy.[47] Cryopreservation of testicular tissue for reimplantation following chemotherapy is still being tested in preclinical studies.[47]

In females of childbearing age, cryopreservation of oocytes is not as successful as sperm banking in men, and egg viability is lost during the freezing process.[43,47] However, in vitro fertilization of the oocyte with the spouse's sperm cells and freezing the resulting embryo could be an option.[43,47] Although preliminary phase II studies exploring the use of LH-RH agonist, Goserelin, every four weeks before and during chemotherapy to protect the oocyte from the effects of chemotherapy were found to be useful in restoring menses following chemotherapy, phase III studies are underway to clearly determine the efficacy of this strategy, not only to restore menses, but also for successful pregnancy outcomes.[47]

Secondary Malignancies

The occurrence of secondary malignancies months to several years following chemotherapy is a vexing problem for patients with brain tumors. Although such a deleterious effect of chemotherapy was described several decades ago, the clinical impact of this problem has only recently been recognized with increasing frequency, partly due to the therapeutic success with the same agents against the primary tumor and, hence, increasing longevity of the affected patients. Secondary malignancies are discussed here in terms of their relation to chemotherapy. Additional information can also be found in the chapter dedicated to secondary malignancies and in the late effects of CNS radiation therapy chapter.

The carcinogenicity of chemotherapeutic agents is based on their ability to cause mutagenic DNA damage through the formation of base adducts, replication errors, strand breaks, and cross-links.[48] The existence of efficient DNA repair mechanisms allows the affected cell to repair the damage or cause cell cycle arrest and apotosis, thus creating a pathway to eliminate the damaged cell.[49] Absent or defective repair mechanisms within the cell lead to persistence of the mutagenic lesion that leads to acquisition of more mutations resulting in secondary cancers.[49] While both leukemias and solid tumors can occur as second malignancies in patients with brain tumors treated with chemo/radiotherapy, the risk of developing secondary myeloid leukemias (AML) and myelodysplastic syndromes (MDS) are much higher, mostly due to the inherent sensitivity of the bone marrow to the toxic and mutagenic effects of chemotherapeutic agents.[49]

Agents that carry a high risk of causing secondary AML and/or MDS include melphalan, mecholorethamine, nitrosureas, epipodophyllotoxins, and azathioprine.[48] Those with moderate risk include anthracyclines, thiotepa, cyclophosphamide, procarbazine, dacarbazine, and cisplatin.[48] The risk with other agents, including bleomycin, taxanes, busulfan, irinotecan, and temozolomide, is currently unknown.[50] Therapy-induced secondary AML can be clearly divided into two groups. One group of patients develops leukemia following topoisomerase inhibitors with a short latency from last therapeutic exposure (usually a few months and up to 5 years) without a preceding myelodysplastic phase, and only one or two molecular alterations in the leukemic cells.[51] The other group is usually following exposure to alkylating agents, including cyclophosphamide, with a latency period of about 2–10 years, with a preceding myelodysplastic phase, and multiple complex chromosomal abnormalities in the leukemic cells.[49] Patients treated with topoisomerase II inhibitors like epipodophyllotoxins, develop double strand DNA breaks in bone marrow stem cells, which in turn undergo faulty repair resulting in specific chromosomal translocations and formation of chimeric proteins that induce abnormal proliferation of the stem cells.[51] Additional mutations (the "second hit") results in leukemic conversion.[49] In therapy-related secondary AML, chromosome 11q23 is frequently involved in translocations and the 5' component of the *MLL* gene in this location is always one of the translocation partners. The *MLL* gene frequently fuses to the gene that encodes for *Cbp* (c-AMP responsive element binding protein) and is frequently found in therapy-related AML.[49] Another pathway of leukemogenesis that occurs with alkylator-related secondary malignancies (leukemia and solid tumors) is through defective DNA repair mechanisms. In general, bone marrow stem cells ($CD34^+$) have low levels of the DNA repair enzyme methyl guanine methyl transferase (MGMT), which removes alkyl groups from the O-6 position of guanine residues following exposure to alkylating agents.[50] Treatment with alkylators will also select for cells that have defective mismatch repair (MMR) capability, and this selection appears to occur preferentially in cells that have low MGMT expression.[49] Thus, bone marrow cells are highly susceptible to the carcinogenic effects of alkylating agents.[49,50]

The risk of secondary cancers associated with chemotherapy has been widely reported in the literature and the incidence is about 8–20%.[48] Secondary AML has been particularly associated with the use of etoposide that is frequently used to treat children with acute lymphoblastic leukemia and brain tumors in combination with other chemotherapy drugs. This secondary leukemia is usually of the FAB M4 or M5 subtype.[48,49] Dose intensity of etoposide is more important in the development of AML than cumulative doses of drug.[48] In a study from the National Cancer Institute comparing the risks of developing AML following exposure to epipodophyllotoxins, the incidence of secondary AML (0.7%–3.3%) did not differ significantly between patients who received cumulative doses between 1.5–5 gm/m^2.[51] The "two hit" model and clinical experience suggests that etoposide is unlikely to be carcinogenic on its own, but requires other toxins like irradiation, alkylating agents (CDDP, cyclophosphamide, bleomycin, or nitrosoureas), or other topoisomerase inhibitors (anthracyclines, mitoxantrone) to induce secondary malignancies.[49] Green et al. reviewed the course of 1,406 children with cancer and found an actuarial risk of 5.6% of developing secondary malignant tumors. The only independent risk factors in this study were exposure to BCNU and doxorubicin.[52] In a large prospective study of 198 infants (<3 years of age) with malignant brain tumors who received one to two years of chemotherapy with vincristine, CDDP, cyclophosphamide, and etoposide +/− craniospinal irradiation, secondary AML (n = 1) or MDS (n = 2) was observed in three children at a interval of 33–92 months from diagnosis.[53] Two other patients developed a sarcoma (in the absence of radiation exposure) and meningioma. The oral methylating agent, temozolomide (Temodar®, Schering Plough Corporation, Kenilworth, NJ) is increasingly used in patients with brain tumors. Given its DNA damaging effects, especially in bone marrow stem cells that lack MGMT, there is an increasing concern for the risk of secondary leukemias in patients exposed to this drug, especially in prolonged schedules.[54] There are only anecdotal reports of occurrence of MDS or AML in adults with malignant glioma or breast cancer who had also previously been treated with other alkylating agents or topoisomerase inhibitors.[54] These clinical studies support the need for counseling and vigilance regarding second malignancies in patients with brain tumors treated with chemotherapy with or without irradiation. There are currently no preventative measures other than avoiding or minimizing exposure to irradiation and certain drugs, including alkylators and epipodophyllotoxins. Such alterations in therapy should be balanced against the risk of diminishing efficacy.

It is rare for solid tumors to occur as second malignancies following chemotherapy only in the absence of radiation exposure. In such cases, it is imperative to evaluate for possible germ line p-53 mutations in both patients and their family members. The role of chemotherapy in the induction of these tumors is unclear and hard to establish, especially in the face of an inherent genetic susceptibility to cancer. However, it is possible that mutagenic effects can be initiated in normal tissues other than bone marrow following prolonged and increased chemotherapy exposure. In a study from St. Jude Children's Research Hospital, 52 patients with acute lymphoblastic leukemia who were treated uniformly with prophylactic irradiation and intensive chemotherapy (including antimetabolite therapy), six developed secondary brain tumors as compared to zero of 101 patients in the same study who did not received cranial irradiation.[55] Three of the six patients were heterozygous or homozygous for thiopurine methyl transferase deficiency that increased their systemic exposure to 6-mercaptopurine and possibly contributed to the development of secondary malignant glioma.[55]

Delayed Neurotoxicity

While cranial irradiation is always blamed for acute and delayed brain damage, chemotherapeutic drugs, especially the highly lipid soluble alkylators and antimetabolites (including methotrexate), can cause neurotoxicity based on dose and route of administration. The use of intra-arterial chemotherapy to improve drug delivery to brain tumors can have some serious consequences on the normal brain. Administration of intra-arterial cisplatin, carboplatin, or BCNU can cause seizures, blindness, and sensorineural hearing loss in 10–15% of patients.[56] Delayed leucoencephalopathy has been observed in patients receiving intra-arterial BCNU and is dependent on the cumulative dose of drug and administration of radiotherapy proximal to this treatment.[56] The alkylating agents used in myeloablative chemotherapy are very lipophilic and enter brain tissue readily. Thus, neurotoxicity is frequently seen in patients treated with these agents, particularly at high doses, and can occur from the time of administration of these agents until approximately three months post-transplant.[1] Factors that contribute to this toxicity include concurrent administration of high volume fluids, sedatives, and narcotics, as well as electrolyte and metabolic imbalances.[1] Neurotoxicity usually manifests as hallucinations, encephalopathy, seizures, or coma.[1] White matter changes in the brain have been noted by neuroimaging studies within six months posttransplant in patients who received high-dose regimens containing carmustine, carboplatin, and cyclophosphamide.[1] The use of intrathecal MTX as prophylaxis or treatment of leptomeningeal disease from brain tumors, especially in patients who also receive cranial irradiation of >20 Gy, can cause delayed neurotoxicity manifested as dementia, limb spasticity or, in more severe cases, coma.[57] Neuroimaging reveals cerebral atrophy, ventricular dilatation, and diffuse intracerebral calcifications.[57] Similarly, high-dose MTX (doses as high as 5–12 gm/m^2) can cause a delayed leucoencephalopathy and severe neurocognitive dysfunction, especially in patients who have already received cranial irradiation.[57]

Summary

The chemotherapeutic era of treatment of patients with brain tumors has certainly seen improvements in survival, but concomitantly caused an increase in both acute and chronic side effects from these systemic poisons that significantly impact the quality of life of these long-term survivors. Although recent advances in treatment have identified promising new agents for patients with brain tumors, none have supplanted or exceeded the efficacy of traditional chemotherapy and/or irradiation. It is likely that we will continue to use chemotherapy for these patients in the near future. It is, therefore, necessary that neuro-oncologists continue to understand and measure the important side effects of the chemotherapy used in the clinic and help minimize toxicities seen in their patients. Continuing research is needed to identify compounds that would negate or minimize the toxicity of chemotherapy drugs on normal tissue and possibly biomarkers that might reliably predict for acute and chronic toxicities in survivors of brain tumors.

References

1. Gururangan S, Friedman HS. Innovations in design and delivery of chemotherapy for brain tumors. *Neuroimaging Clin N Am*. 2002;12:583–597.
2. Duffner PK, Horowitz ME, Krischer JP, et al. Postoperative chemotherapy and delayed radiation in children less than three years of age with malignant brain tumors. *N Eng J Med*. 1993;328:1725–1731.
3. Packer RJ, Goldwein J, Nicholson HS, et al. Treatment of children with medulloblastomas with reduced-dose craniospinal radiation therapy and adjuvant chemotherapy: A Children's Cancer Group Study. *J Clin Oncol*. 1999;17:2127–2136.
4. Kretschmar CS, Warren MP, Lavally BL, Dyer S, Tarbell NJ. Ototoxicity of preradiation cisplatin for children with central nervous system tumors. *J Clin Oncol*. 1990;8:1191–1198.
5. Kushner BH, Budnick A, Kramer K, Modak S, Cheung NK. Ototoxicity from high-dose use of platinum compounds in patients with neuroblastoma. *Cancer*. 2006;107:417–422.
6. Li Y, Womer RB, Silber JH. Predicting cisplatin ototoxicity in children: the influence of age and the cumulative dose. *Eur J Cancer*. 2004;40:2445–2451.
7. Schell MJ, McHaney VA, Green AA, et al. Hearing loss in children and young adults receiving cisplatin with or without prior cranial irradiation. *J Clin Oncol*. 1989;7:754–760.
8. Skinner R, Pearson AD, Amineddine HA, Mathias DB, Craft AW. Ototoxicity of cisplatinum in children and adolescents. *Br J Cancer*. 1990;61:927–931.
9. Rybak LP, Whitworth CA, Mukherjea D, Ramkumar V. Mechanisms of cisplatin-induced ototoxicity and prevention. *Hear Res*. 2007;226:157–167.
10. Brock PR, Bellman SC, Yeomans EC, Pinkerton CR, Pritchard J. Cisplatin ototoxicity in children: a practical grading system. *Med Pediatr Oncol*. 1991;19:295–300.
11. Kohn S, Fradis M, Pratt H, et al. Cisplatin ototoxicity in guinea pigs with special reference to toxic effects in the stria vascularis. *Laryngoscope*. 1988;98:865–871.
12. Freilich RJ, Kraus DH, Budnick AS, Bayer LA, Finlay JL. Hearing loss in children with brain tumors treated with cisplatin and carboplatin-based high-dose chemotherapy with autologous bone marrow rescue. *Med Pediatr Oncol*. 1996;26:95–100.
13. Bokemeyer C, Berger CC, Hartmann JT, et al. Analysis of risk factors for cisplatin-induced ototoxicity in patients with testicular cancer. *Br J Cancer*. 1998;77:1355–1362.
14. Kennedy BJ, Torkelson JL. Familial hearing loss and cisplatin therapy. *Cancer Invest*. 1998;16:213–216.
15. Gaynon PS, Ettinger LJ, Moel D, et al. Pediatric phase I trial of carboplatin: a Children's Cancer Study Group report. *Cancer Treat Rep*. 1987;71:1039–1042.
16. Skinner R. Best practice in assessing ototoxicity in children with cancer. *Eur J Cancer*. 2004;40:2352–2354.
17. Block KI, Gyllenhaal C. Commentary: the pharmacological antioxidant amifostine – implications of recent research for integrative cancer care. *Integr Cancer Ther*. 2005;4:329–351.
18. Fisher MJ, Lange BJ, Needle MN, et al. Amifostine for children with medulloblastoma treated with cisplatin-based chemotherapy. *Pediatr Blood Cancer*. 2004;43:780–784.
19. Marina N, Chang KW, Malogolowkin M, et al. Amifostine does not protect against the ototoxicity of high-dose cisplatin combined with etoposide and bleomycin in pediatric germ-cell tumors: a Children's Oncology Group study. *Cancer*. 2005;104:841–847.
20. Doolittle ND, Muldoon LL, Brummett RE, et al. Delayed sodium thiosulfate as an otoprotectant against carboplatin-induced hearing loss in patients with malignant brain tumors. *Clin Cancer Res*. 2001;7:493–500.
21. Skinner R. Preventing platinum-induced ototoxicity in children-is there a potential role for sodium thiosulfate? *Pediatr Blood Cancer*. 2006;47:120–122.
22. Armstrong T, Almadrones L, Gilbert MR. Chemotherapy-induced peripheral neuropathy. *Oncol Nurs Forum*. 2005;32:305–311.
23. Postma TJ, Benard BA, Huijgens PC, Ossenkoppele GJ, Heimans JJ. Long-term effects of vincristine on the peripheral nervous system. *J Neuro-oncol*. 1993;15:23–27.

24. Verstappen CC, Heimans JJ, Hoekman K, Postma TJ. Neurotoxic complications of chemotherapy in patients with cancer: clinical signs and optimal management. *Drugs.* 2003;63:1549–1563.
25. Kesari S, Schiff D, Doherty L, et al. Phase II study of metronomic chemotherapy for recurrent malignant gliomas in adults. *Neuro Oncol.* 2007;9:354–363.
26. Mileshkin L, Stark R, Day B, Seymour JF, Zeldis JB, Prince HM. Development of neuropathy in patients with myeloma treated with thalidomide: patterns of occurrence and the role of electrophysiologic monitoring. *J Clin Oncol.* 2006;24:4507–4514.
27. Kintzel PE. Anticancer drug-induced kidney disorders. *Drug Saf.* 2001;24:19–38.
28. Hanigan MH, Devarajan P. Cisplatin nephrotoxicity: Molecular mechanisms. *Cancer Ther.* 2003;1:47–61.
29. Cornelison TL, Reed E. Nephrotoxicity and hydration management for cisplatin, carboplatin, and ormaplatin. *Gynecol Oncol.* 1993;50:147–158.
30. Skinner R. Chronic ifosfamide nephrotoxicity in children. *Med Pediatr Oncol.* 2003;41:190–197.
31. Womer RB, Pritchard J, Barratt TM. Renal toxicity of cisplatin in children. *J Pediatr.* 1985;106:659–663.
32. Brock PR, Koliouskas DE, Barratt TM, Yeomans E, Pritchard J. Partial reversibility of cisplatin nephrotoxicity in children. *J Pediatr.* 1991;118:531–534.
33. Hensley ML, Schuchter LM, Lindley C, et al. American Society of Clinical Oncology clinical practice guidelines for the use of chemotherapy and radiotherapy protectants. *J Clin Oncol.* 1999;17:3333–3355.
34. Gururangan S, Friedman HS. Recent advances in the treatment of pediatric brain tumors. *Oncology* (Williston Park, NY). 2004;18:1649–1661; discussion 62, 65–66, 68.
35. Schacht RG, Feiner HD, Gallo GR, Lieberman A, Baldwin DS. Nephrotoxicity of nitrosoureas. *Cancer.* 1981;48:1328–1334.
36. Prasad VK, Lewis IJ, Aparicio SR, et al. Progressive glomerular toxicity of ifosfamide in children. *Med Pediatr Oncol.* 1996;27:149–155.
37. Jakacki RI, Schramm CM, Donahue BR, Haas F, Allen JC. Restrictive lung disease following treatment for malignant brain tumors: a potential late effect of craniospinal irradiation. *J Clin Oncol.* 1995;13:1478–1485.
38. Limper AH. Chemotherapy-induced lung disease. *Clin Chest Med.* 2004;25:53–64.
39. Mertens AC, Yasui Y, Liu Y, et al. Pulmonary complications in survivors of childhood and adolescent cancer. A report from the Childhood Cancer Survivor Study. *Cancer.* 2002;95:2431–2441.
40. O'Driscoll BR, Kalra S, Gattamaneni HR, Woodcock AA. Late carmustine lung fibrosis. Age at treatment may influence severity and survival. *Chest.* 1995;107:1355–1357.
41. O'Driscoll BR, Hasleton PS, Taylor PM, Poulter LW, Gattameneni HR, Woodcock AA. Active lung fibrosis up to 17 years after chemotherapy with carmustine (BCNU) in childhood. *N Eng J Med.* 1990;323:378–382.
42. Bedrossian CW, Miller WC, Luna MA. Methotrexate-induced diffuse interstitial pulmonary fibrosis. *South Med J.* 1979;72:313–318.
43. Schilsky R. Infertility after cancer chemotherapy. In: Chabner BA, Longo DL, eds. *Cancer Chemotherapy & Biotherapy..* 3rd ed. Philadelphia, PA: Lippincott Williams & Wilkins; 2001:50–66.
44. Schmiegelow M, Lassen S, Poulsen HS, et al. Gonadal status in male survivors following childhood brain tumors. *J Clin Endocrinol Metab.* 2001;86:2446–2452.
45. Larsen EC, Muller J, Schmiegelow K, Rechnitzer C, Andersen AN. Reduced ovarian function in long-term survivors of radiation- and chemotherapy-treated childhood cancer. *J Clin Endocrinol Metab.* 2003;88:5307–5314.
46. Clayton PE, Shalet SM, Price DA, Jones PH. Ovarian function following chemotherapy for childhood brain tumours. *Med Pediatr Oncol.* 1989;17:92–96.

47. Lee SJ, Schover LR, Partridge AH, et al. American Society of Clinical Oncology recommendations on fertility preservation in cancer patients. *J Clin Oncol.* 2006;24:2917–2931.
48. Erlichman C, Moore M. Carcinogenesis: A late complication of cancer chemotherapy. In: Chabner BA, Longo DL, eds. *Cancer Chemotherapy & Biotherapy.* 3rd ed. Philadelphia, PA: Lippincott Williams & Wilkins; 2001:67–84.
49. Allan JM, Travis LB. Mechanisms of therapy-related carcinogenesis. *Nat Rev Cancer.* 2005;5:943–955.
50. Gerson SL. MGMT: its role in cancer aetiology and cancer therapeutics. *Nat Rev Cancer.* 2004;4:296–307.
51. Smith MA, Rubinstein L, Anderson JR, et al. Secondary leukemia or myelodysplastic syndrome after treatment with epipodophyllotoxins. *J Clin Oncol.* 1999;17:569–577.
52. Green DM, Zevon MA, Reese PA, et al. Second malignant tumors following treatment during childhood and adolescence for cancer. *Med Pediatr Oncol.* 1994;22:1–10.
53. Duffner PK, Krischer JP, Horowitz ME, et al. Second malignancies in young children with primary brain tumors following treatment with prolonged postoperative chemotherapy and delayed irradiation: a Pediatric Oncology Group study. *Ann Neurol.* 1998;44:313–316.
54. Gururangan S, Fisher MJ, Allen JC, et al. Temozolomide in children with progressive low-grade glioma. *Neuro Oncol.* 2007;9:161–168.
55. Relling MV, Rubnitz JE, Rivera GK, et al. High incidence of secondary brain tumours after radiotherapy and antimetabolites. *Lancet.* 1999;354:34–39.
56. Dropcho EJ. Intra-arterial chemotherapy for malignant gliomas. In: Berger MS, Wilson CB, eds. *The Gliomas.* Philadelphia, PA: W.B.Saunders Company; 1999:537-547.
57. Messmann RA, Allegra CJ. Antifolates. In: Chabner BA, Longo DL, eds. *Cancer Chemotherapy & Biotherapy.* 3rd ed. Philadelphia, PA: Lippincott Williams & Wilkins; 2001:139–184.

Chapter 5
Late Effects of Stem Cell Transplantation in Brain Tumor Survivors

Karina Danner-Koptik, David A. Jacobsohn, and Kimberley J. Dilley

Introduction

Children with malignant central nervous system tumors have begun to benefit from slightly improved outcomes in recent years. There is improved five-year disease free survival for children diagnosed with standard risk medulloblastoma and other primitive neuroectodermal tumors (PNET).[1]

Conventional therapeutic strategies continue to include surgery, radiation, and chemotherapy for children diagnosed with malignant brain tumors. However, outcomes can remain poor especially when surgical intervention is not a therapeutic option, or when there is neuroaxial dissemination, metastatic or recurrent tumors in the very young pediatric patient.[2] Also, patients whose tumors recur despite aggressive initial therapy can have unfortunate results. Attempts to improve the outlook for these patients have resulted in therapeutic strategies including high-dose chemotherapy administration followed by autologous hematopoietic stem cell transplantation (HSCT).[1]

High-dose chemotherapy followed by autologous HSCT has been a treatment modality since the mid- to late 1990s for children with recurrent and high risk brain tumors. Studies have illustrated that this treatment modality is feasible and safe, and survival outcomes early on showed promise, which has led to increased numbers of young patients being enrolled on these treatment protocols.[3,4]

Autologous HSCT has been used as a way to improve tumor-free survival, delay the use of radiotherapy in the very young pediatric patient's central nervous system, consolidate total therapy, and avoid the hematopoietic toxicity of high-dose chemotherapy in the treatment of pediatric CNS tumors.[5–9]

While high-dose chemotherapy with autologus HSCT has been a treatment modality employed for children with brain tumors, its use in the adult

K. Danner-Koptik (✉)
Advanced Practice Nurse, Hematology/Oncology/Stem Cell Transplant, Children's
Memorial Medical Center, Chicago, IL 60614-3394, USA
e-mail: kdannerkoptik@childrensmemorial.org

S. Goldman, C.D. Turner (eds.), *Late Effects of Treatment for Brain Tumors*,
Cancer Treatment and Research 150, DOI 10.1007/b109924_5,
© Springer Science+Business Media, LLC 2009

population has been limited. Some studies have shown this to be a feasible treatment modality in the adult setting with malignant gliomas, as well as recurrent brain tumors, such as medulloblastomas, ependymomas, germ cell tumors, intracranial rhabdomyosarcomas, and primitive neuroectodermal tumors.[10] While some individual adult patients have achieved a prolonged disease-free survival, the toxic morbidity and mortality can be substantial[10,11] and many patients go on to develop progressive or recurrent disease. Future trials might prove effective if the toxicity due to the high-dose chemotherapy regimens could be reduced, without sacrificing efficacy, to improve the survival for a larger cohort of adults with brain tumors.[10,12,13]

Hematopoietic Stem Cell Transplantation (HSCT) Specific Late Effects

It must be restated that the cumulative effects of all therapies received in this patient population prior to HSCT can lead to significant long-term sequellae. The impacts of late effects linked to autologous HSCT are based upon the preparative/conditioning regimen used and the exposure to a single or tandem transplant modality.

As described, autologous HSCT has been used as a treatment modality in the pediatric brain tumor population since the mid-1990s. Whether single versus tandem HSCT will afford improved outcomes for these patients is still under investigation. However, increased toxicities and the development of long-term sequellae related to the chemotherapeutic agents used for the HSCT conditioning may be increased if multiple exposures are incurred.

Autologous HSCT conditioning regimens for the pediatric brain tumor population have historically included chemotherapeutic agents, such as alkylating agents (cyclophosphamide, thiotepa, busulfan, melphalan), heavy metal agents (cisplatin, carboplatin) and epipodophyllotoxins (etoposide).[9] All of these agents cross the blood-brain barrier, and sensitivity of brain tumors has been described with cisplatin, carboplatin, etoposide, as well as thiotepa. Cyclophosphamide and melphalan have long been effective agents as part of myeloablative conditioning regimens in HSCT. Clinical trials for pediatric brain tumor patients have described these agents used in varied combinations for autologous HSCT, such as thiotepa/cyclophosphamide, busulfan/melphalan, thiotepa/carboplatin, thiotepa/etoposide, and cyclophosphamide/carboplatin.[5,14-17]

Complications in the peritransplant period arising from conditioning regimen chemotherapy for autologous HSCT include neutropenia, infections, mucositis, and multiorgan system failure (MOSF).[18]

The major peritransplant toxicity common to all of these agents is hematopoietic, causing pancytopenia. Late effects incurred from these agents are more commonly associated by their agent classification (see Table 5.1).

Table 5.1 Potential late-effects of chemotherapy agents commonly used in stem cell transplant

Chemotheraputic class	Potential late effects

Alkylating Agents:
  Melphalan
  Thiotepa
  Busulfan
  Cyclophosphamide
	1) Gonadal dysfunction (ovarian & testicular)
	  – hypogonadism
	  – delayed/arrested puberty
	  – infertility
	  – Female premature menopause
	  – Male oligo/azospermia
	2) Acute Myeloid leukemia
	3) Myelodysplasia

Special concerns: Busulfan	pulmonary fibrosis, cataracts
Cyclophosphamide	Urinary Tract Toxicity (hemorrhagic cystitis, bladder fibrosis, dysfunctional voiding, vesicoureteral reflux, hydronephrosis, secondary bladder malignancy)

Heavy Metals:
  Carboplatin
  Cisplatin
	1) Gonadal dysfunction
	  (ovarian, testicular)
	  – hypogonadism
	  – delayed/arrested puberty
	  – infertility
	  – Female premature menopause
	  – Male oligo/azospermia
	2) Acute Myeloid leukemia
	3) Myelodysplasia
	4) Ototoxicity
	5) Peripheral sensory neuropathy
	6) Renal toxicity
	7) Dyslipidemia

Epipodophyllotoxins: Etoposide	1) Acute Myeloid Leukemia

General Health and Well-Being

Children who have undergone autologous HSCT for brain tumors often struggle with cumulative sequellae that affect nutrition, body weight, physical activity, and overall health. The effects of the brain tumor's location and the therapeutic modalities used may play a role in altering general health for these survivors. Good nutrition and regular exercise offer many benefits to childhood cancer and HSCT survivors.

Education related to general health promotion can empower patients to take charge by promoting healing of tissues and organs damaged by cancer and its treatment, building strength and endurance, reducing the risk of certain types of adult cancers and other diseases, and decreasing stress and providing a feeling of well-being.

Recommendations from both the National Cancer Institute and the American Cancer Society promote daily moderate to vigorous physical activity for this patient population.[19,20]

Many childhood brain tumor survivors have special mobility needs, and the help of physical and/or occupational therapy may be needed to adapt the activity for success. A social worker may be able to help find insurance coverage or other resources for special equipment. Specialized programs for individuals with special needs, organizations and other resources are often available through your health care center, in your local community, and at The National Center on Physical Activity and Disability www.ncpad.org.[21]

Ototoxicity

The incidence of high frequency hearing loss is significant with protocols using cisplatin and carboplatin as part of the HSCT conditioning regimen. However, this is similar to results of other clinical trials that used this agent for brain tumors in children.[15]

Types of hearing loss include conductive hearing loss, which is hearing loss due to a problem in transmission of sound from the air to the inner ear, or sensorineural hearing loss which results from damage to the inner ear or auditory nerve. Conductive hearing loss may improve over time, but sensorineural hearing loss is usually permanent.[22] Symptoms of hearing loss may include ringing or tinkling sounds in the ear, difficulty hearing in the presence of background noises, not paying attention to sounds (such as voices, environmental noises), and general school/academic problems.

Hearing loss impacts how children interface with their surrounding environment and learn. Younger children are at higher risk for school, learning, and social difficulties, and problems with language development. It is, therefore, crucial to have hearing evaluated while on therapy and thereafter.

Risk Factors

Chemotherapy from the "platinum" group, such as cisplatin or high doses of carboplatin; high doses of radiation (30 Gy or 3000 cGy/rads or higher) to the head or brain; surgery involving the brain, ear or auditory (eighth cranial) nerve; and certain antibiotics and diuretics can cause hearing loss.

Recommendations

An audiogram or Brainstem Auditory Evoked Response (BAER) should be performed by an experienced audiologist at least once after completion of therapy. Additional testing is dependent upon the type and dosage of cancer treatments that were used. Patients should have an audiologic evaluation as a baseline upon entry into a long-term follow up porgram. If hearing loss is found, testing should be repeated yearly or as advised by an audiologist.[22]

Cochlear implants may be an option for people with profound hearing loss who are unable to benefit from hearing aids. After the cochlear implant is installed, auditory training is given for a period of time to teach the individual to recognize and interpret sounds.

Other available options for the pediatric stem cell transplant survivor with hearing loss, include hearing aids, auditory trainers (also known as "FM trainers"), and other assistive devices including telephone amplifiers and tele-typewriters (TTYs –Telephone Devices for the Deaf or TDDs).

Community and educational resources in the United States include services through local public school districts or referral agencies (available under the IDEA legislation, PL 105-17), such as intensive speech therapy and auditory trainers for classroom use. Special accommodations, such as seating in the front of the classroom, can also benefit the child, but this usually requires the parent to request an Individualized Education Plan (IEP) for the child through the school district. The Americans with Disabilities Act (ADA, PL 101-336) guar-antees people with hearing loss equal access to public events, spaces and opportunities, including text telephones and telephone amplifiers in public places, and assistive listening devices in theaters.

Neurocognitive/Educational Late Effects

Children and adolescents who have been treated with autologous HSCT for malignant brain tumors often exhibit effects on educational progress related to surgical interventions, chemotherapy, and radiation therapies. HSCT condi-tioning regimens that include methotrexate, cisplatin, carboplatin, and cytara-bine, in addition to the cumulative effects of all previous chemo- or radiotherapy received, can have the most deleterious effects on learning, especially when administered at younger ages.[23]

Many educational issues and effects on memory and learning abilities may not arise until years after the completion of therapy. Common problem areas include: handwriting, spelling, reading, vocabulary, math, concentration, atten-tion span, staying on-task, memory, processing and prioritization, planning, organization, problem-solving, and social skills.

Risk Factors

Factors that may place children and teens at increased risk for difficulties in school are not only related to the therapies and surgical interventions received, but also impacted by prolonged school absences. The diagnosis of a brain tumor at a very young age, chemotherapeutic agents including methotrexate (high-dose IV and intrathecal), cytarabine, cisplatin, carboplatin, radiation therapy to the central nervous system, and surgery involving the brain can lead to deleterious neurocognitive late effects. It must also be understood that a history of learning difficulties before the brain tumor diagnosis could well lead to increased neurocognitive difficulties.

Recommendations

Any young person who has had any of the above therapies, or who is having difficulties in school, should undergo a specialized evaluation by a pediatric psychologist and neuropsychological testing. This should occur, if possible, at the time of entry into a long-term follow-up program.

This type of testing will measure IQ and school-based skills, along with more detailed information about how the child processes and organizes information. It is recommended that serial neuropsychological testing be performed, especially at times when more academic challenges are likely, such as entry into elementary school, middle school, high school, and during pre-college planning.[22,24]

Special accommodations or services can be requested via the child's educational system if academic issues are identified. It is crucial that the child's family work closely with the school/educational institution to develop a specialized educational plan. Caregivers, parents, and educators need to be aware of potential educational problems that may be related to these treatments so that children and teens at risk can be watched closely and given extra help if the need arises.

Specific accommodations can be made for these children including special seating in the classroom, minimizing the amount of written work required and using a computer keyboard, allowing the use of tape-recorded textbooks and lectures, and use of a calculator for math. These students may also benefit from modification of test requirements (extra time, oral instead of written exams), a classroom aide assigned to them, and extra help with math, spelling, reading, and organizational skills. Access to an elevator, along with extra time for transition between classes, and a duplicate set of textbooks to keep at home can help these students achieve their potential. (10)

Within the United States, there are several laws which protect the rights of students who have undergone treatment for any type of cancer therapy. These laws are reviewed in detail in Chapter 24 and can be most helpful to this patient population post HSCT.

Endocrine/Gonadal Dysfunction

Endocrine dysfunction in pediatric brain tumor survivors who have undergone HSCT is a major long-term risk due to the cumulative effects of therapies received. The incidence is as high as 43%, according to the CCSS (Childhood

Cancer Survivor Study).[23] Since the endocrine system regulates many body functions including growth, puberty, energy level, urine production, and stress response, dysfunction has widespread effects in the growing and developing child.

Pediatric survivors of brain tumors after HSCT can exhibit vast hormonal dysfunction. The pituitary gland is often affected by the cumulative effects of therapies received in these patients. Hypopituitarism, the decrease or lack of one or more of the pituitary hormones, or panhypopituitarism, the lack of three or more of the pituitary hormones, can affect multiple hormonal pathways in the developing child.

Pediatric brain tumor survivors post HSCT can develop endocrine late effects including growth hormone (GH) deficiency, adrenocorticotropic hormone deficiency, thyroid stimulating hormone deficiency, and gonadal failure related to gonadotropin deficiency.

Risks

Gonadal failure post HSCT is linked to the alkylating and heavy metal chemotherapeutic agents. These chemotherapeutic agents which cross the blood-brain barrier, radiation therapy to the brain, eye or orbit, ear or infratemporal region, and nasopharynx, especially in excess of 3,000 cGy, and surgery to the brain, notably at the suprasellar or central region (pituitary gland location), can dramatically increase the risk of endocrine dysfunction, especially in the young patient.

Recommendations

All survivors should have a yearly physical examination that includes height and weight measurements, assessment of their progression through puberty, and assessment of overall well-being. Slowing of growth (height) is one of the most obvious signs of GH deficiency in children.

A GH deficient child usually grows less than two inches per year. Children with GH deficiency are smaller and tend to look younger than children their same age, but they usually have normal body proportions. If hypopituitarism or GH deficiency is suspected, further tests may be done with referral to an endocrinologist.

Children who received radiation in a dose of 40 Gy (4,000 cGy/rads) or higher to the central area of the brain (hypothalamic-pituitary axis) should have the cortisol level evaluated. This test should be done yearly for at least 15 years since this complication can occur many years after radiation.[22]

Pulmonary Fibrosis

Pulmonary toxicity is a possibility following high dose chemotherapy for CNS tumors, and pulmonary fibrosis can certainly be noted in patients having received busulfan as part of their conditioning regimens for HSCT.

Risks

This exposure, in addition to prior exposures to anthracyclines, bleomycin, BCNU, and CCNU, along with radiation therapy, can lead to pulmonary fibrosis, recurrent pneumonias, bronchitis, bronchiolitis obliterans, and restrictive/obstructive lung disease.[22]

Again, the cumulative exposure to these agents cannot be underestimated, along with younger age at diagnosis and treatment, history of pulmonary injury prior to therapy initiation, such as asthma, and any use of tobacco or exposure to secondhand smoke. A patient/family report of becoming easily fatigued, episodes of shortness of breath, or exercise intolerance can be an early symptom of lung damage.

Recommendations

All survivors should have an annual medical evaluation. At least two years after completion of the HSCT a chest X-ray and pulmonary function testing (PFT), including diffusion of CO_2 (DLCO) and spirometry, may show lung problems that are not apparent during a checkup.

Other recommendations include the patient receiving the pneumococcal (pneumonia) vaccine; yearly influenza vaccines; avoid SCUBA diving; avoid smoking and secondhand smoke; avoid breathing toxic fumes from chemicals, solvents, and paints; participate in regular physical exercise, and follow all safety rules in your workplace per Occupational Safety and Health Administration (OSHA) guidelines, such as the use of protective ventilators in some work environments.[22]

Peripheral Sensorineural Neuropathy (PSN)

Damage to the nerves is often caused by a breakdown of the myelin sheath or there may be direct damage to the nerve cells from pressure or trauma (for example from a tumor or surgery) causing peripheral neuropathies. Symptoms can include burning, tingling, or prickling sensation usually in the hands or feet, numbness or sensitivity to pain or temperature, extreme sensitivity to touch, sharp shooting pain, poor balance or coordination, loss of reflexes, muscle weakness, and ataxia. Symptoms typically start during treatment and persist, and are not late in onset, but for some survivors symptoms may persist for months or years.

Risks

Peripheral neuropathy is a potential side effect of chemotherapy drugs including vincristine, cisplatin and carboplatin and may cause the hands or feet to hurt, tingle, and feel numb or weak. Those who have received higher doses of these drugs or combinations of these drugs are at higher risk of developing a PSN.

Recommendations

Since there is no treatment that can cure or reverse nerve damage, treatment is directed toward symptom management: supportive care, pain management, and evaluation of Raynaud's Phenomenon. Certain prescription medications including birth control pills, some heart and blood pressure medicines, and specific over-the-counter medications containing pseudoephedrine (such as Actifed®, Chlor-Trimeton®, and Sudafed®) can heighten symptoms and should be avoided.

Physical therapy is often helpful in providing exercises to improve strength, balance, and coordination. Occupational therapy can help to improve hand/eye coordination and other skills needed for daily life. Additionally, orthotic devices can often be helpful to improve walking in these youngsters.[22]

Urinary Tract/Renal Toxicity

Urinary tract and renal toxicities can occur following the administration of both alkylating as well as heavy metal chemotherapeutic agents used in HSCT conditioning regimens. Specifically, alkylating agents can cause hemorrhagic cystitis, bladder fibrosis, dysfunctional voiding patterns, and secondary bladder malignancies. Glomerular and tubular toxicities, Fanconi's syndrome, and hypophosphatemic rickets can also lead to sustained late nephrotoxic effects after HSCT. Clinical manifestations can include phosphaturia, hypophosphatemia, glycosuria, aminoaciduria, elevated serum alkaline phosphatase, hypokalemia, renal tubular acidosis, defective concentrating capacity, and reduced glomerular filtration rate.[23]

Risks

Persistent deficits in renal function have been shown to exist many years after therapy is completed. Any renal dysfunction or combined nephrotoxic therapy, such as aminoglycoside administration, can increase the risk of urinary and renal toxicities, specifically during the time period that alkylating and heavy metal agents are administered. Adequate hydration must be maintained during the conditioning therapy to help prevent acute and chronic toxicities.[22,23]

Recommendations

General consequences of renal impairment, inclusive of hypertension, altered growth, bone demineralization, and reduced renal drug excretion can be ongoing to late effects post HSCT. Annual blood pressure screening along with renal chemistry screening at entry into a long-term follow-up program is a baseline for this survivor group. Patients with persistent electrolyte wasting should be educated on dietary and hydration considerations.[22,23]

Dyslipidemia

Childhood brain tumor survivors following stem cell transplant have an increased risk of developing hypothalamic-pituitary deficiencies related to the cumulative chemo-radiotherapies and surgical interventions. Dyslipidemias and, subsequently, cardiovascular disease related to the neuroendocrine deficiencies from this panhypopituitary picture can occur.[23,25]

Risks

The risks of cardiovascular disease are elevated due to dyslipidemia, central obesity, and elevated systolic blood pressure, especially in the growth hormone deficient survivors.[23] Family history of dyslipidemia will potentially compound the risk.

Recommendations

A fasting lipid profile should be obtained at entry into a long-term follow-up program. Heart healthy diet and exercise education needs to be initiated early on as this will be the first treatment modality for patients with dyslipidemia. Early referral to Cardiology may also be helpful in comprehensive assessment, as well as the consideration of pharmacologic intervention.

Secondary Malignancy

Childhood cancer survivors have a higher risk of developing a secondary cancer compared to people their same age in the general population. Given the high doses of chemotherapy used in HSCT, this risk is thought to be even higher in HSCT survivors. Specific agents and the cumulative exposures to chemo- and radiotherapy, along with a younger age at diagnosis and genetic and family history can contribute to the development of a secondary malignancy.

Risks

The development of acute myeloid leukemia (AML) after treatment can occur within the first 10 years following treatment. The risk of developing a secondary leukemia is increased for patients treated with high doses of alkylating agents (such as cyclophosphamide) and epipodophyllotoxins (such as etoposide or teniposide) that are commonly used in many standard HSCT conditioning regimens. Alkylator-associated AML is typically characterized by a mean latency of five to seven years, a prodromal myelodysplastic phase, and abnormalities of chromosomes 5 and 7.[23]

Radiation therapy, especially given at a younger age, increases the risk of developing a secondary solid CNS tumor. The risk of developing a secondary solid tumor is increased when radiation is delivered at high doses and over large fields to children at a young age. Specific secondary CNS malignancies include meningiomas and glial tumors.[23]

Recommendations

Ongoing comprehensive annual monitoring is a key component to these survivors. Cancer screening evaluations should be tailored to be appropriate for age, sex, and treatment history. Patients should be educated to monitor and report easy ecchymosis, petechiae, pallor, fatigue, pain, lymphadenopathy, sores that do not heal, hematuria, shortness of breath, persistent cough, bloody sputum, stool changes/gastrointestinal bleeding, persistent headaches, visual changes, and persistent early morning vomiting.

Patients and families should be educated to avoid cancer-promoting habits, such as smoking or chewing tobacco, and to practice healthy diet and exercise behaviors to help keep the risk of second cancers to a minimum.

Long-Term Survivorship

Long-term survival in pediatric brain tumor patients having received high-dose chemotherapy and autologous HSCT is improving. Survival in these patients can be measured by progression-free survival (PFS), and event-free survival (EFS). There are many compounding variables when addressing the outcomes for these patients, such as tumor type and grade, risk group, CNS extension into the spinal column, metastatic sites, minimal residual disease, surgical interventions, radiation therapies, and single versus tandem autologous HSCT. The late effects that these survivors may experience are dependent upon the cumulative chemo- and radiotherapy, surgical interventions, as well as HSCT therapy received. Treatment options for those who recur post-autologous HSCT, given as salvage therapy, can further the cumulative effect of therapies previously given and must also be taken into consideration when assessing long-term sequellae for these patients.[22]

Pediatric brain tumor survivors post-autologous HSCT need lifelong long-term management to assess, evaluate, and manage complications. A comprehensive, central approach to survivor care is needed to help these patients maintain healthy growth and development and assess for potential long-term risks.

The Children's Oncology Group (COG) has developed survivorship guidelines for all pediatric cancer survivors. These guidelines have been designed to incorporate potential late effects directly related to the type of chemotherapy, radiation therapy, surgical intervention, and transplant type received.[22] These guidelines are available on the Children's Oncology Group website at www.survivorshipguidelines.org.

Again, it is important to consider the neurological and neurocognitive effects that the patient may have experienced at diagnosis and primary therapy as part of the cumulative effects of all therapies received. In that light, it is key to address all potential late effects that the pediatric brain tumor patient may endure after autologous HSCT. Ongoing management of survivorship issues is best performed in a long-term follow-up program for survivors of childhood cancer. Long-term follow-up programs screen for late effects and educate survivors about ways to lower the risk of health problems after cancer therapy and stem cell transplant. Long-term follow-up programs will provide a complete health evaluation, but are not typically designed to meet the everyday health care needs of survivors. Therefore, it is very important that each patient has a primary health care provider to care for their general medical needs.

The basic tenets of health care for childhood cancer and HCST survivors include longitudinal care that is designed as a continuum from cancer diagnosis and all therapeutic modalities through adulthood, and continuity of that care with a "partnership" between the survivor and the health care provider to coordinate services. A comprehensive, proactive approach to care that includes a systematic method of prevention and surveillance, caring for the whole person, and acknowledging the patient's sensitivity to the issues of the cancer experience is fundamental to the establishment of a good patient-provider relationship. Additionally, a multidisciplinary team approach with communication and facilitation of required care between the provider of late effects-focused care, the primary health care provider, and subspecialty services, is essential.[23]

References

1. Finlay JL. The role of high-dose chemotherapy and stem cell rescue in the treatment of malignant brain tumors: a reappraisal. *Pediatr Transplant*. 1999;3(Suppl 1):87–95.
2. Perez-Martinez A, Quintero V, Vicent MG, et al. High-dose chemotherapy with autologous stem cell rescue as first line of treatment in young children with medulloblastoma and supratentorial primitive neuroectodermal tumors. *J Neurooncol*. 2004;67:101–106.
3. Cohn SL, Moss TJ, Hoover M, et al. Treatment of poor-risk neuroblastoma patients with high-dose chemotherapy and autologous peripheral stem cell rescue. *Bone Marrow Transplant*. 1997;20:543–551.
4. Graham ML, Herndon JE, 2nd, Casey JR, et al. High-dose chemotherapy with autologous stem-cell rescue in patients with recurrent and high-risk pediatric brain tumors. *J Clin Oncol*. 1997;15:1814–1823.
5. Finlay JL, Goldman S, Wong MC, et al. Pilot study of high-dose thiotepa and etoposide with autologous bone marrow rescue in children and young adults with recurrent CNS tumors. The Children's Cancer Group. *J Clin Oncol*. 1996;14:2495–2503.

6. Kremens B, Wieland R, Reinhard H, et al. High-dose chemotherapy with autologous stem cell rescue in children with retinoblastoma. *Bone Marrow Transplant.* 2003;31:281–284.

7. Sung KW, Yoo KH, Cho EJ, et al. High-dose chemotherapy and autologous stem cell rescue in children with newly diagnosed high-risk or relapsed medulloblastoma or supratentorial primitive neuroectodermal tumor. *Pediatr Blood Cancer.* 2007;48:408–415.

8. Thorarinsdottir HK, Rood B, Kamani N, et al. Outcome for children <4 years of age with malignant central nervous system tumors treated with high-dose chemotherapy and autologous stem cell rescue. *Pediatr Blood Cancer.* 2007;48:278–284.

9. Wolff JE, Finlay JL. High-dose chemotherapy in childhood brain tumors. *Onkologie.* 2004;27:239–245.

10. Abrey LE, Rosenblum MK, Papadopoulos E, et al. High dose chemotherapy with autologous stem cell rescue in adults with malignant primary brain tumors. *J Neurooncol.* 1999;44:147–153.

11. Bay JO, Linassier C, Biron P, et al. Does high-dose carmustine increase overall survival in supratentorial high-grade malignant glioma? An EBMT retrospective study. *Int J Cancer.* 2007;120:1782–1786.

12. Abrey LE, Childs BH, Paleologos N, et al. High-dose chemotherapy with stem cell rescue as initial therapy for anaplastic oligodendroglioma: long-term follow-up. *Neuro Oncol.* 2006;8:183–188.

13. Brandes AA, Palmisano V, Pasetto LM, et al. High-dose chemotherapy with bone marrow rescue for high-grade gliomas in adults. *Cancer Invest.* 2001;19:41–48.

14. Chen B, Ahmed T, Mannancheril A, et al. Safety and efficacy of high-dose chemotherapy with autologous stem cell transplantation for patients with malignant astrocytomas. *Cancer.* 2004;100:2201–2207.

15. Foreman NK, Schissel D, Le T, et al. A study of sequential high dose cyclophosphamide and high dose carboplatin with peripheral stem-cell rescue in resistant or recurrent pediatric brain tumors. *J Neurooncol.* 2005;71:181–187.

16. Gururangan S, McLaughlin C, Quinn J, et al. High-dose chemotherapy with autologous stem-cell rescue in children and adults with newly diagnosed pineoblastomas. *J Clin Oncol.* 2003;21:2187–2191.

17. Perez-Martinez A, Lassaletta A, Gonzalez-Vicent M, et al. High-dose chemotherapy with autologous stem cell rescue for children with high risk and recurrent medulloblastoma and supratentorial primitive neuroectodermal tumors. *J Neurooncol.* 2005;71:33–38.

18. Mason WP, Grovas A, Halpern S, et al. Intensive chemotherapy and bone marrow rescue for young children with newly diagnosed malignant brain tumors. *J Clin Oncol.* 1998;16:210–21.

19. American Cancer Society. Available at: www.cancer.org. Accessed April 2007.

20. National Cancer Institute. Available at: www.cancer.gov. Accessed April 2007.

21. The National Center on Physical Activity and Disability. Available at: www.ncpad.org. Accessed April 2007.

22. Children's Oncology Group's Long-Term Follow-Up Guidelines for survivors of childhood, adolescent, and young adult cancers. Available at: http://www.survivorshipguidelines.org. Accessed April 17, 2007.

23. Oeffinger KC, Hudson MM. Long-term complications following childhood and adolescent cancer: foundations for providing risk-based health care for survivors. *CA Cancer J Clin.* 2004;54:208–236.

24. Mitby PA, Robison LL, Whitton JA, et al. Utilization of special education services and educational attainment among long-term survivors of childhood cancer: a report from the Childhood Cancer Survivor Study. *Cancer.* 2003;97:1115–1126.

25. Heikens J, Ubbink MC, van der Pal HP, et al. Long term survivors of childhood brain cancer have an increased risk for cardiovascular disease. *Cancer.* 2000;88:2116–2121.

Chapter 6
Effect of Cancer Treatment on Neural Stem and Progenitor Cells

Jörg Dietrich and Santosh Kesari

Introduction

Cancer therapy can target the central and peripheral nervous system, and neurotoxic adverse reactions include both acute and delayed treatment complications. This is particularly a concern for long-term survivors, such as children treated with chemotherapy and radiation. While both radiation treatment and chemotherapy alone can be associated with significant long-term toxicity, the combination of radiation and chemotherapy may be particularly harmful to the nervous system. Along with the use of more aggressive treatment regimens and prolonged survival of cancer patients, neurological complications have been observed with increasing frequency.

Neurotoxic complications may result from direct toxic effects of the drug or radiation on the cells of the nervous system, or indirectly through metabolic abnormalities, inflammatory processes, or vascular adverse effects. Interestingly, in contrast to the large number of clinical studies and reports documenting both acute and prolonged neurotoxicity following radiation and chemotherapy, surprisingly little is known about the cellular mechanisms underlying such damage to the nervous system.

The identification and characterization of neural stem cells and precursor cell populations in the adult mammalian central nervous system (CNS) have allowed for the study of the effects of radiation and chemotherapy on specific cellular populations and lineages. Most recent studies suggest that neural progenitor cells and oligodendrocytes are highly vulnerable to cancer treatment, and damage to these cells may play a key role for the frequently observed long-term neurotoxic side effects in cancer patients, such as cognitive impairment and white matter disease.

J. Dietrich (✉)
Department of Neurology, Brigham and Women's Hospital, 75 Francis Street, Boston, MA 02115; Massachusetts General Hospital, MA 02114, USA
e-mail: jdietrich1@partners.org

S. Goldman, C.D. Turner (eds.), *Late Effects of Treatment for Brain Tumors*,   81
Cancer Treatment and Research 150, DOI 10.1007/b109924_6,
© Springer Science+Business Media, LLC 2009

   This chapter will focus on the current understanding of the potential effects of cancer treatment on the normal cellular compartments of the CNS with special emphasis on neural progenitor cells and neural stem cells.

Cells and Lineages of the CNS

Cancer therapy might be harmful to a wide range of normal cell types within the nervous system. As with any other organ system, damage to immature cell types, such as to stem cells and progenitor cells, will have a different impact on cellular plasticity and long-term outcome than damage on the level of mature and differentiated cell types. For example, high-dose chemotherapy may result in severe myelosuppression secondary to progenitor and stem cell toxicity.[1]

   In order to understand cancer treatment-related neurotoxicity on a cellular level, it is important to be familiar with the current concept of the various cell types and their lineage relationships within the CNS, including neural stem and progenitor cells, mature glia cells and neurons.

   Stem cells and their progeny orchestrate the development and regeneration of mammalian tissues. They are found in most organ systems, including the brain. Neural stem cells (NSCs) are defined by their self-renewal potential, their ability to proliferate extensively, and their multipotentiality, reflecting their capability to differentiate into multiple neuroectodermal lineages.[2–4] Through the hierarchical generation of intermediate glial and neuronal progenitor cells,[5,6] NSCs are able to generate all major cell types of the CNS – neurons, astrocytes and oligodendrocytes (Fig. 6.1). In contrast to NSCs, neural progenitor cells are restricted in their differentiation potential, although they still may give rise to more than one lineage. For example, glial-restricted progenitor cells are able to give rise to both oligodendrocytes and astrocytes.[6,7] Progenitor cells also have the ability for self-renewal, but this capacity is limited compared to NSCs.

   NSCs and neural progenitor cells do play an integral part in normal brain development. They also appear to be critical components in the physiology and integrity of the adult mammalian brain. NSCs persist throughout a person's lifetime within specifically organized neurovascular niches,[8–12] where they support ongoing neurogenesis and gliogenesis. During development, stem cells are found in the ventricular zone of the CNS. In the adult brain, NSCs are primarily restricted to two brain areas, the subependymal zone of the lateral ventricles and the subgranular zone of the dentate gyrus within the hippocampus.[4,11,13] In the rodent brain, progeny of neural stem cells from the subventricular zone migrate along the rostral migratory stream to the olfactory bulb to differentiate into local interneurons.[14,15] In the human brain, migration of neuroblasts towards the olfactory bulb is orchestrated differently and appears to occur via

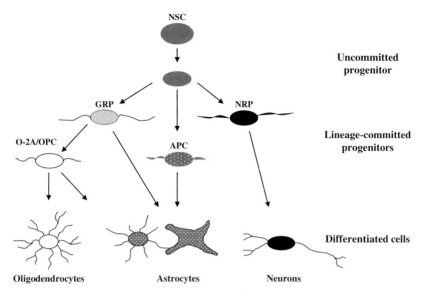

Fig. 6.1 Overview of the complex lineage relationships between both immature and mature cell types in the CNS. Multipotent neural stem cells (NSCs) give rise to neurons, astrocytes and oligodendrocytes through the generation of intermediate or lineage-committed progenitor cell populations. Tripotential glial-restricted precursor cells (GRP) have the potential to differentiate both into astrocytes and oligodendrocytes through the generation of bipotential oligodendrocyte type 2 astrocyte (O-2A) cells (also known as oligodendrocyte precursor cells (OPC)). Mature astrocytes may be derived from astrocyte precursor cells (APC), and mature neurons may be generated via neuron-restricted precursor cells (NRP). There may be additional lineage-committed cell populations, such as putative oligodendrocyte–neuron precursor cells, that are not represented in this diagram

alternate routes.[11,12,16] In the hippocampus, NSCs give rise to new granule cells that are functionally integrated in the existing neuronal network.[17–21]

In addition to the main germinal zones of the CNS – the lateral subventricular zone and the hippocampus – small numbers of NSCs have also been identified in other brain regions, such as the subcortical white matter,[22] cerebral corte[23,24] and retina.[25] It has been suggested that different NSC populations exist in the CNS, and both cell intrinsic and local environmental signals contribute to the presence of regionally different NSC populations.[26–28]

There is increasing evidence that the persistence of NSCs in the adult mammalian brain reflects their role for endogenous repair mechanisms and maintenance of normal brain functions (for review, see e.g.[29]). While under physiological circumstances NSCs comprise a relatively quiescent cell population, these cells have the potential to proliferate and migrate extensively, characterizing the adult brain as a surprisingly dynamic organ system.

Glial and neuronal progenitor cells derived from multipotent stem cells will eventually differentiate into mature cell types of the CNS to replace existing astrocytes, oligodendrocytes and neurons.[30–32] Consequently, the disruption of neural stem and progenitor cell function in the adult mammalian brain might result in critical impairment of neurological function. There is growing evidence that this assumption may be the answer for many neurological diseases and syndromes, including chemotherapy- and radiation-induced long-term neurological adverse effects, such as cognitive impairment, white matter degeneration and cerebral atrophy.[29,33–35] The remaining sections in this chapter will summarize the current understanding of cellular toxicity and vulnerability to both radiation and chemotherapy, and will discuss how specific cellular toxicity might be linked to commonly seen long-term neurologic complications of cancer treatment.

The Spectrum of Neurological Adverse Effects Following Cancer Treatment

Cancer treatment usually involves various therapeutic modalities. In case of solid tumors, surgery is commonly followed by radiation therapy and chemotherapy. Hematologic malignancies typically are treated with chemotherapy alone or in combination with radiation therapy. In addition, hormonal agents, steroids and other novel drug treatments (e.g., small molecules, such as angiogenesis inhibitors, designed to target growth signaling pathways) are used invariantly in cancer patients. Survival commonly depends on an aggressive and combined treatment approach. Many patients may, therefore, be exposed to multiple chemotherapeutic regimens applied sequentially in response to recurrent disease. As both radiation and chemotherapy are associated with significant dose-limiting neurotoxicity, the use of multimodal treatment approaches and the application of multiple chemotherapeutic regimens significantly increase the risk of developing severe neurotoxic adverse reactions.

Radiation-Induced CNS Toxicity

The harmful effects of brain radiation have been well-recognized for decades and include a spectrum of acute, subacute and chronic side effect[36,37] as discussed in Chapter 3. Common complications consist of acute or subacute encephalopathy, cognitive decline, radiation necrosis, leukoencephalopathy, dementia and cerebral atrophy.[38–40] The most prominent and debilitating long-term consequence of cranial radiation therapy is cognitive impairment. Cognitive decline typically is progressive and involves deficits in short-term memory, visual motor processing, and attention. Hippocampal dysfunction appears to be a prominent component of this syndrome.[41]

Radiation necrosis and leukoencephalopathy may occur with delayed onset of months to years.[42–46] Leukoencephalopathy may result from radiation or chemotherapy alone, but is more common after combined treatment. Tissue analysis of diffuse leukoencephalopathy shows loss of white matter, reactive gliosis, and scattered foci of necrosis. The most severe form consists of a disseminated necrotizing leukoencephalopathy with confluent necrotic foci followed by diffuse cerebral atrophy.[45,47–50]

The exact etiology of these long-term side effects is not known. While acute toxicities may be the result of vascular toxicity, blood-brain barrier disruption, fluid and electrolyte shifts,[49,51] the mechanisms of chronic radiation damage are likely related to long-term toxicity to normal neural cell types, including stem and progenitor cells in combination with metabolic derangements, immune and inflammatory responses.[34,52–54]

Cellular Basis of Radiation Induced Neurotoxicity

The cellular mechanisms for cognitive decline and other structural changes, including brain atrophy and white matter changes, have long been obscure. Recent advances in studying neurogenesis and gliogenesis in animal models have revealed a high degree of sensitivity of neural stem cells and progenitor cell populations to radiation treatment.[33,52,54–58] Moreover, it has been shown that disruption of hippocampal neurogenesis may play a key role in the pathogenesis of cognitive impairment following cranial radiation.[33,34,59,60] Brain radiation results in decreased cell proliferation in the subgranular zone of the hippocampus and increased cell death as measured by apoptosis in a radiation dose-dependent manner.[56,59] The radiation-induced decline in hippocampal neurogenesis appears to be largely mediated by chronic inflammatory processes and changes in the neurovascular microenvironment.[33] Consequently, nonsteroidal anti-inflammatory drugs, such as indomethacin, were shown to partially restore hippocampal neurogenesis.[60]

Neurogenesis depends on a permissive neurovascular environment, and learning and memory functions are strongly influenced by hippocampal plasticity.[8,21,61,62] Thus, radiation-impaired hippocampal dysfunction and neurogenesis offer an attractive explanation for delayed cognitive decline in patients undergoing cranial radiation.

As predicted by animal models, a recent study revealed that hippocampal neurogenesis, as measured by the number of doublecortin-positive immature neurons, was drastically reduced in patients treated with cranial radiation for brain cancer.[63] The decrease in the number of immature neurons was associated with inflammatory changes and microglia activation at least in one patient who underwent hippocampal radiation just two months prior.

In addition to decreased hippocampal neurogenesis, radiation-associated toxicity also involves damage to glial cell populations.[33,52,53] It has been shown that radiation results in impaired glial progenitor cell proliferation in multiple brain regions, including cortex, subcortical white matter, hippocampus and corpus callosum.[64] Similar to impairment of neuronal progenitor cell proliferation, glial progenitor cell toxicity occurs in a radiation dose-dependent manner.[33,64,65] Moreover, surviving glial progenitor cells appear to be functionally impaired[65] and unable to differentiate into mature oligodendrocytes in vitro (Dietrich et al., unpublished observations).

Taken together, there is increasing evidence that cranial radiation results in disruption of neural stem and progenitor cell function in the hippocampus and other brain regions. These effects are largely medicated via inflammatory responses. Progenitor and stem cell toxicity has provided a compelling explanation for prolonged and delayed cognitive decline in patients undergoing radiation therapy. The use of anti-inflammatory drugs has offered an interesting target to minimize radiation-induced progenitor cell toxicity. Clinical trials are currently in progress to study the neuroprotective effects of nonsteroidal anti-inflammatory drugs in patients undergoing brain radiation.

Chemotherapy-Induced Neurotoxicity

A wide spectrum of chemotherapy-induced neurotoxic adverse effects is seen in cancer patients, and survival is commonly associated with the price of long-term neurological complications.[66-68] Similar to radiation-induced toxicity, neurotoxic syndromes following chemotherapy may present as acute, subacute, or delayed effects – even years after cessation of treatment. Frequently encountered delayed neurologic complications include cognitive impairment, white matter disease, difficulties with gait and coordination, cerebral atrophy and dementia (see Table 6.1).[50,68-71]

Some agents, such as methotrexate or carmustine, are well-known to cause a leukoencephalopathy syndrome, especially when administered at a high dose, intrathecally, or in combination with cranial radiotherapy.[72-75] Non-enhancing, confluent, periventricular white matter lesions, necrosis, ventriculomegaly, and cortical atrophy characterize this syndrome. While progressive cognitive deficits are frequently present clinically, white matter abnormalities seen

Table 6.1 Chemotherapeutic agents that have clearly been associated with delayed neurologic side effects, including cognitive decline, white matter abnormalities and cerebral atrophy

- Carmustine (BCNU)
- Carmofur
- Cisplatin
- Cyclophosphamide
- Cytosine arabinoside (Ara-C)
- Fludarabine
- 5-FU
- Ifosfamide
- Levamisole
- Methotrexate

on neuroimaging do not necessarily correlate with the degree of cognitive deficits.[76,77]

Additionally, adverse neurological effects have been observed with virtually all categories of chemotherapeutic agents,[67,68,78–80] including antimetabolites (e.g., cytosine arabinoside, 5-FU, and methotrexate), DNA cross-linking agents (e.g., carmustine and cisplatin), mitotic inhibitors (e.g., vincristine) and anti-hormonal agents.

The detailed mechanisms for the wide spectrum of long-term neurological adverse effects following chemotherapy have been largely unknown until most recently. While some drugs may be more harmful to the nervous system than others, there is now compelling evidence that many chemotherapeutic agents directly target the normal cells of the nervous system (Table 6.2). Methotrexate, for example, is associated with a relatively high frequency of neurotoxicity, which may be severe and progressive, especially if the drug is administered after radiation therapy. Given the large number of cancer patients receiving chemotherapy, it is not clear, however, why certain patients are more affected by CNS toxicity than others, suggesting that beside direct drug effects on cellular viability, other mechanisms appear to play important roles in compromising CNS function and integrity.

Table 6.2   Chemotherapeutic agents that have been shown in animal studies to target neural progenitor cells and oligodendrocytes

- Carmustine (BCNU)
- Cisplatin
- Cyclophosphamide
- Cytosine arabinoside (Ara-C)
- 5-Fluorouracil (5-FU)
- Ifosfamide
- Methotrexate
- Misonidazole
- Thiotepa

Cellular Basis of Chemotherapy-Induced Neurotoxicity

The majority of cancer treatments affect a diverse range of normal cell types, resulting in a broad spectrum of toxicities to multiple organ systems. While treatment-related toxicities have probably been most extensively studied in the hematopoietic system, there is no comparable level of analysis for most other organ systems. Strikingly, despite a large number of reports documenting both acute and prolonged neurotoxicity following chemotherapy, surprisingly little is known about the cellular mechanisms underlying the damage seen in the CNS. The conventional view has been that cytotoxic drugs preferentially target rapidly dividing cells, such as glia cells and endothelial cells. More recent studies indicate, however, that the mechanisms of neurotoxicity are far more complex than simply toxic effects on proliferating cells alone.

Morphological studies of rats exposed to methotrexate and misonidazole suggested that glial progenitor cells might be particularly vulnerable to cytotoxic agents.[81] Single dose application of methotrexate into the ventricles of rats was associated with ventricular dilatation, edema and visible destruction of the ependymal cell layer lining the ventricles and the surrounding brain tissue. Numerous glial cells with pycnotic nuclei were observed in the gray and white matter, with increased numbers of microglial cells. There was also a rapid reduction in the number of nuclei per unit area in the rostral extension of the subependymal plate, with a 30% reduction seen 1–2 days after methotrexate administration. A similar reduction was seen in the number of mitotic cells. Other experimental studies suggested that exposure to numerous cytotoxic agents, including cyclophosphamide, cisplatin, ifosfamide and thiotepa, is associated with significant and dose-dependent neurotoxicity, evident in cortex, basal ganglia and hippocampus in seven-day-old animals.[82] These studies, however, did not provide a lineage-based analysis of neurotoxicity following chemotherapy. Based on the observation that oligodendrogliomas and astrocytomas typically show a differential response to chemotherapy, Nutt et al. provided initial experimental evidence that the oligodendroglial lineage might be particularly vulnerable to alkylating agents when compared with the sensitivity profile of astrocytic cells.[83]

Most recent studies reveal detailed insight into the biological basis for CNS toxicity following systemic chemotherapy. It has been shown that dividing neural progenitor cells, which are the direct ancestors of all differentiated cell types of the CNS, and the nondividing oligodendrocytes (the myelin-forming cells of the CNS), are the most vulnerable cell populations to the effects of multiple chemotherapeutic agents.[35] Alarmingly, the degree of sensitivity of normal progenitor cells and oligodendrocytes surpassed the sensitivity of most cancer cells tested when applied at drug dosages commonly achieved in humans. In contrast, dividing astrocytes and mature neurons were less vulnerable when compared with the degree of sensitivity of oligodendrocytes and neural progenitor cells. In vitro results were predictive of in vivo effects. Systemic application of BCNU, cisplatin and cytosine arabinoside into mice was associated with significant apoptosis of oligodendrocytes and neural progenitor cell populations. Single exposure to chemotherapeutic agents resulted in significant post-treatment impairment of cell proliferation and increased apoptosis, followed by a marked rebound in cell proliferation in the subventricular zone, the dentate gyrus and corpus callosum. However, repetitive drug exposure resulted in long-term suppression of cell division in the CNS.

Other groups reported similar findings after systemic application of thiotepa[84] and methotrexate.[85] Systemic application of these drugs was associated with a dose-dependent inhibition of hippocampal cell proliferation in vivo. In addition, methotrexate has been shown to result in impaired cognitive performance in animal models.[85,86]

Damage on the level of neural progenitor cells offers a compelling explanation for the frequently seen delayed toxicities in patients, such as progressive dementias and leukoencephalopathies. It is conceivable that long-term and progressive cognitive decline in cancer survivors are the result of a combination of decreased proliferation of neural progenitor cells, impaired hippocampal neurogenesis, and damage to oligodendroglial cells and white matter tracts.

Many open questions remain, however, regarding the effects of chemotherapy on the brain. For example, many patients are repeatedly exposed to a number of different drugs. It is not known how multiple drugs given concomitantly influence the integrity of the blood-brain barrier to allow other, less lipophilic drugs to penetrate the CNS. It is also not known why certain individuals are much more affected than others by the devastating toxic adverse effects of cancer treatment. Next to direct toxic effects of chemotherapeutic compounds on the cells of the CNS, there are likely other factors critically important in influencing the degree of neurotoxicity. Several candidate mechanisms have been identified in recent years that possibly modulate neurotoxicity in individual patients undergoing cancer treatment. For example, genetic polymorphisms have been shown to influence the efficiency of DNA repair mechanisms and drug efflux pump systems.[87–91] Furthermore, therapy-induced production of reactive oxygen species and subsequent changes in cellular redox balance are likely to influence the profile and extent of toxic side effects.[92–94] Many chemotherapeutic agents have oxidizing character and are associated with profound changes in antioxidant levels[95,96] that may persist even for years after cessation of treatment.[97] Oxidative balance is a critically important factor that influences key cellular functions in stem and progenitor cells, such as proliferation and differentiation.[98] Thus, pro-oxidative states following anticancer treatment are likely to influence normal cellular functions and protein metabolism in progenitor cells and postmitotic cells. Chemotherapy has also been shown to shorten telomere length and to decrease the lifespan of a dividing cell by senescence and apoptosis.[99,100] This effect may critically interfere with the normal cellular physiology and function of stem and progenitor cells.[101]

Summary and Future Perspectives

There has been increasing evidence that anticancer treatment, including radiation and chemotherapy, is directly toxic to progenitor cells and oligodendrocytes in the CNS. Damage on the level of neural progenitor cells has offered a compelling explanation for delayed toxicities, such as progressive dementias, cerebral atrophies and white matter disease. Next to the direct cellular toxicity, however, there are likely a number of cofactors and mechanisms that determine an individual patient's risk and degree of developing neurotoxicity.

Several novel anticancer agents have been introduced in recent years to complement conventional chemotherapeutic regimens. Many of these agents designed to target small molecules and growth factor signaling pathways have not been available long enough to have gathered sufficient understanding about their long-term effects on the nervous system. For example, by targeting FGF, PDGF and VEGF signaling pathways, all of which are critically important in normal neural stem cell physiology, serious complications due to stem and progenitor cell toxicity need to be anticipated.

Future studies need to identify the risk factors of developing CNS toxicity, to design and optimize individual therapies in order to avoid unnecessary toxicities, and to closely monitor individuals at highest risk of developing neurotoxicity using longitudinal neurocognitive assessments and sophisticated neuroimaging methods. When compared with the hematopoietic system, where the use of certain growth factors (e.g., GM-CSF, G-CSF, Erythropoietin, etc.) has enabled patients to rapidly recover from serious treatment-related myelosuppression, there are currently no neuroprotective strategies available to enhance endogenous CNS repair. Increasing our understanding about the differential vulnerability of neural cell populations to anticancer therapy will allow us to develop means for selective neuroprotection. Thus, one of the most important goals of future cancer therapies will be the identification of neuroprotective strategies along with the development of tumor-specific therapies to avoid unnecessary toxicities, and to promote endogenous nervous system repair in case temporary toxicity is unavoidable.

References

1. Carey PJ. Drug-induced myelosuppression: diagnosis and management. *Drug Saf.* 2003;26:691–706.
2. Reynolds BA, Weiss S. Generation of neurons and astrocytes from isolated cells of the adult mammalian central nervous system. *Science.* 1992;255:1707–1710.
3. Temple S, Alvarez-Buylla A. Stem cells in the adult mammalian central nervous system. *Curr Opin Neurobiol.* 1999;9:135–141.
4. Gage FH. Mammalian neural stem cells. *Science.* 2000;287:1433–1438.
5. Mayer-Proschel M, Kalyani AJ, Mujtaba T, Rao MS. Isolation of lineage-restricted neuronal precursors from multipotent neuroepithelial stem cells. *Neuron.* 1997;19: 773–785.
6. Rao MS, Noble M, Mayer-Proschel M. A tripotential glial precursor cell is present in the developing spinal cord. *Proc Natl Acad Sci USA.* 1998;95:3996–4001.
7. Dietrich J, Noble M, Mayer-Proschel M. Characterization of A2B5+ glial precursor cells from cryopreserved human fetal brain progenitor cells. *Glia.* 2002;40:65–77.
8. Palmer TD, Willhoite AR, Gage FH. Vascular niche for adult hippocampal neurogenesis. *J Comp Neurol.* 2000;425:479–494.
9. Shen Q, Goderie SK, Jin L, et al. Endothelial cells stimulate self-renewal and expand neurogenesis of neural stem cells. *Science.* 2004;304:1338–1340.
10. Alvarez-Buylla A, Lim DA. For the long run: maintaining germinal niches in the adult brain. *Neuron.* 2004;41:683–686.

11. Sanai N, Tramontin AD, Quinones-Hinojosa A, et al. Unique astrocyte ribbon in adult human brain contains neural stem cells but lacks chain migration. *Nature*. 2004;427:740–4.
12. Quinones-Hinojosa A, Sanai N, Soriano-Navarro M, et al. Cellular composition and cytoarchitecture of the adult human subventricular zone: a niche of neural stem cells. *J Comp Neurol*. 2006;494:415–434.
13. Eriksson PS, Perfilieva E, Bjork-Eriksson T, et al. Neurogenesis in the adult human hippocampus. *Nat Med*. 1998;4:1313–1317.
14. Luskin MB. Restricted proliferation and migration of postnatally generated neurons derived from the forebrain subventricular zone. *Neuron*. 1993;11:173–189.
15. Lois C, Garcia-Verdugo JM, Alvarez-Buylla A. Chain migration of neuronal precursors. *Science*. 1996;271:978–981.
16. Curtis MA, Kam M, Nannmark U, et al. Human neuroblasts migrate to the olfactory bulb via a lateral ventricular extension. *Science*. 2007;315:1243–1249.
17. Altman J, Das GD. Autoradiographic and histological evidence of postnatal hippocampal neurogenesis in rats. *J Comp Neurol*. 1965;124:319–335.
18. Kuhn HG, Dickinson-Anson H, Gage FH. Neurogenesis in the dentate gyrus of the adult rat: age-related decrease of neuronal progenitor proliferation. *J Neurosci*. 1996;16:2027–2033.
19. Hastings NB, Seth MI, Tanapat P, Rydel TA, Gould E. Granule neurons generated during development extend divergent axon collaterals to hippocampal area CA3. *J Comp Neurol*. 2002;452:324–333.
20. Cameron HA, McKay RD. Adult neurogenesis produces a large pool of new granule cells in the dentate gyrus. *J Comp Neurol*. 2001;435:406–417.
21. van Praag H, Schinder AF, Christie BR, Toni N, Palmer TD, Gage FH. Functional neurogenesis in the adult hippocampus. *Nature*. 2002;415:1030–1034.
22. Nunes MC, Roy NS, Keyoung HM, et al. Identification and isolation of multipotential neural progenitor cells from the subcortical white matter of the adult human brain. *Nat Med*. 2003;9:439–447.
23. Marmur R, Mabie PC, Gokhan S, Song Q, Kessler JA, Mehler MF. Isolation and developmental characterization of cerebral cortical multipotent progenitors. *Dev Biol*. 1998;204:577–591.
24. Arsenijevic Y, Villemure JG, Brunet JF, et al. Isolation of multipotent neural precursors residing in the cortex of the adult human brain. *Exp Neurol*. 2001;170:48–62.
25. Coles BL, Angenieux B, Inoue T, et al. Facile isolation and the characterization of human retinal stem cells. *Proc Natl Acad Sci USA*. 2004;101:15772–15777.
26. Temple S. The development of neural stem cells. *Nature*. 2001;414:112–117.
27. Hitoshi S, Tropepe V, Ekker M, van der Kooy D. Neural stem cell lineages are regionally specified, but not committed, within distinct compartments of the developing brain. *Development*. 2002;129:233–244.
28. Shen Q, Wang Y, Dimos JT, et al. The timing of cortical neurogenesis is encoded within lineages of individual progenitor cells. *Nat Neurosci* 2006;9:743–751.
29. Dietrich J, Kempermann G. Role of endogenous neural stem cells in neurological disease and brain repair. *Adv Exp Med Biol*. 2006;557:191–220.
30. Goldman JE, Zerlin M, Newman S, Zhang L, Gensert J. Fate determination and migration of progenitors in the postnatal mammalian CNS. *Dev Neurosci*. 1997;19:42–48.
31. Marshall CA, Suzuki SO, Goldman JE. Gliogenic and neurogenic progenitors of the subventricular zone: who are they, where did they come from, and where are they going? *Glia*. 2003;43:52–61.
32. Lie DC, Song H, Colamarino SA, Ming GL, Gage FH. Neurogenesis in the adult brain: new strategies for central nervous system diseases. *Annu Rev Pharmacol Toxicol*. 2004;44:399–421.
33. Monje ML, Mizumatsu S, Fike JR, Palmer TD. Irradiation induces neural precursor-cell dysfunction. *Nat Med*. 2002;8:955–962.

34. Monje ML, Palmer T. Radiation injury and neurogenesis. *Curr Opin Neurol.* 2003;16: 129–134.
35. Dietrich J, Han R, Yang Y, Mayer-Proschel M, Noble M. CNS progenitor cells and oligodendrocytes are targets of chemotherapeutic agents in vitro and in vivo. *J Biol.* 2006;5:22.
36. Sheline GE, Wara WM, Smith V. Therapeutic irradiation and brain injury. *Int J Radiat Oncol Biol Phys.* 1980;6:1215–1228.
37. Packer RJ, Meadows AT, Rorke LB, Goldwein JL, D'Angio G. Long-term sequelae of cancer treatment on the central nervous system in childhood. *Med Pediatr Oncol.* 1987;15:241–253.
38. DeAngelis LM, Delattre JY, Posner JB. Radiation-induced dementia in patients cured of brain metastases. *Neurology.* 1989;39:789–796.
39. Duffner PK. Long-term effects of radiation therapy on cognitive and endocrine function in children with leukemia and brain tumors. *Neurologist.* 2004;10:293–310.
40. Perry A, Schmidt RE. Cancer therapy-associated CNS neuropathology: an update and review of the literature. *Acta Neuropathol.* 2006;111:197–212.
41. Abayomi OK. Pathogenesis of irradiation-induced cognitive dysfunction. *Acta Oncol.* 1996;35:659–663.
42. Oppenheimer JH, Levy ML, Sinha U, et al. Radionecrosis secondary to interstitial brachytherapy: correlation of magnetic resonance imaging and histopathology. *Neurosurgery.* 1992;31:336–343.
43. Morris JG, Grattan-Smith P, Panegyres PK, O'Neill P, Soo YS, Langlands AO. Delayed cerebral radiation necrosis. *Q J Med.* 1994;87:119–129.
44. Chong VE, Fan YF. Radiation-induced temporal lobe necrosis. *AJNR Am J Neuroradiol.* 1997;18:784–785.
45. Lai R, Abrey LE, Rosenblum MK, DeAngelis LM. Treatment-induced leukoencephalopathy in primary CNS lymphoma: a clinical and autopsy study. *Neurology.* 2004;62: 451–456.
46. Fouladi M, Chintagumpala M, Laningham FH, et al. White matter lesions detected by magnetic resonance imaging after radiotherapy and high-dose chemotherapy in children with medulloblastoma or primitive neuroectodermal tumor. *J Clin Oncol.* 2004;22: 4551–4560.
47. Robain O, Dulac O, Dommergues JP, et al. Necrotising leukoencephalopathy complicating treatment of childhood leukemia. *J Neurol Neurosurg Psychiatry.* 1984;47:65–72.
48. Asai A, Matsutani M, Kohno T, et al. Subacute brain atrophy after radiation therapy for malignant brain tumor. *Cancer.* 1989;63:1962–1974.
49. Rubin P, Gash DM, Hansen JT, Nelson DF, Williams JP. Disruption of the blood-brain barrier as the primary effect of CNS irradiation. *Radiother Oncol.* 1994;31:51–60.
50. Omuro AM, Ben-Porat LS, Panageas KS, et al. Delayed neurotoxicity in primary central nervous system lymphoma. *Arch Neurol.* 2005;62:1595–1600.
51. Behin A, Delattre JY. Complications of radiation therapy on the brain and spinal cord. *Semin Neurol.* 2004;24:405–417.
52. Belka C, Budach W, Kortmann RD, Bamberg M. Radiation induced CNS toxicity – molecular and cellular mechanisms. *Br J Cancer.* 2001;85:1233–1239.
53. Noble M, Dietrich J. Intersections between neurobiology and oncology: tumor origin, treatment and repair of treatment-associated damage. *Trends Neurosci.* 2002;25:103–7.
54. Fike JR, Rola R, Limoli CL. Radiation response of neural precursor cells. *Neurosurg Clin N Am.* 2007;18:115–27, x.
55. Parent JM, Tada E, Fike JR, Lowenstein DH. Inhibition of dentate granule cell neurogenesis with brain irradiation does not prevent seizure-induced mossy fiber synaptic reorganization in the rat. *J Neurosci.* 1999;19:4508–4519.
56. Tada E, Parent JM, Lowenstein DH, Fike JR. X-irradiation causes a prolonged reduction in cell proliferation in the dentate gyrus of adult rats. *Neuroscience.* 2000;99:33–41.

57. Fukuda H, Fukuda A, Zhu C, et al. Irradiation-induced progenitor cell death in the developing brain is resistant to erythropoietin treatment and caspase inhibition. *Cell Death Differ.* 2004;11:1166–1178.
58. Limoli CL, Giedzinski E, Rola R, Otsuka S, Palmer TD, Fike JR. Radiation response of neural precursor cells: linking cellular sensitivity to cell cycle checkpoints, apoptosis and oxidative stress. *Radiat Res.* 2004;161:17–27.
59. Mizumatsu S, Monje ML, Morhardt DR, Rola R, Palmer TD, Fike JR. Extreme sensitivity of adult neurogenesis to low doses of X-irradiation. *Cancer Res.* 2003;63:4021–7.
60. Monje ML, Toda H, Palmer TD. Inflammatory blockade restores adult hippocampal neurogenesis. *Science.* 2003;302:1760–1765.
61. Palmer TD. Adult neurogenesis and the vascular Nietzsche. *Neuron.* 2002;34:856–858.
62. Wurmser AE, Palmer TD, Gage FH. Neuroscience. Cellular interactions in the stem cell niche. *Science.* 2004;304:1253–1255.
63. Monje ML, Vogel H, Masek M, Ligon KL, Fisher PG, Palmer TD.Impaired human hippocampal neurogenesis after treatment for central nervous system malignancies. *Ann Neurol.* 2007;62(5):515–520.
64. Moore AH, Noble M, O'Banion MK, Dietrich J. Evaluation of cell proliferation, apoptosis and gliosis following neonatal brain irradiation. In: Proceedings of the Society for Neuroscience; 2004:940.12.
65. Chari DM, Huang WL, Blakemore WF. Dysfunctional oligodendrocyte progenitor cell (OPC) populations may inhibit repopulation of OPC depleted tissue. *J Neurosci Res.* 2003;73:787–793.
66. Posner JB. Side effects of chemotherapy. In: Posner JB, ed. *Neurologic Complications of Cancer.* Philadelphia: F.A. Davis; 1995:282–310.
67. Keime-Guibert F, Napolitano M, Delattre JY. Neurological complications of radiotherapy and chemotherapy. *J Neurol.* 1998;245:695–708.
68. Dietrich J, Wen P. *Neurologic Complications of Chemotherapy.* 2. edition ed. Totowa, New Jersey: Humana Press Inc.; 2008.
69. Schagen SB, van Dam FS, Muller MJ, Boogerd W, Lindeboom J, Bruning PF. Cognitive deficits after postoperative adjuvant chemotherapy for breast carcinoma. *Cancer.* 1999;85:640–650.
70. Brezden CB, Phillips KA, Abdolell M, Bunston T, Tannock IF. Cognitive function in breast cancer patients receiving adjuvant chemotherapy. *J Clin Oncol.* 2000;18:2695–2701.
71. Duffner PK. The long term effects of chemotherapy on the central nervous system. *J Biol* 2006;5:21.
72. Shapiro WR, Chernik NL, Posner JB. Necrotizing encephalopathy following intraventricular instillation of methotrexate. *Arch Neurol.* 1973;28:96–102.
73. Bashir R, Hochberg FH, Linggood RM, Hottleman K. Pre-irradiation internal carotid artery BCNU in treatment of glioblastoma multiforme. *J Neurosurg.* 1988;68:917–919.
74. Rosenblum MK, Delattre JY, Walker RW, Shapiro WR. Fatal necrotizing encephalopathy complicating treatment of malignant gliomas with intra-arterial BCNU and irradiation: a pathological study. *J Neurooncol.* 1989;7:269–281.
75. Newton HB. Intra-arterial chemotherapy of primary brain tumors. *Curr Treat Options Oncol.* 2005;6:519–530.
76. Fliessbach K, Helmstaedter C, Urbach H, et al. Neuropsychological outcome after chemotherapy for primary CNS lymphoma: a prospective study. *Neurology.* 2005;64:1184–1188.
77. Neuwelt EA, Guastadisegni PE, Varallyay P, Doolittle ND. Imaging changes and cognitive outcome in primary CNS lymphoma after enhanced chemotherapy delivery. *AJNR Am J Neuroradiol.* 2005;26:258–265.
78. Dropcho EJ. Neurotoxicity of cancer chemotherapy. *Semin Neurol.* 2004;24:419–426.

79. Minisini A, Atalay G, Bottomley A, Puglisi F, Piccart M, Biganzoli L. What is the effect of systemic anticancer treatment on cognitive function? *Lancet Oncol.* 2004;5:273–282.
80. Wefel JS, Lenzi R, Theriault RL, Davis RN, Meyers CA. The cognitive sequelae of standard-dose adjuvant chemotherapy in women with breast carcinoma: results of a prospective, randomized, longitudinal trial. *Cancer.* 2004;100:2292–2299.
81. Morris GM, Hopewell JW, Morris AD. A comparison of the effects of methotrexate and misonidazole on the germinal cells of the subependymal plate of the rat. *Br J Radiol.* 1995;68:406–412.
82. Rzeski W, Pruskil S, Macke A, et al. Anticancer agents are potent neurotoxins in vitro and in vivo. *Ann Neurol.* 2004;56:351–360.
83. Nutt CL, Noble M, Chambers AF, Cairncross JG. Differential expression of drug resistance genes and chemosensitivity in glial cell lineages correlate with differential response of oligodendrogliomas and astrocytomas to chemotherapy. *Cancer Res.* 2000;60:4812–4818.
84. Mignone RG, Weber ET. Potent inhibition of cell proliferation in the hippocampal dentate gyrus of mice by the chemotherapeutic drug thioTEPA. *Brain Res.* 2006;1111:26–29.
85. Seigers R, Schagen SB, Beerling W, et al. Long-lasting suppression of hippocampal cell proliferation and impaired cognitive performance by methotrexate in the rat. *Behav Brain Res.* 2008;186:168–175.
86. Winocur G, Vardy J, Binns MA, Kerr L, Tannock I. The effects of the anti-cancer drugs, methotrexate and 5-fluorouracil, on cognitive function in mice. *Pharmacol Biochem Behav.* 2006;85:66–75.
87. Hoffmeyer S, Burk O, von Richter O, et al. Functional polymorphisms of the human multidrug-resistance gene: multiple sequence variations and correlation of one allele with P-glycoprotein expression and activity in vivo. *Proc Natl Acad Sci USA.* 2000;97: 3473–3478.
88. Muramatsu T, Johnson DR, Finch RA, et al. Age-related differences in vincristine toxicity and biodistribution in wild-type and transporter-deficient mice. *Oncol Res.* 2004;14:331–343.
89. Jamroziak K, Balcerczak E, Cebula B, et al. Multi-drug transporter MDR1 gene polymorphism and prognosis in adult acute lymphoblastic leukemia. *Pharmacol Rep.* 2005;57:882–888.
90. Linnebank M, Pels H, Kleczar N, et al. MTX-induced white matter changes are associated with polymorphisms of methionine metabolism. *Neurology.* 2005;64:912–913.
91. Fishel ML, Vasko MR, Kelley MR. DNA repair in neurons: so if they don't divide what's to repair? *Mutat Res.* 2007;614:24–36.
92. Kaya E, Keskin L, Aydogdu I, Kuku I, Bayraktar N, Erkut MA. Oxidant/antioxidant parameters and their relationship with chemotherapy in Hodgkin's lymphoma. *J Int Med Res.* 2005;33:687–692.
93. Papageorgiou M, Stiakaki E, Dimitriou H, et al. Cancer chemotherapy reduces plasma total antioxidant capacity in children with malignancies. *Leuk Res.* 2005;29:11–16.
94. Kennedy DD, Ladas EJ, Rheingold SR, Blumberg J, Kelly KM. Antioxidant status decreases in children with acute lymphoblastic leukemia during the first six months of chemotherapy treatment. *Pediatr Blood Cancer.* 2005;44:378–385.
95. Weijl NI, Hopman GD, Wipkink-Bakker A, et al. Cisplatin combination chemotherapy induces a fall in plasma antioxidants of cancer patients. *Ann Oncol.* 1998;9:1331–1337.
96. Conklin KA. Dietary antioxidants during cancer chemotherapy: impact on chemotherapeutic effectiveness and development of side effects. *Nutr Cancer.* 2000;37:1–18.
97. Gietema JA, Meinardi MT, Messerschmidt J, et al. Circulating plasma platinum more than 10 years after cisplatin treatment for testicular cancer. *Lancet.* 2000;355:1075–1076.
98. Smith J, Ladi E, Mayer-Proschel M, Noble M. Redox state is a central modulator of the balance between self-renewal and differentiation in a dividing glial precursor cell. *Proc Natl Acad Sci USA.* 2000;97:10032–10037.

99. Schroder CP, Wisman GB, de Jong S, et al. Telomere length in breast cancer patients before and after chemotherapy with or without stem cell transplantation. *Br J Cancer*. 2001;84:1348–1353.
100. Lahav M, Uziel O, Kestenbaum M, et al. Nonmyeloablative conditioning does not prevent telomere shortening after allogeneic stem cell transplantation. *Transplantation* 2005;80:969–976.
101. Cheng A, Shin-ya K, Wan R, et al. Telomere protection mechanisms change during neurogenesis and neuronal maturation: newly generated neurons are hypersensitive to telomere and DNA damage. *J Neurosci*. 2007;27:3722–3733.

Chapter 7
The Pediatric Brain Tumor Late Effects Clinic

Kimberley J. Dilley and Barbara Lockart

Introduction

Childhood brain tumor patients are surviving at ever increasing rates. In the time period from 1973 to 1994 the incidence of brain tumors increased while the annual mortality rate has decreased from 1 to 0.78 deaths per 100,000.[1] The survival rate for pediatric brain tumors is now 50%, compared to 80% overall survival rates for pediatric malignancies. The National Coalition for Cancer Survivorship states that a person is considered a cancer survivor at the time of diagnosis. Included in this definition of survivor are the family and community supporting the survivor.[2]

Lifelong surveillance for delayed effects of chemotherapy, radiation and surgery is needed for all patients treated for a brain tumor. For many patients with a brain tumor the experience is more chronic than terminal in nature. Each generation surviving treatment will face new challenges and health care issues as treatments evolve with changing medical technology. Both of these factors influence the health care needs of brain tumor survivors. As the patients' health care needs change from curing cancer to monitoring for late effects, the medical expertise required to manage health care issues is also different. Oeffinger and Robison described the importance of risk-based health care of survivors. "Such an approach should be longitudinal, proactive, and anticipatory and should include a systematic plan of prevention and surveillance based on risks associated with the previous cancer, cancer therapy, genetic predispositions, lifestyle behaviors and comorbid health conditions".[3]

Up to 80% of pediatric brain tumor survivors experience significant, lifelong sequelae from treatment.[4] Radiation therapy and surgery have been implicated as important treatment factors for the development of long-term

K.J. Dilley (✉)
Director, STAR Program, Children's Memorial Hospital, Division of Hematology/
Oncology/Transplant, Assistant Professor of Pediatrics, Northwestern University
Feinberg School of Medicine, Chicago, IL 60614, USA
e-mail: kdilley@childrensmemorial.org

S. Goldman, C.D. Turner (eds.), *Late Effects of Treatment for Brain Tumors*,
Cancer Treatment and Research 150, DOI 10.1007/b109924_7,
© Springer Science+Business Media, LLC 2009

health issues, especially neurocognitive and endocrine dysfunction. The complexity of the health care issues experienced by many brain tumor survivors requires that services be coordinated between multiple disciplines that few health care providers have experience providing. The treating team or the primary care physician may not have the time or expertise to follow survivors with more chronic medical issues. Health care providers in other medical specialty areas such as cardiology, gynecology and endocrinology may lack sufficient experience or education regarding the unique health care needs of childhood cancer survivors.[5] Thus, as the number of brain tumor survivors continues to grow many centers have begun to develop multidisciplinary late effects clinics that specialize in cancer survivors.

The focus of a late effects clinic is to monitor the patient for both long-term and late effects of treatment, as well as referring survivors to appropriate subspecialists. Maintaining the health of this patient should focus on monitoring for late effects, monitoring mental and social functioning and well-being, and providing health education specific to the individual and treatment received. Finally, anticipatory guidance for issues regarding insurance, schooling and career is also under the domain of the late effects clinic.[6]

Scope of the Problem

Cancer survivors are at risk for late effects affecting any organ system in the body. The occurrence of late effects is caused by numerous factors including treatment, dosage received, age at the time of treatment, method of treatment delivery, gender and genetic make-up. Treatment sequelae might be subtle, such as a high frequency hearing loss, or quite apparent, such as a gross motor deficit. A 2006 study showed that 20% of adult survivors of a childhood malignancy face a late effect that interferes with activities of daily living. It is clear that brain tumor survivors experience more long-term health issues than survivors of other pediatric malignancies.[7]

Educating the survivor should include a discussion of all treatments the individual received and the relative risk for potential late effects. This includes evaluation for secondary malignancies or relapse of disease, monitoring for late effects and education on healthy lifestyle.[5] Regardless of the survivor's age, the survivor should be included in the discussion of diagnosis, treatment received and general health. As the survivor matures the focus of the education should deal with developmentally appropriate concerns. Counseling a teenager on the effects of chemotherapy or radiation on sexual development should also include a discussion on sexually transmitted diseases and pregnancy prevention. Counseling for adults should be appropriate to the functional level and include issues pertaining to vocational and family needs.

Research done by Kadan-Lottick et al. found that, when compared to survivors of other pediatric malignancies, CNS tumor survivors are less likely to know their diagnosis.[8] Health care providers are often unaware of the late consequences of chemotherapy, radiation and surgery. Childhood cancer survivors are often faced with the challenge of educating adult health care providers about the unique health care needs of survivors. One-third of adult survivors participating in the Childhood Cancer Survivors' Study report they were not confident in their primary care physician's ability to manage a late effect.[9] To properly advocate for appropriate follow-up and surveillance the survivor and/or family must first be aware of the importance of regular medical follow-up and then be prepared to advocate for health care. The complexity of the health care needs of brain tumor survivors may be staggering. Brain tumor survivors face a multitude of potential late effects, including endocrine, cardiac, musculoskeletal, reproductive and cognitive. Coordinating care between subspecialties is often overwhelming and confusing for the brain tumor survivor, as they may experience cognitive difficulties that make organizing care challenging. Often, family members are needed to assist the survivor to manage a complex health care system.

Psychological consequences from diagnosis of a CNS tumor may result in social and academic difficulties. Depression, post-traumatic stress disorder, anxiety and risk taking behaviors are seen in childhood cancer survivors. Females are more likely than males to report post-traumatic stress related to their cancer experience.[10] Research has shown that the survivor's belief about the experience is more predictive of post-traumatic stress than the diagnosis or treatment received.[11]

Unfortunately, these issues also affect career and personal relationships into adulthood. Finding and maintaining meaningful employment may be challenging due to issues such as cognitive delays, fatigue and social difficulties. Coordination of services between the school system, medical team and social services agencies is often needed to maximize the survivor's potential for success in adulthood. Ideally, these issues are faced when the survivor is young so that inventions to improve school and job performance may be implemented early.

School Age Children

Coordinating services between the school system, the survivor and the health care team is vital to academic success. Brain tumor survivors may face a myriad of physical and cognitive challenges in the school system. Most require either a 504 plan, which provides individuals with a medical diagnosis, or disability classroom accommodations. The purpose of the accommodations is to allow successful functioning at school. Students needing special education services usually require an Individual Education Plan.[12] The full scope and range of educational services available are beyond the scope of this chapter, but detailed information can be found in Chapter 24. It is important to point out in this chapter that the late effects team expertise may be needed to assist the family and school system in providing appropriate education services.

Additionally, neurocognitive testing is an integral part of the academic evaluation process. The goal of neurocognitive testing is to identify the survivor's strengths and weaknesses to maximize academic performance. The Children's Oncology Group's Late Effects Screening Guidelines recommends that neurocognitive testing be performed when the patient is more likely to experience academic difficulties or school transition periods, for example elementary school to middle school. Further testing is recommended any time the patient is experiencing any new academic difficulties.[13,14] Neurocognitive testing may be performed by the school district or a pediatric psychologist, preferably affiliated with the late effects clinic. Students' education rights are protected through the Americans with Disabilities Act, the Rehabilitation Act of 1973 – Section 504 or the Individuals with Disabilities Education Act. Those individuals requiring special education services are eligible for services from three to 21 years of age. Families should be informed of their child's educational rights at each late effects visit.[13] Please refer to Chapter 24 for more details about these and other laws important to brain tumor survivors.

Adult Survivors

Vocational counseling through the school system, state government agency or a rehabilitation facility may benefit the survivor. The goal of vocational counseling is to provide the survivor with the tools and knowledge to find appropriate and meaningful employment.[12] Ideally, these services begin in high school and continue through adulthood. Any survivor with a cognitive or physical impairment should contact their state's Department of Rehabilitation or Department of Vocational Services to see what assistance can be provided to the survivor. Job training, coaching and internships can be provided to qualified survivors. Additionally, the vocational counselor will be able to provide information regarding workplace rights and responsibilities of both the employer and employee.

Obtaining insurance coverage may be difficult for the survivor, especially as an adult. Insurance is often tied to employment status and employment may be limited as a result of physical or cognitive challenges in the survivor. Issues surrounding fatigue, motor deficits or cognitive limitations may limit the survivor's employment options. Each survivor should receive counseling regarding what and when health information should be disclosed to any employer. This is another area where we believe that a multidisciplinary team approach, as found in a late effects clinic that includes social workers and vocation counselors, will benefit the survivor.

Benefits of a Dedicated Late Effects Clinic

Late effects clinics provide the survivor and family with a perspective that is different than the treating oncology team or neurosurgery team. The focus of a late effects clinic visit is health promotion rather than monitoring for disease reoccurrence. Health care providers who are primarily responsible for on-therapy treatment may find this change in philosophy difficult. Additionally, on-therapy patients' needs are more acute in nature than the survivors', resulting in a prioritizing of patients that may deem survivors' issues as less important.[6]

Transitioning to a prevention model of care may also be difficult for families. Clinic visits in the acute care setting focus on scan and laboratory results and it may be challenging for families to shift to a prevention mode. Concerns about tumor reoccurrence are always paramount in patients' and families' minds. Discussion regarding prevention of osteoporosis, cataracts or other health issues that affect the general population may appear to be less important to brain tumor survivors and their families. The challenge of the late effects clinic visit is to identify the risk factors unique to each patient based upon treatment, lifestyle choices, and family history, and translate that into pertinent patient education.

Guidelines from the National Cancer Institute and the Children's Oncology Group state that all member institutions of the Children's Oncology Group must have follow-up clinics.[13,15] This guideline is open to interpretation and not all member institutions have programs which encompass the vast and unique needs of the survivor population. Four integral pieces of care have been identified by the National Cancer Institute. These include: (1) psychological services to families; (2) academic support throughout the educational process; (3) resources to counsel families regarding insurance and workplace issues, and (4) integration of the pediatric cancer survivor into the adult health care system.[15]

The Clinic Visit

The late effects team should provide the survivor with the most current information available, assist with identifying community resources and coordinate care between subspecialties. The complexity of potential medical issues for the brain tumor patient requires a significant amount of preparation time and clinic time on the part of the health care providers. The Children's Oncology Group recommends that each visit include a summary that will provide the survivor with diagnosis, date of diagnosis, treatment received, including start and end dates and date(s) of relapse. Results of pertinent laboratory and radiograph studies and information on all known late effects should also be included in the summary (see Fig. 7.1).[13]

Each patient visit to the long-term clinic should be crafted for individual, risk-based follow-up and education. Needed laboratory and radiological evaluation should be determined according to the treatment the patient received. COG has developed screening and follow-up guidelines for management of survivors of pediatric malignancies. The guidelines are not disease-based, but rather exposure-based. The rationale for this method also takes into consideration that the patient's age at the time of treatment, standards of treatment at the time and long-term sequelae from treatment impact the overall health of the survivor.[13] The goal of the COG guidelines are "to increase quality of life and decrease complication-related healthcare costs of pediatric cancer survivors by providing standardized and enhanced follow-up care throughout the lifespan that (a) promotes healthy lifestyles, (b) provides for ongoing monitoring of health status, (c) facilitates early identification of late effects, and (d) provides timely intervention for late effects."[13]

Personnel requirements for a brain tumor late effects clinic will vary according to clinic location, population served and institution resources. At a minimum, there

Survivor's Taking Action & Responsibility
Children's Memorial Hospital Pediatric "STAR" Program
Division of Hematology/Oncology
2300 Children's Plaza, Box#30
Chicago, IL 60614
Coordinator/Appointments:
Nurse Practitioner:
Stem Cell Transplant Advanced Practice Nurse:
Director,
Visit Date:

Children's
Memorial Hospital
Where kids come first.™

Name: MR#:   DOB:
Sex: Race:
Diagnosis:
Date of Diagnosis: Date of Last Visit:
Presenting Symptoms & Findings:

PMH:

FH:

Prognostic Factors: **Leukemia**   **Solid Tumors**
                             Age: Stage:
                             WBC: Primary Site:
                             CNS Status: Metastatic Site:
                             Lineage: Other:
                             Cytogen/Other:
                             Risk Group:

PRIMARY THERAPY
Treatment Protocol: Date Initiated:
Chemotherapy: Cumulative Drug Dosage

Radiation Therapy?   Date Off Therapy:
RELAPSED THERAPY (If applicable)
Treatment Protocol: Date Initiated:
Chemotherapy: Cumulative Drug Dosage

Radiation Therapy?   Date Off Therapy:
BONE MARROW TRANSPLANT (If applicable)
Treatment Protocol: Date Initiated:
Chemotherapy: Cumulative Drug Dosage

Transplant Immune Suppression: Start: Stop:

Radiation Therapy?   Date Off Therapy:
Total Anthracycline Dose: mg/m²

Radiation

Date (From –To)	Site	Dose

Procedures/Surgeries:
Acute Complications:

Fig. 7.1 Survivors' Summary Sheet used at Children's Memorial Hospital, Chicago, IL

Name: **MR#:**   **DOB:**

PSYCHOSOCIAL/NEUROCOGNITIVE:

Martial Status	Pregnancies:
Employed?	Viable Offspring:
Occupation:	Education-Highest Level:
Insurance?	Special Education:

KNOWN LATE EFFECTS:

□ Growth	□ Hepatic	□ Ortho	□ Pulmonary
□ Renal	□ Muscular	□ Obesity/FTT	□ 2nd Malignancy
□ Neurological	□ Dermatological	□ Immunologic	□ Malig-1st Rel
□ Cognitive	□ Endocrine	□ a/c GVHD	□ Malig-2nd Rel
□ Psychological	□ GI	□ Dental	□ Neurology
□ Ophthal	□ Cardio-vasc	□ ENT	□

REVIEW OF SURVEILLANCE TESTING:

CARDIAC	DATE	RESULTS
Echocardiogram		
Echocardiogram		
EKG		

PULMONARY	DATE	RESULTS
PFT's		
Chest X-Ray		

ENDOCRINE	DATE	RESULTS
LH		
FSH		
IGF-1		
IGF-BP3		
Estradiol		
Testosterone		
T^4		
TSH		

RENAL	DATE	RESULTS
Chemistry Panel/Chem 14		
U/A		
BUN		
Creatinine		

HEMATOLOGY	DATE	RESULTS
CBC w/ Diff		
ESR		

OTHER	DATE	RESULTS
Hep-C		
Hep-C AB-Elisa		
Hep-C PCR Quantative		
LFT's/GGT		
PT/PTT		
Ultrasound		
MRI		
CT		

TESTING	DATE	RESULTS
Audiogram		
Neuropsych Evaluation		

Fig. 7.1 (continued)

SPECIALTY	SPECIALIST NAME	DATE LAST SEEN	FINDINGS
PCP			
Cardiology			
Dentistry			
Endocrinology			
Ophthalmology			
Otolaryngology			
Psychiatry			
PT/OT			
Dermatology			

_____
_____
_____
_____
_____
_____
_____
_____
_____
_____
_____
_____
_____
_____

Reviewed by:
Date:
Updated:

Fig. 7.1 (continued)

must be a medical director responsible for the care provided in the clinic. Direct patient care may be provided by a physician, nurse practitioner or physician assistant.[12] Additionally, there is a great deal of patient care coordination required for a successful late effects clinic. A nurse is needed to coordinate visits, manage referral to subspecialties and communicate with the patient, health care providers, schools, etc. Social work is a vital component to the success of a late effects clinic.[15] The skills and knowledge of social work are needed to assist families with school, employment, financial and insurance concerns. There is often an overlap of care and expertise among the health care team members. For instance, all providers seeing a school-aged patient should be asking questions regarding school performance. The clinician may make the referral to the neuropsychologist for cognitive testing and the social worker can assist the family and school to develop an IEP.

Assistance with daily operational needs such as correspondence, medical record management, billing issues and patient follow-up is needed. Each institution will need to determine where these services should be located, i.e., oncology, neuro-oncology, brain tumor clinic, etc.[12] Access to additional personnel and resources must also be considered. For instance, many brain tumor survivors have endocrine issues requiring ongoing follow-up. Is it feasible to coordinate clinic visits or to have an endocrinologist at a late effects clinic to facilitate patient care? Are there health care providers in the community with an interest in caring for this unique population who can facilitate or expedite care from a referring institution? For example, an adult reproductive gynecologist may not be on staff at a pediatric hospital, but is willing to accept referrals from a pediatric late effects clinic.

Patient education is a large part of the clinic visit and is often the lengthiest period of the visit. This integral part of the visit should be undertaken by all members of the late effects clinic team and should encompass physical, emotional and psychosocial aspects of the patient's and family's well-being. Successful patient education includes not just the survivor, but also family members, school or job, other health care providers and, sometimes, even the patient's social networks.[12]

Coordination of Care Within the Health Care Community

Brain tumor survivors often face myriad health care issues that require coordination of services between specialties. The burden of the coordination often falls upon the late effects team. As the conductor of the orchestra, it is often the late effects team who is called upon to manage and coordinate care, educational and psychosocial issues. Primary care providers in pediatrics, family practice or internal medicine may not be comfortable acting as overseer of a brain tumor survivor's health care needs, but may be better suited to provide routine physicals, immunizations and manage common illnesses. To successfully meet the health care needs of the survivor two-way communication must exist between the late effects team and all other health care providers.[5,12]

It may be the patient's or family's preference to have the late effects team act as the primary care provider for the survivor. Each late effects clinic must decide how issues regarding physicals, immunizations, and other primary care issues should be dealt with and where optimal care for such services should be obtained. Does the late effects clinic maintain adequate immunization records for patients? Management of routine illnesses is usually best handled by the primary care provider. Survivors may not understand the importance of maintaining a relationship with a provider in their community and may need to be educated about the role and responsibility of the late effects team.

Given the complexity of health care needs for brain tumor survivors and their long-standing relationships with the neuro-oncologist, neurosurgeon and other treating team members, some families find transitioning to a late effects clinic difficult. To ease the transition, some clinics choose to integrate the late effects clinic into the brain tumor clinic.[12] The benefit to this is that families continue to see their treatment team in addition to the late effects team. Unfortunately, this model inhibits some survivors and families from "graduating" mentally to survivor status. Families may also find sharing clinic space with patients on treatment emotionally difficult and continued visits with the treatment team may be traumatizing. Some centers with large brain tumor populations have developed specific neuro-oncology late effects clinics.

Some brain tumor survivors choose to sever ties with the treatment team and obtain health care in the community. The decision to seek care in the community may be due to insurance issues, relocation of the survivor, post-traumatic stress disorder or other factors. Unfortunately, many health care providers have not been educated in the numerous health issues facing brain tumor survivors.[5,12] This lack of knowledge often translates into less than adequate care for the survivor. A primary care provider may only have five to seven cancer survivors in a practice.[9] Additionally, health care for brain tumor survivors is unique based upon treatment received, and guidelines for care are updated frequently. Knowledge of treatment-specific sequelae, in addition to lack of easy access to diagnostic resources and research, places an extra burden on the community health care provider. Managing the health of a brain tumor survivor may prove to be too taxing on a primary care provider.[6]

Another model of care for survivors is the cancer center and community health care providers working together to maintain the health of the survivor. This model of care requires more coordination of services between the health care teams and the survivor, and places a greater responsibility on the survivor to coordinate services and advocacy.[12] Determining which health care provider is responsible for providing what aspect of care may not be clear-cut in all cases. For those survivors with complex medical needs or cognitive delays this model may not provide optimal care.[6]

Research

Research has played a vital role in improving childhood cancer survivor rates. Approximately 50% to 60% of patients diagnosed with a pediatric malignancy will be enrolled in a clinical trial. This has helped to establish standards of care for all aspects of diagnosis and treatment.[15] In addition, treatment plan's focus for some childhood cancers has shifted to look at ways to maximize cure rates while minimizing long-term effects of treatment. For instance, clinical trials studied lowering cranial radiation doses to prevent or reduce long-term endocrine dysfunction in brain tumor patients with the goal of maintaining or improving survival rates.

Because some effects of treatment are not evident until 15 to 20 years after completion of therapy, longitudinal study of patients is necessary. This is difficult to accomplish due to a highly mobile society, the cost of studies, allocation of resources, and survivor interest in participating in studies.[16,17] Brain tumor survivors' participation in research studies evaluating physiological, psychological, social and academic functioning are vital to continuing with the goal of improving outcomes. Often, cooperative group studies are necessary to obtain significant numbers for evaluation of late effects.[17] The Childhood Cancer Survivor Study is looking at large groups of patients and their siblings to study treatment-related effects. The Children's Oncology Group has a Late Effects Committee responsible for establishing follow-up recommendations and conducting research on childhood cancer survivors. Follow-up in a late effects clinic promotes capturing patients to participate in studies and should be a focus of the late effects team.[12]

Transitioning Pediatric Survivors to Adult Health Care

Research shows that the longer a survivor is from diagnosis the less likely he or she is to have been seen by a health care provider.[7] In a study of adult childhood cancer survivors, participants stated they did not have information regarding diagnosis and treatment received. Several barriers to optimal health care were identified, including primary care provider's lack of knowledge regarding the unique health care needs of survivors and less than adequate communication between the treating team and the primary care team.[18] Other barriers to obtaining health care in the adult arena may include lack of insurance, lack of knowledge as to where to obtain health care, lack of resources, perceived time constraints and neurocognitive issues. Inadequacy or absence of insurance coverage is an important barrier to receiving health care, especially as an adult. Research from the Childhood Cancer Survivor Study demonstrated that significant discrepancy in insurance coverage between a survivor and their siblings exists. Childhood cancer survivors are more likely than their siblings to remain on their parents' health care policy or to be covered by Medicaid.[14] For those who have their own health care insurance coverage, the policies written for them are more likely to include exclusions to coverage based upon preexisting conditions when compared to their siblings.

Childhood cancer survivors desire information regarding their overall health and health maintenance, which takes into consideration their medical history and the resources available to them.[18] Part of the challenge to delivering care is that adult primary care providers and subspecialty providers must be educated about the health care needs of brain tumor survivors.[5] Patients and their families must be prepared to advocate for medical, vocational and social needs. "Pediatric cancer survivors must have knowledge of their disease and the treatment they received; they must be able to advocate for themselves in medical situations. Pediatric centers must carefully prepare young adults for this transition by allowing adequate time for this process to occur relatively seamlessly".[19]

Transitioning patients and their families to adult health care may be challenging. Therefore, the transition process should start years before the patient is transitioned to an adult health care setting. The patient, family and health care providers should all be working together to make this a smooth process. Communication and coordination of health care between several medical subspecialties may complicate the issue of transitioning the young adult to appropriate health care providers. A written health care summary is necessary to facilitate the transition process and make it as seamless as possible. This will provide the medical team and the survivor with pertinent information for health risks and screening.[12,15]

A limited number of centers offer a transition program for adult survivors of pediatric cancers. This type of program may employ a primary care provider as well as a provider with expertise in childhood malignancies. The benefit to this type of care is the patient's ability to access experts in both primary and oncology care at one visit.[20] Unfortunately, this model of care may be limited to large, urban academic centers due to resource allocation.[12,20]

Summary

Survivorship is a unique phase of health care for all cancer patients. While survivors of all types of cancer face myriad late effects, the survivorship issues faced by brain tumor survivors are often some of the most complex and long lasting of any of other type of cancer. Brain tumor survivors are often faced with ongoing health, psychological and social challenges throughout the lifespan. Meeting the ongoing needs of the survivor, as well as family, requires evaluation of medical and psychosocial needs. The expertise and resources of an experienced late effects clinic cannot only assist the patient and family with maintaining health, but also provide the patient and family with needed tools and resources to reach the patient's full potential.

References

1. SEER Pediatric Monograph, pp 57, www.seer.cancer.gov/publications/childhood/cnspdf
2. www.canceradvocacy.org/about/org
3. Oeffinger K, Robison L. Childhood Cancer Survivors. Late effects and a new model for understanding survivorship. *JAMA*. 2007; 297(24):2762–2764
4. Geenan M, Cardous-Ubbink M, Kremer L, et al. Medical assessment of adverse health outcomes in long-term survivors of childhood cancer. *JAMA*. 2007;297(24):2705–2715.
5. Landier W, Wallace H, Hudson M. Long-term follow-up of pediatric cancer survivors: education, surveillance, and screening. *Pediatr Blood Cancer*. 2006;46:149–158.
6. Friedman D., Freyer D, Levitt G. Models of Care for Survivors of Childhood Cancer. *Pediatr Blood Cancer*. 2006;46:159–168.
7. Oeffinger K, Mertens A, Sklar C, et al. Chronic Health Conditions in Adult Survivors of Childhood Cancer. *N Engl J Med*. 2006;355:1572–1582.
8. Kadan-Lottick N, Robison L, Gurney J, et al. Childhood Cancer Survivors' Knowledge About Their Past Diagnosis and Treatment. Childhood Cancer Survivor Study. *JAMA*. 2002;287 (14):1832–1839.
9. Oeffinger K, Wallace H. Barriers to Follow-up Care of Survivors in the United States and the United Kingdom. *Pediatric Blood Cancer*. 2006;46:135–142.
10. Langeveld N, Grootenhuis M, Voute P, de Haan. Posttraumatic Stress Symptoms in Adult Survivors of Childhood Cancer. *Pediatr Blood Cancer*. 2004;42 (7):604–610
11. Rourke M, HObbie W, Schwartz L, Kazak A, Posttraumatic Stress Disorder (PTSD) in Young Adult Survivors of Childhood Cancer. *Pediatr Blood Cancer*. 2007;49:177–182
12. Curesearch, Children's Oncology Group. Establishing and Enhancing Services for Childhood Cancer Survivors, Long-Term Follow-up Program Resource Guide. Children's Oncology Group; 2007.

13. Children's Oncology Group, Long-Term Follow-Up Guidelines for Survivors of Child-hood, Adolescent and Young Adult Cancers. Version 2.0. CureSearch Children's Oncol-ogy Group; 2006.
14. Mitby P, Robison L, Whitton J, et al. Utilization of Special Education Services and Educational Attainment among Long-Term Survivors of Childhood Cancer. *Cancer.* 2003;97:1115–1125
15. Weiner S, Simone J, Hewitt, M. *Childhood Cancer Survivorship: Improving Care and Quality of Life, Institute of Medicine, National Research Council of the National Acade-mies.* Washington D.C.: The National Academies Press; 2003:4, 102
16. Park E, Li F, Liu Y, et al. Health Insurance Coverage in Survivors of Childhood Cancer: The Childhood Cancer Survivor Study. *J Clin Oncol.* 2005;23:9187–9197
17. Hawkins M, Robison L. Importance of clinical and Epidemiological Research in Defin-ing the Long-Term Clinical Care of Pediatric Cancer Survivors. *Pediatr Blood Cancer.* 2006;46:174–178
18. Zebreck B, Eshelman D, Hudson M, et al. Health Care for Childhood Cancer Survivors. Insights and Perspectives from a Delphi Panel of Young Adult Survivors of Childhood Cancer. *Cancer.* 2004;100:843–850.
19. Ginsberg J, Hobbie W, Carlson C, Meadows A. Delivering Long-Term Follow-up care to Pediatric Cancer Survivors: Transitional Care Issues. *Pediatr Blood Cancer.* 2006;46:169–173
20. Bhatia S, Meadows A. Long-term Follow-Up of Childhood Cancer Survivors: Future Directions for Clinical Care and Research. *Pediatr Blood Cancer.* 2006;46143–46148.

Part II
Medical Late Effects of Brain Tumor Treatment

Chapter 8
Neurological Complications in Adults

Michelle Monje and Patrick Y. Wen

Introduction

Structure and function are intimately linked in the nervous system. However, normal functioning of the nervous system depends not only on the structural integrity of the brain, spinal cord and peripheral nerves, but also on several dynamic physiological processes. While the majority of the nervous system is formed during development, many cell types continue to divide and regenerate throughout life. Astrocytic and oligodendroglial populations replenish themselves continually, as do the endothelial cells that comprise the neurovasculature. These support cells are necessary for normal neuronal physiology and normal function of the peripheral nerves. Newborn neurons, particularly the dentate granule cell neurons of the hippocampus, are constantly generated throughout life. This process of adult hippocampal neurogenesis is thought to be crucial to proper memory function. These dynamic cell populations are vulnerable to the cytostatic and mutagenic actions of cancer therapies. Mindfulness of these physiological processes may elucidate many incompletely understood mechanisms of neurotoxicity from cancer therapies. In the following chapter, the neurological complications of oncologic therapies in adults will be reviewed, with a focus on radiotherapy and chemotherapy.

Complications of Radiotherapy

Radiation therapy is one of the most important causes of neurotoxicity in patients with cancer. It may affect the nervous system by: (1) direct injury to neural structures included in the radiation portal or (2) indirectly by damaging blood

P.Y. Wen (✉)
Director, Division of Neuro-Oncology, Center for Neuro-Oncology, Dana-Farber/
Brigham and Women's Cancer Center, SW430, 44 Binney St, Boston, MA 02115, USA
e-mail: pwen@partners.org

S. Goldman, C.D. Turner (eds.), *Late Effects of Treatment for Brain Tumors*,
Cancer Treatment and Research 150, DOI 10.1007/b109924_8,
© Springer Science+Business Media, LLC 2009

vessels or endocrine organs necessary for functioning of the nervous system or by producing tumors. Radiation injury may occur acutely, but more commonly occurs after a delay of months or years. Many factors determine whether radiation injury will occur. These include the radiation dose, fraction size, duration of treatment, the volume treated, the length of survival following radiation therapy and the presence of other therapies and systemic diseases.

The complications of radiotherapy are classically categorized in terms of acute, early-delayed and late-delayed form[1] (see Table 8.1). Radiation toxicity occurs in all parts of the nervous system: brain, spinal cord and peripheral nerve.

Table 8.1 Summary of neurologic complications in nervous system

Neurologic complications of radiation therapy to the brain

Direct effects of radiation therapy

Acute reactions (hours or days)
– Cerebral edema: headaches, nausea, vomiting, lethargy
  Early delayed reactions (2 weeks to 4 months)
    – Drowsiness, increased cognitive dysfunction, exacerbation of neurologic deficits
  Late delayed reactions (4 months to several years)
    – Mild to moderate cognitive decline
    – Dementia
    – Cerebral necrosis
    – Leukoencephalopathy
  Normal pressure hydrocephalus

Indirect effects of radiation therapy

Cerebrovascular disorders
    – Large and small vessel disease, Moyamoya, telangiectasias, cavernomas, angiomatous malformations, aneurysms
Radiation-induced neoplasms
    – Meningiomas, sarcomas, gliomas, schwannomas
Endocrine dysfunction
    – Hypothyroidism, hypogonadism, growth hormone deficiency, hypoadrenalism

Neurologic complications of radiation therapy to the spinal cord

Early-delayed radiation myelopathy
Late-delayed radiation myelopathy
    – Delayed radiation myelopathy (DRM)
    – Radiogenic lower motor neuron disease
    – Spinal vasculopathy and hemorrhage

Neurologic complications of radiation therapy to the brachial plexus

Early-delayed brachial plexopathy
Late-delayed brachial plexopathy

Neurologic complications of radiation therapy to peripheral nerves

Cranial Neuropathies
Peripheral Neuropathy
Nerve Sheath tumor

Late-Delayed Effects of Radiotherapy on the Brain

Radionecrosis

Radiation necrosis has been reported in the treatment of both intracranial and extracranial tumors, such as nasopharyngeal carcinoma (see Fig. 8.1). Radiation necrosis typically occurs 1–2 years after radiation, but latency as short as three months and as long as 30 years have been reported.[2,3] Radiographically, it can be difficult to distinguish from a recurrent tumor. Recognition of the risk factors for radiation necrosis has resulted in a decrease in incidence. *Radiation total dose and fraction size are important risk factors*, and a total external beam dose of 55–60 Gy delivered in 1.8–2.0 Gy fraction constitute the upper limits of "safe" dose. Other risk factors include lesion volume and location, old age, associated chemotherapy and vascular risk factors such as diabetes. Therapies that attempt to increase the dose of radiation delivered to the tumor volume, such as interstitial brachytherapy and stereotactic radiosurgery, also result in an increased incidence of radiation necrosis.[4] Radiation necrosis can result in devastating clinical consequences. Patients present with focal neurological symptoms, often recapitulating the presenting symptoms of the patient's initial disease in the case of primary brain tumors, severe cognitive deficits, signs and symptoms of increased intracranial pressure and/or seizures. About one-half of patients present with seizure as the first sign. Imaging characteristics of radiation necrosis are very similar to recurrent tumor. CT reveals hypodensity and variable contrast enhancement. MRI shows T1 hypointensity and T2

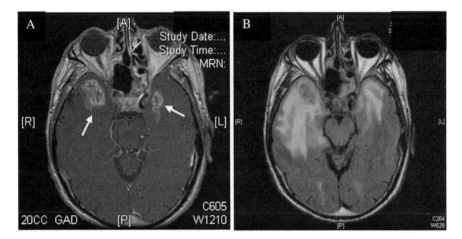

Fig. 8.1 Forty-nine-year-old man with T4 squamous cell carcinoma of the paranasal sinuses treated with radiotherapy six years previously presenting with confusion and memory loss. (**A**) T1-weighted axial MRI with gadolinium showing enhancing necrotic areas in both temporal lobes (*white arrows*); (**B**) Axial FLAIR MRI showing edema around necrotic areas. FDGPET scan showed no uptake, suggesting that the areas of enhancement were necrosis

hyperintensity predominantly involving white matter. Lesions frequently enhance with gadolinium.[5] Mass effect may be present. PET or SPECT imaging and MR spectroscopy may be employed to differentiate radiation necrosis from malignancy.[6] In one series, a (201)T1-SPECT technique yielded diagnostic sensitivity of 0.88 and a specificity of 0.83, compared to routine neuroanato-mincal imaging (CT and MRI), which was found to have a sensitivity of 0.63 and a specificity of 0.59.[6] However, biopsy remains the only definitive means of diagnosis. Histopathologically, the lesions of radiation necrosis predominantly affect white matter. Vascular changes include vessel wall hyalinization, thickening and fibrinoid necrosis, fibrinous exudates, vascular hemorrhage and thrombosis. These changes affect the small arteries and arterioles. Demyelination is also evident.

The etiology of radiation necrosis is not yet clear. Histopathology reveals vascular damage and demyelination, implicating the vascular cells and/or oligodendrocytes as the targets of radiation injury. Classically, radiation injury has been attributed to either the vascular hypothesis or the glial hypothesis. The *vascular hypothesis* states that radiation-induced vasculopathy and the resultant ischemic necrosis account for radiation injury. The *glial hypothesis* proposes that radiation-induced damage to oligodendrocytes and their precursors is the underlying cause of radiation injury. However, the lesions of radiation necrosis are not typical of either pure vascular or demyelinating disease, and neither hypothesis seems sufficient alone to account for radiation necrosis.[7]

Treatment of radiation necrosis involves surgical excision and steroid therapy. Additional therapies have been proposed, including anticoagulants,[8] hyperbaric oxygen[9] and alpha-tocopherol[10] but their clinical utility has yet to be proven.

Leukoencephalopathy

Diffuse white matter changes may occur as a late-delayed effect of radiation alone, a combination of radiotherapy and chemotherapy or, more rarely, after chemotherapy alone. Clearly, radiation and chemotherapy have a synergistic effect. In addition to concomitant chemotherapy such as methotrexate, risk factors for radiation-induced leukoencephalopathy include higher radiation dose[11] and age greater than 60 years.[12] This diffuse white matter injury is an entity distinct from radiation necrosis. As patients are surviving longer after cancer therapies, radiation-induced leukoencephalopathy is an increasingly important complication of treatment. Histopathology reveals rarefication of white matter, reactive astrogliosis and foci of necrosis.[13,14] In the most severe form, disseminated necrotizing leukoencephalopathy, necrotic foci become confluent and a prominent axonopathy is noted ultrastructurally.[15] Neuroimaging reveals hypodensity on CT scans and increased T2/FLAIR signal in the white matter. Diffuse atrophy is often seen. MR spectroscopy reveals loss of NAA, choline and creatine, implying axonal and membrane damage in the abnormal-appearing white matter.[16]

Dementia

Associated with diffuse leukencephalopathy, with or without radionecrosis, is a devastating dementia syndrom.[17] (see Fig. 8.2). The dementia is typically a subcortical dementia characterized by deficits in memory, attention and intellectual function. Gait disturbance, urinary incontinence and personality changes may occur. Cortical functions such as apraxis and language are relatively spared. Typical onset is within two years of radiation exposure, and the course is usually progressive. A large meta-analysis of the literature found an incidence of post-radiation dementia to be 12%.[18] Risk factors are the same as for leukencephalopathy, including radiation dose, fractions size, volume of brain irradiated, older age and concomitant chemotherapy. Methylphenidate.[19] and anticholinesterases such as donepezil[20] are sometimes used for symptomatic relief. As the survival of brain tumor patients improves, an increasing number develop impairment of normal cerebrospinal fluid reabsorption through the arachnoid granulations. This leads to a communicating hydrocephalus with cognitive impairment, gait unsteadiness and urinary symptoms. Some of these patients may benefit from placement of a ventriculoperitoneal shunt.[21]

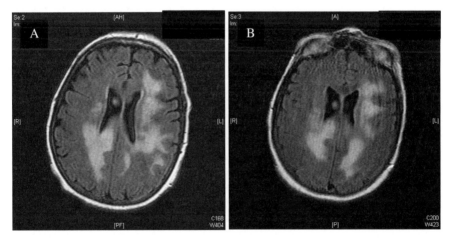

Fig. 8.2 Seventy-year-old woman with CNS lymphoma treated with methotrexate and radiation therapy. Axial FLAIR MRI of the brain showing increased periventricular leucoencephalopathy

Mild to Moderate Cognitive Impairment

Cognitive dysfunction, characterized by prominent dysfunction of short-term memory, is perhaps the most common sequelae of radiotherapy. Cranial radiotherapy causes a debilitating cognitive decline in both children[22–24] and adults.[18,25–28] Months to years after cranial radiation exposure, patients exhibit progressive deficits in short-term memory, spatial relations, visual motor processing, quantitative skills and attention.[29] Hippocampal dysfunction is a prominent feature of these neuropsychological sequelae. In fact, the severity of the cognitive deterioration appears to depend upon the radiation dosage delivered to the medial temporal lobes.[30]

The incidence of treatment–induced impairment in cognition has been very well described in children. It is estimated that, when the whole brain is irradiated at less than seven years of age, nearly 100% of children require special education; after age seven approximately 50% of children require special education. Some degree of memory dysfunction is thought to occur in the majority of children. The incidence of memory dysfunction in adult patients has been difficult to quantify, largely due to a lack of uniformity in neuropsychometic testing in the literature. However, as adults are surviving longer after treatment and the long-term consequences of radiation are becoming more important for this population, an extremely high rate of cognitive dysfunction of varying degrees has been recognized.

Mild to moderate cognitive dysfunction is inconsistently associated with radiological findings, and frequently occurs in patients with normal-appearing neuroimaging.[31] Clinically significant memory deficit in the absence of radiological findings implicates damage to a subtle process with robust physiological consequences.

One such process is hippocampal neurogenesis. Studies in animal models have demonstrated that therapeutic doses of cranial irradiation virtually ablates neurogenesis[7,32–34] and that this inhibition of neurogenesis correlates with impaired performance on hippocampal-dependent memory tests.[35] Surprisingly, irradiation does not simply deplete the stem cell population, but rather disrupts the microenvironment that normally supports hippocampal neurogenesis.[33] This microenvironmental perturbation is largely due to irradiation-induced microglial inflammation, and anti-inflammatory therapy with the nonsteroidal anti-inflammatory agent indomethacin partially restores hippocampal neurogenesis and function.[34] Human trials are currently underway to evaluate the clinical utility of anti-inflammatory therapy during cranial radiotherapy.

Additional possible mechanisms underlying mild to moderate cognitive dysfunction include subtle white matter dysfunction and altered regional blood flow due to microvascular disease.

Radiotherapy-Induced Tumors

Criteria for defining a radiation-induced tumor include a long latency (years to decades) to occurrence of the second tumor, and the location of the tumor within the radiation portal. Although uncommon, secondary tumors do occur following cranial irradiation, particularly meningiomas, gliomas (see Fig. 8.3), and sarcomas. The relative proportion of secondary cranial tumors is roughly 70%, 20% and 10%, respectively. In an Israeli study of 10,834 patients exposed in childhood to an average dose of only 1.5 Gy for tinea capitis, the relative risk of developing a neural tumor was found to be 6.9. In patients receiving 2.5 Gy,

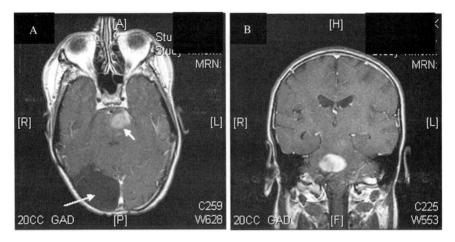

Fig. 8.3 Twenty-five-year-old with a history of right parietal cerebral neuroblastoma at age three treated with surgical resection and radiotherapy who presented with a two month history of ataxia, headaches and drowsiness. (**A**) Axial and (**B**) coronal T1-weighted MRI with gadolinium shows enhancing brain stem lesion. The right parietal surgical cavity from his prior surgery for neuroblastoma is visible (*longer arrow*). Biopsy showed anaplastic astrocytoma, presumably induced by prior radiotherapy

the relative risk was 20.[36] After cranial irradiation for childhood leukemia, one series found a relative risk for secondary tumor of 22.[37]

More than 300 cases of radiation-induced meningiomas have been reported.[38] Authors frequently differentiate between low-dose (< 10 Gy) irradiation and high-dose (> 20 Gy) irradiation-induced meningiomas. The latency from time of treatment to meningioma development ranges from one to three decades.[39,40] There is an increased incidence of cellular atypia and aggressive subtypes following irradiation.[40,41] A cytogenetic study of radiation-induced meningiomas revealed consistent abnormalities involving chromosome 1p.[42]

More than 100 case of secondary gliomas have been reported (see Fig. 8.3); of these, approximately 40% are glioblastomas.[11] Gliomas arise after a mean latency of 9.6 years.[43] To date, four cases of gliomas at sites of previous radiosurgery have also been reported.[43,44] Prognosis is often poor in secondary gliomas relative to spontaneous forms, due either to a more aggressive behavior or because treatment options are limited by previous exposures.

Rarely, sarcomas involving the skull base, calvaria or dura may occur. Osteosarcoma, fibrosarcoma and chondrosarcoma have been reported. Extensive discussion on secondary malignancies can also be found in Chapter 14.

Vasculopathy

Large Vessel Atherosclerosis

Radiation of head and neck cancers or lymphoma can cause accelerated atherosclerosis of the carotid arteries.[45] Intracranial accelerated atherosclerosis also occurs.[46] Treatment involves aggressive control of vascular risk factors, such as hyperlipidemia and hypertension. Carotid endarterectomy may be pursued when indicated, but may be more complicated due to vascular fibrosis and post-radiation skin changes that may impair healing and increase risk of infection.

Moyamoya Pattern

Progressive cerebral arterial occlusive disease, also known as moyamoya disease, is a stenosis or occlusion of large and intermediate cerebral arteries, abnormal netlike vessels and transdural anastomoses. Consequences include TIA, stroke and seizure. Cranial irradiation is a rare cause of secondary moyamoya disease, particularly radiation for tumors of the optic chiasm, suprasellar region and brain stem during childhood and in patients with neurofibromatosis.[47,48]

Vascular Malformations

Radiation-induced vascular malformations occur more frequently in children than in adults, and carry a significant risk of hemorrhage. In one series, 20% of children who had undergone cranial irradiation exhibited radiological evidence of at least one new telangiectasia, defined as small low-signal intensity foci on T2 MR images.[49] In another series, five out of 20 patients with post-irradiation telangectesias developed hematoma formation at the site of previously identified T2 shortening.[50] Postmortem histopathology reveals thin-walled vessels surrounded by hemosiderin and gliosis.[50] Radiation-induced retinal telangeiectasias and microaneurysms have also been reported.[51] Cavernous angiomas also develop after cranial irradiation, particularly when radiation exposure occurs during childhood. The reported latency between irradiation and diagnosis ranges from three to 41 years.[52,53] Radiation-induced cavernomas may appear as contrast enhancing masses and may mimic tumor radiogaphically.[54] These lesions are of great concern given their hemorrhagic potential.

Small Vessel Disease

Radiation injury to the microvasculature has been extensively described. A mineralizing microangiopathy occurs more frequently in children than in adults, resulting in calcifications in the basal ganglia, subcortical white matter or dentate nuclei.[55] The etiology is radiation-induced intimal injury to small vessels, subsequent tissue ischemia and dystrophic calcification. Lacunar infarctions have also been reported to be a consequence of cranial irradiation. The burden of lacunar disease increases with time from irradiation. The most significant risk factor for developing lacunar disease in this series was age younger than five years at the time of irradiation.[56]

Neuroendocrine Dysfunction

The hypothalamic-pituitary axis is exquisitely sensitive to irradiation.[57] Endocrine disorders can be the consequence of direct irradiation of an endocrine gland (e.g. 50% of patients developing hypothyroidism within 20 years follow-ing radiotherapy for Hodgkin's disease as a result of irradiation of the thyroid gland) or as a result of hypothalamic-pituitary dysfunction secondary to cranial irradiation.[57] In children, the most common endocrinopathy is growth hor-mone deficiency. Gonadotrophin deficiency and secondary and tertiary hypothyroidism occur less frequently. In adults, although growth hormone deficiency is common, it is rarely symptomatic. Approximately 67% of adult males experience sexual difficulties, usually decreased libido and impotence, within two years of radiotherapy. These problems are thought to result from gonadotrophin deficiency from hypothalamic damage. Hypothyroidism and hypoadrenalism occur less commonly and may require hormonal replacement. Hyperprolactinemia may also occur.[58,59]

Late Effects of Radiation Therapy to the Spinal Cord

The spinal cord may be affected by radiotherapy for primary spinal tumors, epidural metastases, tumors of the head and neck or tumors near the spinal cord, such as Hodgkin's lymphoma.

Late-Delayed Radiation Myelopathy

Late-delayed myelopathy takes two main forms – a progressive radiation mye-lopathy and a rare radiogenic lower motor neuron disease. In comparison to the early-delayed myelopathy, the late forms of myelopathy carry a poor prognosis.

Delayed Radiation Myelopathy (DRM)

This complication occurs six months to 10 years after radiation exposure. Risk factors include higher doses, larger fraction sizes, previous radiation exposure (therapeutic or incidental), old age, concurrent radiosensitizing chemotherapies and radiation sites in the lower thoracic and lumbar spine.[60] Clinical presenta-tion may be acute or insidious at onset, progressing to paraparesis or quad-riparesis with variable sensory disturbances, bowel and bladder dysfunction or diaphragmatic weakness in the case of high cervical lesions. Patients may present with a Brown-Sequard hemicord syndrome or a transverse myelitis. Pathology reveals findings similar to cerebral radionecrosis, with areas of focal necrosis, hyalinization and fibrinoid necrosis of the vasculature, demyelination and telangeictasias with focal hemorrhage. As in cerebral radiation injury, the etiology is thought to be either radiation-induced vascular and/or glial injury, but the pathogenesis is incompletely understood. MRI often shows cord edema and enhancement early in the course, and atrophy late in the course, but imaging may also be normal at very early or intermediate stages.[61] Cyst forma-tion has also been reported.[62] Prognosis is poor. There is no effective treatment, although hyperbaric oxygen, anticoagulation and steroid therapies have been suggested.[8,63,64] To minimize risk of this terrible complication, radiation to the spinal cord is generally limited to 4,500 cGy in 22–25 fractions.

Radiogenic Lower Motor Neuron Disease

A lower motor neuron syndrome is a rare complication of radiotherapy to the spinal cord or paraspinal tumors.[65,66] This complication predominately affects the lower extremities; in one series of 47 patients, only one had upper extremity weakness.[67] Patients tend to be adolescent to young adults and there's a male predominance.[67] Reported latency from irradiation to presentation ranges from four to 312 months.[67] There is no apparent dose-dependence, and authors have suggested that the etiology of radiogenic lower motor neuron disease may be multifactorial.[67] Based on electrophysiologic data and the absence of sensory findings, the anterior horn cell has been implicated as the target cell; however, damage to motor nerve roots is also a possibility.[68]

Vascular Changes

Rarely, spinal cord hemorrhage may occur. This is likely to be related to formation of spinal telangiectesias or cavernous malformations.[69]

Cranial Neuropathies

The optic nerve (strictly speaking, part of the central nervous system) is the most frequently affected cranial nerve. Other cranial nerves affected by radiotherapy include the olfactory nerve (also part of the central nervous system), hypoglossal nerve and the spinal accessory nerve. Multiple cranial neuropathies are also possible. Involvement of the occulomotor, trochlear and abducens nerves are rare.

Complications of Chemotherapy

Chemotherapy-Induced Cognitive Impairment

Chemotherapy-induced cognitive impairment, known amongst cancer patients and oncologists as "chemofog" or "chemobrain," and characterized by deficits in memory function and concentration is an increasingly recognized complication.[70–74] A recent meta-analysis estimates that mild cognitive impairment occurs in 10–40% of breast cancer survivors.[74] In contrast to the cognitive dysfunction that follows cranial irradiation, chemotherapy-induced deficits in memory and concentration appear to be transient, but may resolve slowly over a number of years.[74]

Additional complications of chemotherapy include acute encephalopathy, seizure, headaches, aseptic meningitis, acute cerebellar syndrome, vasculopathy and stroke, neuropathy, visual loss, myelopathy, reversible posterior leukoencephalopathy syndrome (RPLES) and dementia. The following section will focus on the drugs that frequently cause neurotoxicity. Neurologic complications of chemotherapy are reviewed in detail in several recent review[75] (see Table 8.2).

Table 8.2 Neurological complications of chemotherapy, biological response modifiers and targeted molecular agents

Acute encephalopathy	Headache	Seizures
• Asparaginase	• Asparaginase	• Amifostine
• 5-Azacytidine	• Capecitabine	– Asparaginase
• BCNU (IA or HD)	• Cetuximab	• BCNU
• Chlorambucil	• Cisplatin	• Busulphan (HD)
• Cisplatin	• Corticosteroids	– Chorambucil
• Corticosteroids	• Cytosine arabinoside	• Cisplatin
– Cyclophosphamide	• Danazol	• Corticosteroids
• Cytosine arabinoside (HD)	• Estramustine	• Cytosine arabinoside
• Dacarbazine	• Etoposide	• Dacarbazine
• Doxorubicin	• Fludarabine	• Etanercept
– Etoposide (HD)	• Gefitinib	• Etoposide
• Fludarabine	• Hexamethylmelamine	– 5-FU
• 5-Fluorouracil (5-FU)	• Interferons	• Ifosfamide
• Hexamethylmelamine	• Interleukins 1, 2, 4	– Interferon
• Hydroxyurea	• Ibritumomab	– Interleukin-2
• Ibritumomab	• Levamisole	• Letrozole
– Ifosfamide	• Mechlorethamine	– Levamisole
– Imatinib	• Methotrexate (IT)	• Mechloramine
– Interferons	• Nelarabine	• Methotrexate
• Interleukins 1 and 2	• Octreotide	• Octreotide
• Mechloramine	• Oprelvekin	• Paclitaxel
• Methotrexate	• Plicamycin	• Pentostatin
• Misonidazole	• Rituximab	• Suramin
• Mitomycin C	• Retinoic acid	• Teniposide
• Nelarabine	• SU5416	• Thalidomide
• Paclitaxel	• Tamoxifen	– Vinca alkaloids
• Pentostatin	• Temozolomide	
• Procarbazine	• Thiotepa (IT)	**Visual loss**
• Tamoxifen	• Topotecan	• BCNU (IA)
• Thalidomide	• Tositumomab	• Cisplatin
• Thiotepa (HD)	• Trastuzumab	• Etanercept
• Tumor necrosis factor	• ZD1839	• Fludarabine
• Vinca alkaloids		• Methotrexate (HD)
• Tipifarnib	**Aseptic meningitis**	• Tamoxifen
	• Cytosine arabinoside (IT)	
Dementia	• Levamisole	**Neuropathy**
• BCNU (IA and HD)	• Methotrexate (IT)	• 5-Azacytidine
• Corticosteroids	• Thiotepa (IT)	• Bortezomib
• Cytosine arabinoside		• Capecitabine
• Dacarbazine	**Myelopathy**	• Carboplatin
• 5-FU + Levamisole	• Cisplatin	• Cisplatin
• Fludarabine	• Cladribine	• Cytosine arabinoside

Table 8.2 (continued)

• Interferon-alpha	• Corticosteroids	• Docetaxel
• Methotrexate	• Cytosine arabinoside	• Etoposide
	• Doxorubicin	• 5-FU
Cranial neuropathy	– DFMO	• Gemcitabine
• BCNU (IA) (ototoxicity)	• Fludarabine	• Hexamethylmelamine
• Cisplatin (ototoxicity)	• Interferon alpha	• Ifosphamide
• Cytosine arabinoside	• Methotrexate (IT)	• Interferon-alpha
• Ifosfamide	• Mitoxantrone (IT)	• Misonidazole
• Methotrexate	• Docetaxel	• Nelarabine
• Nelarabine	• Thiotepa (IT)	• Oprelvekin
• Vincristine (extraocular	• Vincristine (IT)	• Oxaliplatin
palsies)		• Paclitaxel
		• Pemetrexed
Acute cerebellar syndrome	**Vasculopathy and stroke**	• Procarbazine
• Cytosine arabinoside	• Asparaginase	• Purine analogs (fludarabine,
• 5-FU	• Bevacizumab	cladribine, pentostatin)
• Hexamethylmelamine	• BCNU (IA)	• Sorafenib
• Ifosfamide	• Bleomycin	• Sunitinib malate
– Interleukin-2	• Carboplatin (IA)	• Suramin
• Procarbazine	• Cisplatin (IA)	• Teniposide (VM-26)
• Tamoxifen	• Doxorubicin	• Thalidomide
• Thalidomide	• Erlotinib	• Tumor necrosis factor
• Vinca alkaloids	• Estramustine	• Vinca alkaloids
• Tipifarnib	• 5-FU	• Tipifarnib
	• Imatinib mesylate	
Leukoencephalopathy	• Methotrexate	**Syncope**
• Capecitabine	• Nelarabine	• Bevacizumab
• Cisplatin	• Tamoxifen	• Erlotinib
• Cytarabine (IT)		• Nelarabine
• 5-FU with levamisole		
• Cyclosporin-A		
• Methotrexate (IT)		
• Nelarabine		
• Sunitinib malate		

Adapted with permission from Medlink Neurology (Wen PY, Kesari S, Grier J. Neurologic complications of chemotherapy 2006)

Antimetabolites

Methotrexate

Methotrexate is a dihydrofolate reductase inhibitor used in the treatment of leukemia, lymphomas (including central nervous system lymphoma), chorio-carcinoma, breast cancer, and leptomeningeal metastases. The manifestations of methotrexate toxicity depend upon the route of administration, dose and the use of other treatment modalities such as irradiation.

Intrathecal methotrexate produces aseptic meningitis in about 10% of patients. Symptoms of headache, nuchal rigidity, back pain, nausea, vomiting, fever and lethargy begin 2–4 hours after the drug is administered into the intrathecal space, and persist for 12–72 hours. Transverse myelopathy is also possible, presenting as back or leg pain, followed by paraplegia, sensory loss

Fig. 8.4 Sixty-one-year-old
man with Burkitt's
lymphoma treated with
intrathecal methotrexate
and Ara-C. Three days after
administration of the third
intrathecal cycle the patient
developed fecal incontinence
and weakness in all
extremities, with relatively
preserved arm strength
compared to leg sagittal T2.
MRI of the cervical spinal
cord reveals diffuse
myelopathy

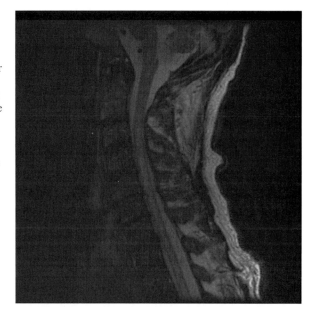

and sphincter dysfunction (see Fig. 8.4). This can occur 30 minutes to up to two weeks later, but typically happens within two days. Variable recovery ensues after methotrexate-induced transverse myelopathy. Rarely, intrathecal methotrexate results in acute encephalopathy, subacute focal neurological deficits, neurogenic pulmonary edema and death. Accidental overdose (more than 500 mg) of intrathecal methotrexate usually results in death.

Low-dose methotrexate toxicity is associated with dizziness, headache and mild cognitive impairment. Symptoms resolve after discontinuation of methotrexate.[76]

High-dose methotrexate toxicity can have acute, subacute and chronic manifestations. Acute toxicity produces somnolence, confusion and seizures within 24 hours of treatment. Subacutely, high-dose methotrexate can cause a subacute stroke-like syndrome, characterized by transient focal neurological deficits, confusion and sometimes seizures that appear within six days of exposure and resolves completely within 72 hours. Chronically, methotrexate can cause leukoencephalopathy, either alone or in combination with radiotherapy (see Fig. 8.2). The manifestations and consequences of leukoencephalopathy were discussed above.

Cytosine Arabinoside (Cytarabine, Ara-C)

Ara-C is a pyrimidine analogue that disrupts DNA synthesis and is used in the treatment of leukemias, lymphomas, and leptomeningeal metastases. Conventional doses do not produce much neurotoxicity. However, at higher doses an acute cerebellar syndrome may develop in 10–25 % of patients, particularly those with renal impairment.[77–79] Widespread loss of Purkinje cells and cerebellar atrophy may ensue. Somnolence is another frequent symptom. Occasionally, high-dose Ara-C produces encephalopathy, seizures, reversible ocular toxicity, lateral rectus syndrome, bulbar and psuedobulbar palsy, Horner's syndrome, aseptic meningitis, anosmia, and/or an extrapyramidal syndrome. The intrathecal administration of liposomal Ara-C may cause significantly more neurotoxicty. In one series, neurotoxicity was reported in five of 31 patients, including cauda equine syndrome and encephalitis.[80]

Alkylating Agents

Cisplatin

Cisplatin produces DNA cross-linking and is used to treat medulloblastoma, head and neck, ovarian, germ cell, cervical, lung, and bladder cancers. Cisplatin produces a neuropathy that affects predominantly large myelinated sensory fibers at the level of the dorsal-root ganglion[81,82] causing proprioceptive loss, numbness and parasthesias. Sural nerve biopsy shows demyelination and axonal loss. The neuropathy typically resolves with time after cessation of treatment. Cisplatin also commonly causes ototoxicity with high-frequency sensorineural hearing loss and tinnitus due to dose-related damage to the hair cells in the organ of Corti. Audiometric hearing loss is present in 74–88% of patients, with symptomatic hearing loss in 16–20% of patients. Irradiation increases the risk of hearing loss.[83,84] Lhermitte's sign occurs in 20–40% of patients receiving cisplatin. Rarely, cisplatin may cause encephalopahty, reversible posterior leukoencephalopathy, late vascular toxicity, taste disturbance and myasthenic syndrome. Oxaliplatin is also associated with a high incidence of neuropathy while neuropathies occur infrequently with carboplatin.

Vincristine

Vincristine is a vinca alkaloid that disrupts microtubules and is used to treat many cancers including leukemia, lymphoma, sarcomas and brain tumors. It causes an axonal neuropathy affecting both sensory and motor fibers in almost all patients. Small sensory fibers are particularly affected. Clinical manifestations include fingertip and foot parasthesias, muscle cramps, foot and wrist drop and sensory loss of varying degrees. Focal neuropathies and cranial neuropathies are also possible. In addition to the sensory and motor neuropathy, vincristine commonly causes an autonomic neuropathy, characterized by gastrointestinal, urinary and/or sexual dysfunction. Rarely, vincristine causes the syndrome of inappropriate antidiuretic hormone (SIADH), resulting in hyponatremia leading to metabolic encephalopathy and seizures.

Vincristine should never be administered intrathecally, and accidental administration of vincristine into the CSF produces a rapidly ascending myelopathy, coma and death.[85,86]

Other vinca alkloids such as vinblastine and vinorlbine are associated with a lower incidence of neuropathies.

Bevacizumab (Avastin)

Bevacizumab and other inhibitors of vascular endothelial growth factor (VEGF) and the VEGF receptor (VEGFR) are associated with Reversible Posterior Leucoencephalopathy syndrome (RPLS).[87,88] RPLS has been reported with various chemotherapeutic and immunosuppressive agents, and typically presents as cortical blindness, headache and confusion. Hypertension may be present, and seizures may occur. Imaging reveals non-enhancing subcortical leukoencephalopathy in a distal vascular distribution. Discontinuing the causative agent usually results in complete resolution of symptoms and signs.

Glucocorticoids

Corticosteroids such as prednisone and dexamethasone are used for a number of reasons in oncological therapy, including cytolytic effect on neoplastic lymphocytes and reduction of peritumoral edema in patients with brain tumors. Corticosteroids have a number of systemic and neurological side effects (see Table 8.3). Common neurological side effects include steroid myopathy and alterations in mood. Steroid psychosis, steroid-induced dementia and

Table 8.3 Neurologic complications of corticosteroids

Common
- Myopathy
- Behavioral changes
- Visual blurring
- Tremor
- Insomnia
- Reduced taste and olfaction
- Cerebral atrophy

Uncommon
- Psychosis
- Hallucinations
- Hiccups
- Dementia
- Seizures
- Dependence
- Epidural lipomatosis

cortical atrophy also occur. Corticosteroids may play an important role in cognitive dysfunction during and after cancer therapy. In animal models, corticosteroids are known to impair the physiology of the developing brain, including hippocampal neurogenesis. In humans, prednisone therapy has been demonstrated to impair verbal memory function[89] and children treated for acute lymphoblastic leukemia exhibited more severe long-term cognitive dysfunction if their regimen included dexamethasone.[90]

Summary

Neurologic complications of oncologic therapies are occurring with increasing frequency in cancer patients. This is a result of the availability of a growing number of treatments associated with neurotoxicities, and prolonged patient survival. Increased understanding of the underlying mechanisms for these neurologic complications, and methods to prevent them, will be an important challenge for the future and will hopefully lead to reduced neurologic morbidity in cancer patients.

Acknowledgments We gratefully acknowledge the support of the James Hagerty Fund

References

1. Sheline GE, Wara WM, Smith V. Therapeutic irradiation and brain injury. *Int J Radiat Oncol Biol Phys*. 1980;6(9):1215.
2. Oppenheimer JH, Levy ML, Sinha U, et al. Radionecrosis secondary to interstitial brachytherapy: correlation of magnetic resonance imaging and histopathology. *Neurosurgery*. 1992;31(2):336.
3. Hoshi M, Hayashi T, Kagami H et al. Late bilateral temporal lobe necrosis after conventional radiotherapy. *Neurol Med Chir* (Tokyo). 2003;43(4):213.
4. Gabayan AJ, Green SB, Sanan A, et al., GliaSite brachytherapy for treatment of recurrent malignant gliomas: a retrospective multi-institutional analysis. *Neurosurgery*. 2006;58(4):701.
5. Kumar AJ, Leeds NE, Fuller GN, et al. Malignant gliomas: MR imaging spectrum of radiation therapy- and chemotherapy-induced necrosis of the brain after treatment. *Radiology*. 2000;217(2):377.
6. Gomez-Rio M, Martinez del Valle Torres D, Rodriguez-Fernandez A, et al. (201)Tl-SPECT in low-grade gliomas: diagnostic accuracy in differential diagnosis between tumour recurrence and radionecrosis. *Eur J Nucl Med Mol Imaging*. 2004;31(9):1237.
7. Monje ML, Palmer T. Radiation injury and neurogenesis. *Curr Opin Neurol*. 2003;16(2):129.
8. Glantz MJ, Burger PC, Friedman AH et al. Treatment of radiation-induced nervous system injury with heparin and warfarin. *Neurology*. 1994;44(11):2020.
9. Leber KA, Eder HG, Kovac H, et al. Treatment of cerebral radionecrosis by hyperbaric oxygen therapy. *Stereotact Funct Neurosurg*. 1998;70(Suppl 1):229.
10. Chan AS, Cheung MC, Law SC, et al. Phase II study of alpha-tocopherol in improving the cognitive function of patients with temporal lobe radionecrosis. *Cancer*. 2004;100(2):398.
11. Behin A and Delattre JY. Complications of radiation therapy on the brain and spinal cord. *Semin Neurol*. 2004;24(4):405.

12. Wassenberg MW, Bromberg JE, Witkamp TD, et al. White matter lesions and encephalopathy in patients treated for primary central nervous system lymphoma. *J Neurooncol.* 2001;52(1):73.
13. Price RA and Jamieson PA. The central nervous system in childhood leukemia. II. Subacute leukoencephalopathy. *Cancer.* 1975;35(2):306.
14. Wang AM, Skias DD, Rumbaugh CL, et al. Central nervous system changes after radiation therapy and/or chemotherapy: correlation of CT and autopsy findings. *AJNR Am J Neuroradiol.* 1983;4(3):466.
15. Perry A and Schmidt RE. Cancer therapy-associated CNS neuropathology: an update and review of the literature. *Acta Neuropathol.* (Berl) 2006;111(3):197.
16. Virta A, Patronas N, Raman R, et al. Spectroscopic imaging of radiation-induced effects in the white matter of glioma patients. *Magn Reson. Imaging.* 2000;18(7):851.
17. DeAngelis LM, Delattre JY, and Posner JB. Radiation-induced dementia in patients cured of brain metastases. *Neurology.* 1989;39(6):789.
18. Crossen JR, Garwood D, Glatstein E, et al. Neurobehavioral sequelae of cranial irradiation in adults: a review of radiation-induced encephalopathy. *J Clin Oncol.* 1994;12(3):627.
19. Meyers CA, Weitzner MA, Valentine AD, et al. Methylphenidate therapy improves cognition, mood, and function of brain tumor patients. *J Clin Oncol.* 1998;16(7):2522.
20. Shaw EG, Rosdhal R, D'Agostino RB Jr, et al. Phase II study of donepezil in irradiated brain tumor patients: effect on cognitive function, mood, and quality of life. *J Clin Oncol.* 2006;24(9):1415.
21. Thiessen B and DeAngelis LM. Hydrocephalus in radiation leukoencephalopathy: results of ventriculoperitoneal shunting. *Arch Neurol.* 1998;55(5):705.
22. Roman DD and Sperduto PW. Neuropsychological effects of cranial radiation: current knowledge and future directions. *Int J Radiat Oncol Biol Phys.* 1995;31(4):983.
23. Anderson VA, Godber T, Smibert E, et al. Cognitive and academic outcome following cranial irradiation and chemotherapy in children: a longitudinal study. *Br J Cancer.* 2000;82(2):255.
24. Moore BD, 3rd, Copeland DR, Ried H, et al. Neurophysiological basis of cognitive deficits in long-term survivors of childhood cancer. *Arch Neurol.* 1992;49(8):809.
25. Abayomi OK. Pathogenesis of irradiation-induced cognitive dysfunction. *Acta Oncol.* 1996;35(6):659.
26. Lee PW, Hung BK, Woo EK, et al. Effects of radiation therapy on neuropsychological functioning in patients with nasopharyngeal carcinoma. *J Neurol Neurosurg Psychiatry.* 1989;52(4):488.
27. Surma-aho O, Niemelä M, Vilkki J, et al. Adverse long-term effects of brain radiotherapy in adult low-grade glioma patients. *Neurology.* 2001;56(10):1285.
28. Kramer JH, Crowe AB, Larson DA, et al. Neuropsychological sequelae of medulloblastoma in adults. *Int J Radiat Oncol Biol Phys.* 1997;38(1):21.
29. Strother DR. Tumors of the Central Nervous System. In: Pizzo PPA and Poplack DG, eds. *Principles and Practice of Pediatric Oncology.* 4th ed. Philadelphia: Lippincott, Williams and Wilkins; 2002:751–824.
30. Abayomi OK. Pathogenesis of cognitive decline following therapeutic irradiation for head and neck tumors. *Acta Oncol.* 2002;41(4):34.
31. Dropcho EJ. Central nervous system injury by therapeutic irradiation. *Neurol Clin.* 1991;9(4):96.
32. Parent JM, Trad E, Fike JR, et al. Inhibition of dentate granule cell neurogenesis with brain irradiation does not prevent seizure-induced mossy fiber synaptic reorganization in the rat. *J Neurosci.* 1999;19(11):450.
33. Monje ML, Mizumatsu S, Fike JR, et al. Irradiation induces neural precursor-cell dysfunction. *Nat Med.* 2002;8(9):955.
34. Monje ML, Toda H, and Palmer TD. Inflammatory blockade restores adult hippocampal neurogenesis. *Science.* 2003;302(5651):1760.

35. Raber J, Rola R, LeFevour A, et al. Radiation-induced cognitive impairments are associated with changes in indicators of hippocampal neurogenesis. *Radiat Res.* 2004;162(1):3.
36. Ron E, Modan B, Boice JD Jr, et al. Tumors of the brain and nervous system after radiotherapy in childhood. *N Engl J Med.* 1988;319(16):1033.
37. Neglia JP, Meadows AT, Robison LL, et al. Second neoplasms after acute lymphoblastic leukemia in childhood. *N Engl J Med.* 1991;325(19):1330.
38. Amirjamshidi A and Abbassioun K. Radiation-induced tumors of the central nervous system occurring in childhood and adolescence. Four unusual lesions in three patients and a review of the literature. *Childs Nerv Syst.* 2000;16(7):390.
39. Nishio S, Morioka T, Inamura T, et al. Radiation-induced brain tumours: potential late complications of radiation therapy for brain tumours. *Acta Neurochir* (Wien.). 1998;140(8):763.
40. Strojan P, Popovic M, and Jereb B. Secondary intracranial meningiomas after high-dose cranial irradiation: report of five cases and review of the literature. *Int J Radiat Oncol Biol Phys.* 2000;48(1):65.
41. Regel JP, Schoch B, Sandalcioglu IE, et al. Malignant meningioma as a second malignancy after therapy for acute lymphatic leukemia without cranial radiation. *Childs Nerv Syst.* 2006;22(2):172.
42. Zattara-Cannoni H, Roll P, Figarella-Branger D, et al. Cytogenetic study of six cases of radiation-induced meningiomas. *Cancer Genet Cytogenet.* 2001;126(2):81.
43. Salvati M, Frati A, Russo N, et al. Radiation-induced gliomas: report of 10 cases and review of the literature. *Surg Neurol.* 2003;60(1):60.
44. McIver JI and Pollock BE. Radiation-induced tumor after stereotactic radiosurgery and whole brain radiotherapy: case report and literature review. *J Neurooncol.* 2004;66(3):301.
45. Murros KE and Toole JF. The effect of radiation on carotid arteries. A review article. *Arch Neurol.* 1989;46(4):449.
46. Laplane D, Carydakis C, Baulac M, et al. Intracranial artery stenoses 44 years after craniofacial radiotherapy. *Rev Neurol.* (Paris) 1986;142(1):65.
47. Kondoh T, Morishita A, Kamei M, et al. Moyamoya syndrome after prophylactic cranial irradiation for acute lymphocytic leukemia. *Pediatr Neurosurg.* 2003;39(5):264.
48. Bitzer M and Topka H. Progressive cerebral occlusive disease after radiation therapy. *Stroke.* 1995;26(1):131.
49. Koike S, Aida N, Hata M, et al. Asymptomatic radiation-induced telangiectasia in children after cranial irradiation: frequency, latency, and dose relation. *Radiology.* 2004;230(1):93.
50. Gaensler EH, Dillon WP, Edwards MS, et al. Radiation-induced telangiectasia in the brain simulates cryptic vascular malformations at MR imaging. *Radiology.* 1994;193(3):629.
51. Bagan SM and Hollenhorst RW. Radiation retinopathy after irradiation of intracranial lesions. *Am J Ophthalmol.* 1979;88(4):694.
52. Jain R, Robertson PL, Gandhi D, et al. Radiation-induced cavernomas of the brain. *AJNR Am J Neuroradiol.* 2005;26(5):1158.
53. Duhem R, Vinchon M, Leblond P, et al. Cavernous malformations after cerebral irradiation during childhood: report of nine cases. *Childs Nerv Syst.* 2005;21(10):922.
54. Olivero WC, Deshmukh P, and Gujrati M. Radiation-induced cavernous angioma mimicking metastatic disease. *Br J Neurosurg.* 2000;14(6):575.
55. Shanley DJ. Mineralizing microangiopathy: CT and MRI. *Neuroradiology.* 1995;37(4):331.
56. Fouladi M, Langston J, Mulhern R, et al. Silent lacunar lesions detected by magnetic resonance imaging of children with brain tumors: a late sequela of therapy. *J Clin Oncol.* 2000;18(4):824.
57. Constine LS, Woolf PD, Cann D, et al. Hypothalamic-pituitary dysfunction after radiation for brain tumors. *N Engl J Med.* 1993;328(2):87.

58. Washburn LC, Carlton JE, and Hayes RL. Distribution of WR-2721 in normal and malignant tissues of mice and rats bearing solid tumors: dependence on tumor type, drug dose and species. *Radiat Res.* 1974;59(2):475.
59. Toogood AA. Endocrine consequences of brain irradiation. *Growth Horm IGF Res.* 2004;14(Suppl A):S118–S124.
60. Rampling R and Symonds P. Radiation myelopathy. *Curr Opin Neurol.* 1998;11(6):627.
61. Wang PY, Shen WC, and Jan JS. MR imaging in radiation myelopathy. *AJNR Am J Neuroradiol.* 1992;13(4):1049.
62. Shindo K, Nitta K, Amino A, et al. A case of chronic progressive radiation myelopathy with cavity formation in the thoracic spinal cord. *Rinsho Shinkeigaku.* 1995;35(9):1012.
63. Udaka F, Tsuji T, Shigematsu K, et al. A case of chronic progressive radiation myelopathy successfully treated with corticosteroid. *Rinsho Shinkeigaku.* 1990;30(4):439.
64. Feldmeier JJ, Lange JD, Cox SD, et al. Hyperbaric oxygen as prophylaxis or treatment for radiation myelitis. *Undersea Hyperb Med.* 1993;20(3):249.
65. Lagueny A, Aupy M, Aupy P, et al. Post-radiotherapy anterior horn cell syndrome. *Rev Neurol* (Paris). 1985;141(3):222.
66. De Carolis P, Montagna P, Cipulli M, et al. Isolated lower motoneuron involvement following radiotherapy. *J Neurol Neurosurg Psychiatry.* 1986;49(6):718.
67. Esik O, Vönöczky K, Lengyel Z, et al. Characteristics of radiogenic lower motor neurone disease, a possible link with a preceding viral infection. *Spinal Cord.* 2004;42(2):99.
68. Bowen J, Gregory R, Squier M, et al. The post-irradiation lower motor neuron syndrome neuronopathy or radiculopathy? *Brain.* 1996;119(Pt 5):1429.
69. Jabbour P, Gault J, Murk SE, et al. Multiple spinal cavernous malformations with atypical phenotype after prior irradiation: case report. *Neurosurgery.* 2004;55(6):1431.
70. Cull A, Hay C, Love SB, et al. What do cancer patients mean when they complain of concentration and memory problems? *Br J Cancer.* 1996;74(10):1674.
71. Ganz PA. Cognitive dysfunction following adjuvant treatment of breast cancer: a new dose-limiting toxic effect? *J Natl Cancer Inst.* 1998;90(3):182.
72. Brezden CB, Phillips KA, Abdolell M, et al. Cognitive function in breast cancer patients receiving adjuvant chemotherapy. *J Clin Oncol.* 2000;18(14):2695.
73. Jansen CE, Miaskowski C, Dodd M, et al. A metaanalysis of studies of the effects of cancer chemotherapy on various domains of cognitive function. *Cancer.* 2005;104(10):2222.
74. Matsuda T, Takayama T, Tashiro M, et al. Mild cognitive impairment after adjuvant chemotherapy in breast cancer patients – evaluation of appropriate research design and methodology to measure symptoms. *Breast Cancer.* 2005;12(4):279.
75. Dietrich J, Wen PY. Neurologic complications of cancer therapy. In Schiff D, Kesari S, Wen PY (ed). Cancer Neurology in Clinical Practice. Humana Press (2nd edition) Totowa, NJ 2007:287–326.
76. Wernick R and Smith DL. Central nervous system toxicity associated with weekly low-dose methotrexate treatment. *Arthritis Rheum.* 1989;32(6):770.
77. Winkelman MD and Hines JD. Cerebellar degeneration caused by high-dose cytosine arabinoside: a clinicopathological study. *Ann Neurol.* 1983;14(5):520.
78. Hwang TL, Yung WK, Estay EH, et al. Central nervous system toxicity with high-dose Ara-C. *Neurology.* 1985;35(10):1475.
79. Herzig RH, Wolff SN, Lazarus HM, et al. High-dose cytosine arabinoside therapy for refractory leukemia. *Blood.* 1983;62(2):361.
80. Jabbour E, O'Brien S, Kantarjian H, et al. Neurologic complications associated with intrathecal liposomal cytarabine given prophylactically in combination with high-dose methotrexate and cytarabine to patients with acute lymphocytic leukemia. *Blood.* 2007;109(8):3214.
81. Roelofs RI, Hrushesky W, Rogin J, et al. Peripheral sensory neuropathy and cisplatin chemotherapy. *Neurology.* 1984;34(7):934.

82. Thompson SW, Davis LE, Kornfeld M, et al. Cisplatin neuropathy. Clinical, electro-
    physiologic, morphologic, and toxicologic studies. *Cancer*. 1984;54(7):1269.
83. Moroso MJ and Blair RL. A review of cis-platinum ototoxicity. *J Otolaryngol*. 1983;12(6):365.
84. Schell MJ, McHaney VA, Green AA, et al. Hearing loss in children and young adults
    receiving cisplatin with or without prior cranial irradiation. *J Clin Oncol*. 1989;7(6):754.
85. Berg RA, Ch'ien LT, Lancaster W, et al. Neuropsychological sequelae of postradiation
    somnolence syndrome. *J Dev Behav Pediatr*. 1983;4(2):103.
86. Gaidys WG, Dickerman JD, Walters CL, et al. Intrathecal vincristine. Report of a fatal
    case despite CNS washout. *Cancer*. 1983;52(5):799.
87. Glusker P, Recht L, and Lane B. Reversible posterior leukoencephalopathy syndrome
    and bevacizumab. *N Engl J Med*. 2006;354(9):980.
88. Ozcan C, Wong SJ, and Hari P. Reversible posterior leukoencephalopathy syndrome and
    bevacizumab. *N Engl J Med*. 2006;354(9):980.
89. Hájek T, Kopecek M, Preiss M, et al. Prospective study of hippocampal volume and
    function in human subjects treated with corticosteroids. *Eur Psychiatry*. 2006;21(2):123.
90. Waber DP, Carpentieri SC, Klar N, et al. Cognitive sequelae in children treated for acute
    lymphoblastic leukemia with dexamethasone or prednisone. *J Pediatr Hematol Oncol*.
    2000;22(3):206.

Chapter 9
Neurological Complications in Children

Sonia Partap and Paul Graham Fisher

Introduction

With advances in surgery, radiation, and chemotherapy, the long-term survival of children with primary brain tumors has improved markedly. Today, the prognosis for children with brain tumors is inherently better than for adults, and has resulted in a growing population of adult survivors.[1] As a result, neurological complications of this cohort are an increasing problem in the daily practice of neurologists, oncologists, and primary care physicians.

Unlike other organ systems, the central nervous system manifests toxicity from the tumor and its therapy in a unique manner. Even though the developing brain is more tolerant to surgical effects due to inherent plasticity, both chemotherapy and irradiation can injure or even devastate the child's neuraxis. In this chapter, the late effects from treating brain tumors in the pediatric nervous system will be discussed.

Seizures

At diagnosis, about 12% of children with brain tumors have seizures.[2,3] While early surgical treatment can often eradicate further seizures, some patients are plagued with recurrent seizures or epilepsy. Specific risk factors contribute to the probability of having seizures postoperatively: residual tumor, vascular injury leading to cerebral infarction, radiation necrosis, and tumor relapse.[4] The risk of developing epilepsy relates also to tumor histology. Children with low-grade gliomas, such as gangliogliomas or grade II astrocytomas, and especially dysembryoblastic neuroepithelial tumors (DNT), have a greater incidence of persistent seizures than those with other tumor types.[5]

S. Partap (✉)
Instructor, Department of Neurology, Stanford University, Stanford Comprehensive Cancer Center, Stanford, CA 94305-5826, USA
e-mail: spartap@stanford.edu

S. Goldman, C.D. Turner (eds.), *Late Effects of Treatment for Brain Tumors*,
Cancer Treatment and Research 150, DOI 10.1007/b109924_9,
© Springer Science+Business Media, LLC 2009

The diagnosis of a seizure depends largely on patient history. If the described symptoms do not correlate with an obvious epileptic etiology, an electroencephalogram may help to confirm the diagnosis or determine the electrical focus of the seizures. Magnetic resonance (MR) imaging with gadolinium contrast is indicated to evaluate for tumor relapse or identify cortical abnormalities, for example gliosis or cavernous malformations, possibly causing the seizures.

Once epilepsy is diagnosed, treatment can be tailored accordingly. The majority of patients will have partial (focal) seizures[6] and can be treated with appropriate antiepileptic drugs, such as oxcarbazepine (20–30 mg/kg divided twice daily), carbamazepine (10–20 mg/kg divided twice daily), valproic acid (30–60 mg/kg divided twice daily), levetiracetam (20–60 mg/kg divided twice daily), or gabapentin (15–45 mg/kg divided three times daily). With specific tumors, as in gangliogliomas, lesionectomy to control epilepsy has been shown to be most effective.[7] When eloquent areas of the brain are involved, surgical resection is not possible and seizure control can remain challenging. Maintaining serum levels of concurrent medications, such as corticosteroids, warfarin, oral contraceptives, and chemotherapeutics which are metabolized by the cytochrome P450 system can be a challenge since many antiepileptic drugs can induce their metabolism. Therefore, using levetiracetam, gabapentin, and other non-enzyme inducing antiepileptics is preferred when patients are concurrently take other medications.[5,8]

Antiepileptic drug withdrawal after a seizure-free period of one and one-half to two years is successfully achieved in the majority of children easily controlled with a single anticonvulsant. However, patients who had either brain tumors at a younger age when myelination was incomplete, aggressive tumor pathology, or treatment with whole-brain radiotherapy carry a higher risk of recurrent seizures when attempting drug withdrawal. The immature brain may be more prone to injury and resultant epilpetogenesis from the effects of chemotherapy, irradiation, and surgery.[9]

Cerebrovascular Disease

Children who have undergone irradiation for intracranial neoplasms have a high risk of cerebrovascular changes with abnormalities in small, intermediate, and large caliber vessels.[10,11] Acquired stenotic vascular changes in the affected large arteries leads to collateralization with small vessels, referred to as moyamoya-like vasculopathy, or moyamoya syndrome. Histologically, the affected vessel wall reveals fibrous thickening of the intimal layer of intermediate and large cerebral arteries, which subsequently leads to collateralization and an increased risk of ischemic stroke.[12]

Moyamoya Syndrome

Cerebral radiation predisposes an individual to moyamoya syndrome. A study of 345 children irradiated for primary brain tumors revealed that 3.5% developed evidence of moyamoya, particularly those children who were younger at diagnosis or did not undergo tumor resection.[13] Patients that received ≤5,000 cGy developed moyamoya at a median of 67 months compared to those treated with >5,000 cGy at 42 months. Those who received radiation near the Circle of Willis and received >5,000 cGy of irradiation were at greatest risk. Thus, children irradiated for parasellar tumors, such as optic gliomas, craniopharyngiomas, and germinomas, are particularly vulnerable to steno-occlusive changes in the field treated.[14]

Patients who have neurofibromatosis type I (NF1) also demonstrate stenotic vascular changes after cranial irradiation that progress more quickly than those without the genetic defect.[13] The NF1 chromosome locus 17q11, which regulates neurofibromin function, is associated with familial moyamoya disease.[15] Since neurofibromin is expressed in both the endothelial and smooth muscle cells of blood vessels, radiation exposure may serve as a "second hit" and promote vascular injury.[13]

Stroke

Stroke, usually ischemic rather hemorrhagic, is another cerebrovascular complication. In a Childhood Cancer Survivor Study of 1,871 brain tumor patients, relative risk of stroke was 29 times that of sibling controls. One-hundred-seventeen (6.3%) patients reported strokes, with 63 reporting stroke after five years at a mean 13.9 years from cancer diagnosis. Again, radiotherapy at a dose of ≥3,000 cGy was significantly predictive of cerebrovascular disease, and stroke risk increased in a dose-dependent fashion, with the highest risk of ischemic stroke after ≥5,000 cGy. Concurrent alkylating agents, but not other chemotherapeutics, further escalated risk.[16]

Vascular Malformations

Cavernous hemangiomas (cavernomas), telangectasias, and aneurysms[17] may also form after cranial irradiation. In a recent study of 297 patients under the age of 16 who had undergone radiotherapy for brain tumor and had no prior vascular abnormalities on neuroimaging, 10 (3.4%) developed cavernomas at a median age of seven years and a median time 37 months after irradiation. This prevalence of cavernomas was six times greater than that previously reported in the literature.[18] Though cavernomas can be benign vascular malformations, they can also cause seizures, mimic tumor recurrence, or hemorrhage.

Apart from large vessel changes, microangiopathic changes may also occur in the form of lacunar infarcts. Lacunar infarcts, a common adult entity, are restricted ischemic infarcts (0.2–15 mm in diameter) in the deep white matter, basal ganglia, or pons. In adults, the significance of lacunes can range from an incidental finding to a significant neuropsychological decline and dementia, and is associated with hypertension and diabetes mellitus.[19] In a St. Jude study of 524 children treated over 10 years for brain tumors, none developed lacunar infarcts if treated with surgery alone. Among the 421 patients who received radiation with or without chemotherapy, 25 developed lacunes detected asymptomatically on surveillance MR imaging. The most significant predictor for lacunes was for patients who were younger than five years at radiotherapy and a median time of two years after radiotherapy. None of the lacunes had clinical significance and all were incidental findings.[20] However, as children with primary brain tumors continue to age, lacunar infarcts may be a harbinger of cognitive or other outcomes, so continued awareness is essential.

Evaluation and Treatment

Since the majority of patients undergo routine surveillance neuroimaging for tumor progression, the caliber of intermediate and large cranial vessels (internal carotid, middle cerebral, and basilar arteries) and white matter changes from radiation can be assessed regularly on T1, FLAIR, and gadolinium-enhanced MR images. FLAIR sequences may be particularly useful in detecting irregularities in blood flow associated with presymptomatic vascular lesions.[13] Other noninvasive techniques, such as carotid and transcranial duplex ultrasound, may also be helpful especially in the presence of a carotid bruit. In a prospective study of carotid duplex ultrasound in patients treated with radiation for head and neck malignancies, 11.7% of 240 patients had stenosis of greater than 70%, which in turn increases the relative risk of stroke. Endarterectomy and stenting procedures have successfully treated radiation-induced carotid stenosis.[21] If clinical suspicion is high for vascular pathology or symptoms are apparent, then MR angiography or conventional cerebral angiography should be performed to detect vascular stenosis or malformations. Neurosurgical interventions for intracranial stenosis with either indirect revascularization with pial synangiosis or direct revascularization with standard extra-intracranial bypass should be considered.[14] Patients with cerebrovascular anomalies should be cognizant of their systemic blood pressure and avoid precipitous variations to reduce the risk of ischemia or hemorrhage. Though many patients are placed on aspirin therapy to reduce the risk of stroke, there is no evidence for the routine use of anticoagulants, platelet inhibitors, or cholesterol modifying agents, such as HMG-CoA reductase inhibitors, in patients with radiation-induced vasculopathy. Such agents may be useful, nonetheless, in patients who develop metabolic syndrome or other risk factors for cerebrovascular disease years after their cancer.

Headaches

Headache is considered an acute rather than late complication in children with brain tumors, as over half of children present with head pain, typically with accompanying signs and symptoms.[22,23] Primary headache or migraine may be an increasingly recognized complication, aside from secondary headache resulting from metastasis or tumor recurrence. Cephalgia can be a product of craniotomy itself; in an adult series, only 4% of patients had uncontrolled headache after one year.[24] Posterior fossa surgery has a higher prevalence of headache, especially with acoustic neuroma resection.[25] Children seldom have significant complaints of postoperative chronic headache.

Cranial radiotherapy can cause headache in all ages. Early onset headache or acute encephalopathy occurs within six months of treatment.[26] Years later, migraine variants have been reported in those treated with cranial irradiation. Patients may present with severe, recurrent headaches, and sometimes prolonged but reversible neurologic deficits, which can be confused with stroke or complicated migraine. Magnetic resonance imaging may reveal a cortical ribbon-like enhancement with gadolinium administration, while electroencephalography shows slowing over the corresponding cerebral region. Common clinical features appear to be posterior tumor location, $\geq 5{,}000$ cGy radiotherapy dose, latency great than a year from irradiation, and repeated episodes.[27] Despite the unknown etiology, stroke-like migraine attacks after radiation therapy (SMART syndrome) are important to recognize to avoid needless interventions which can be both cost-ineffective and potentially harmful. No therapy has been found to be completely effective, but conventional treatments with anticonvulsants used for migraine prophylaxis (e.g., carbamazepine and topiramate), calcium channel blockers, as in verapamil, and the β-receptor blocker propranolol have been helpful in some patients. Others will start aspirin therapy or even anticoagulation with warfarin as prophylaxis against potential cerebrovascular attacks, despite the lack of evidence.[27,28]

As for all primary headaches, appropriate treatment includes lifestyle modification with regular exercise, avoidance of triggers, appropriate hydration and diet, and adequate sleep. Medications for acute relief like sumatriptan have not been studied in brain tumor patients. Prophylactic agents as in β-receptor blockers, tricyclic antidepressants, and antiepileptics should be considered.[29,30] In many cases, relaxation techniques, biofeedback, or cognitive behavioral therapy may be a reasonable and beneficial option.[31]

Leukoencephalopathy

Leukoencephalopathy is a diffuse change or degeneration of white matter, most commonly identified by MR imaging or sometimes indicated by subcortical calcifications on computed tomography. Leukoencephalopathy can be associated with cognitive changes, learning disabilities, or dementia, and rarely can be asymptomatic. Leukoencephalopathy appears to be less common today in brain tumor patients because of decreased usage of methotrexate, but renewed interest in its use for infant medulloblastoma and adult primary central nervous system lymphoma continues to make leukoencephalopathy an important topic.

Methotrexate, whether administered intrathecally or intravenously, has long been a well-documented cause of leukoencephalopathy in the pediatric population when used to treat acute lymphoblastic leukemia.[32] Risk of leukoencephalopathy and its severity increase with the coadministration of radiotherapy and methotrexate, particularly when methotrexate was given following irradiation. Children with medulloblastoma treated with both radiation and methotrexate have lower intelligence quotient scores than those treated without methotrexate.[33] The specific mechanism of toxicity is unclear. Methotrexate may inhibit methylation and, therefore, myelin protein synthesis, or possibly with the loss of blood-brain barrier integrity from radiation effects, intrathecal methotrexate levels may become excessive.[34] Other chemotherapeutics such as BCNU and cytarabine have also been implicated in causing leukoencephalopathy, but their effect on intelligence is unknown.[35] Radiation alone can produce leukoencephalopathy, but more commonly leads to white matter changes in the specific region of the brain treated most intensively with radiation. No therapy or prevention is known for leukoencephalopathy. Methylphenidate and other stimulants have been used to mitigate the symptoms of leukoencephalopathy.[36]

Sleep Disturbances

Brain injury has long been associated with specific sleep problems, such as apnea, insomnia, general sleepiness, or loss of circadian rhythms. Sleep can be disrupted by primary cerebral neoplasms as well. Fatigue, coined as somnolence syndrome, is a well-recognized subacute side effect of radiation, with its sedation and anorexia weeks after a large field of radiation treatment. However, late complications are now becoming more apparent. A retrospective case series reviewed 14 children with varied complaints of sleep disturbance at a mean 42 months after therapy for a brain tumor. Nine complained of excessive daytime sleepiness with five of them having evidence of narcolepsy on polysomnography. The remaining children had hypoxia and fatigue, and one suffered from seizures. Obstructive sleep apnea and obesity were not factors. No obvious relationship with specific treatments and sleep disturbance was found, but there was a correlation with sustained damage to the hypothalamic-pituitary axis by tumor, surgery, hydrocephalus, whole-brain radiation or focal radiation. Respiratory drive issues were correlated with medullary damage from tumor or treatment.[37] Hypersomnolence has been associated with hypothalamic lesions with a mean sleep latency time in the patients that was significantly shorter than in control patients. A deficiency of orexin (hypocretin), produced by the hypothalamus, may be causal, but cerebrospinal fluid levels have not been shown to be significantly deficient.[38]

Patients should be evaluated for late-onset fatigue with detailed sleep histories, sleep logs, and polysomnography if appropriate. Stimulant medications, such as methylphenidate or dextroamphetamine, may help regulate the necessary sleep cycles in these disorders and are essential in narcolepsy. Clinical trials are underway to assess the wake promoting-agent modafinil in patients with fatigue and decreased attention following radiation or chemotherapy.

Superficial Siderosis

Superficial siderosis is a rare, late complication caused by recurrent hemorrhage into the subarachnoid space. Patients present with cerebellar ataxia, sensorineural hearing loss, and myelopathy years after successful surgical resection of brain and spinal tumors.[39,40] The chronic subarachnoid hemorrhage leads to an accumulation of ferritin and hemosiderin in subpial tissues, which in turn triggers the proliferation of astrocytes and microglia in the brain stem, cerebellum, vestibulocochlear nerves and other parts of the nervous system.[41] Symptoms are delayed in onset and are very insidious in nature, with one case presenting 37 years after surgery.[40] Other neurologic complaints are upper motor neuron signs, optic neuropathies, dysarthria, nystagmus, and cognitive impairment. Cerebrospinal fluid contains erythrocytes, a high protein concentration, and a mild lymphocytic pleocytosis.[38,42] Gradient echo and T2-weighted MR imaging shows a hypointense rim of iron coating the affected surfaces.[38] Treatment strategies include iron chelation with desferoxamine and surgical intervention to cease the bleeding, though evidence is lacking.[40]

Neuropathy

Numbness, tingling, burning, and pain are common sensory symptoms of peripheral neurotoxicity. All vinca alkaloids cause peripheral neuropathy, with vincristine being the most neurotoxic.[43] The neuropathy is thought to be related to impairment of the function of microtubules involved in axonal transport.[44] Pain and small-fiber sensory loss predominate early, usually occurring at four to five weeks.[45] Clinically, patients complain of paresthesias and dysesthesias in the tip of the fingers and toes that may progress to bilateral wrist and foot drop. Other effects may include vocal changes and bilateral ptosis. Almost all patients develop areflexia and side effects appear to correlate with total administered dose.[46] Children appear to tolerate vincristine better than adults with better resolution of neuropathy. However, years later many pediatric patients still complain of dysesthesias, foot cramping, and inability to dorsiflex their ankles.

Platinating agents, such as cisplatin, can also cause neuropathy. Cisplatin neuropathy manifests with numbness, paresthesias, and occasionally pain in the distal extremities, with loss of deep tendon reflexes and position sense.[47] Patients will first present with symmetric dysesthesias.[48] Cisplatin affects large myelinated fibers, thereby affecting vibration and proprioception and sparing pain and temperature sensation. Patients will have averaged cumulative doses between 300 and 600 mg/m^2 before symptoms emerge.[49] Again, most symptoms are reversible, but may take longer to improve than vincristine neuropathies. Platinum drugs also have the unfortunate common side effect of ototoxicity. As a variant of peripheral neuropathy, hearing loss is initially in high-frequency ranges. Usually seen with cisplatin, but also with high doses of carboplatin (50 mg/kg), hearing effects are from cumulative exposure and are magnified by irradiation.[49] Regular audiologic screening may help identify patients with decrements early to ensure proper language development and maximize school performance. Patients should receive yearly screenings for five years if they received platinum drugs or radiation near the cochlear, or if hearing loss is detected during treatment if necessary.

Treatment and prevention for chemotherapy-induced neuropathy remains controversial. Prevention of cisplatin neuropathy by amifostine has been studied in limited trials and, to date, has not been proven effective.[50] Other investigated agents including glutathione in cisplatin-induced neuropathy, glutamic acid in vincristine-induced neuropathy, and Org-2766 in both and vincristine- and cisplatin-induced neuropathy have had inconclusive results.[51] A randomized controlled trial of 31 adult patients treated with cisplatin and treated prophylactically with vitamin E at 300 mg twice daily proved beneficial to control patients.[52] To ease neuropathic pain, anticonvulsants such as gabapentin, topiramate, and carbamazepine are frequently used, although randomized placebo-controlled trials have shown them to be ineffective in spite of anecdotal declarations.[51]

Conclusion

The neurological complications from primary brain tumors in the pediatric population have become more evident as survivorship improves. Other late effects on cognition and endocrine function, along with the evolution of secondary neoplasms from radiation and chemotherapy, have a significant impact on both patient and society. Hydrocephalus can also be a lasting neurological problem. These topics are described in other chapters of this book and other resources. For the physicians caring for a childhood brain tumor survivor, it is important to recognize and understand the scope of changes to the brain and the long-term challenges when caring for these patients.

References

1. Legler JM, Ries LA, Smith MA, et al. Cancer surveillance series: brain and other central nervous system cancers: recent trends in incidence and mortality. *J Natl Cancer Inst.* 1999;91:1382–1390.
2. Ibrahim K, Appleton R. Seizures as the presenting symptom of brain tumours in children. *Seizure.* 2004;13:108–112.
3. Khajavi K, Comair YG, Wyllie E, et al. Surgical management of pediatric tumor-associated epilepsy. *J Child Neurol.* 1999;14:15–25.
4. Khan RB, Boop FA, Onar A, et al. Seizures in children with low grade tumors: outcome after tumor resection and risk factors for uncontrolled seizures. *J Neurosurg.* 2006;104: 377–382.
5. van Breemen MS, Vecht CJ. Optimal seizure management in brain tumor patients. *Curr Neurol Neurosci Rep.* 2005;5:207–213.
6. Hildebrand J, Lecaille C, Perennes J, et al. Epileptic seizures during follow-up of patients treated for primary brain tumors. *Neurology.* 2005;65:212–215.
7. Giulioni M, Gardella E, Rubboli G, et al. Lesionectomy in epileptogenic gangliogliomas: seizure outcome and surgical results. *J Clin Neurosci.* 2006;13:529–535.
8. Vecht CJ, van Breemen M. Optimizing therapy of seizures in patients with brain tumors. *Neurology.* 2006;67:S10–S13.
9. Khan RB, Onar A. Seizure recurrence and risk factors after antiepilepsy drug withdrawal in children with brain tumors. *Epilepsia.* 2006;47:375–379.
10. Bitzer M, Topka H. Progressive cerebral occlusive disease after radiation therapy. *Stroke.* 1995;26:131–136.
11. Brant-Zawadzki M, Anderson M, DeArmond SJ, et al. Radiation-induced large intracranial vessel occlusive vasculopathy. *AJR Am J Roentgenol.* 1980;134:51–55.
12. Nishimoto A, Takeuchi S. Moyamoya disease. In: Vinken PJ, Bruyn GW, eds. *Handbook of Clinical Neurology.* Amsterdam, Netherlands: North Holland; 1972;12:352–383.
13. Ullrich NJ, Robertson R, Kinnamon DD, et al. Moyamoya following cranial irradiation for primary brain tumors in children. *Neurology.* 2007;68:932–938.
14. Horn P, Pfister S, Bueltmann E, et al. Moyamoya-like vasculopathy (moyamoya syndrome) in children. *Childs Nerv Syst.* 2004;20:382–391.
15. Yamauchi T, Tada M, Houkin K, et al. Linkage of familial moyamoya disease (spontaneous occlusion of the circle of Willis) to chromosome 17q25. *Stroke.* 2000;31:930–935.
16. Bowers DC, Liu Y, Leisenring W, et al. Late-occurring stroke among long-term survivors of childhood leukemia and brain tumors: a report from the Childhood Cancer Survivor Study. *J Clin Oncol.* 2006;24:5277–5282.
17. Sciubba DM, Gallia GL, Recinos P, et al. Intracranial aneurysm following radiation therapy during childhood for a brain tumor. Case report and review of the literature. *J Neurosurg.* 2006;105:134–139.
18. Burn S, Gunny R, Phipps K, et al. Incidence of cavernoma development in children after radiotherapy for brain tumors. *J Neurosurg.*2007;106:379–383.
19. Fisher CM. Lacunar strokes and infarcts: a review. *Neurology.* 1982;32:871–876.
20. Fouladi M, Langston J, Mulhern R, et al. Silent lacunar lesions detected by magnetic resonance imaging of children with brain tumors: a late sequela of therapy. *J Clin Oncol.* 2000;18:824–831.
21. Rogers LR. Cerebrovascular complications in cancer patients. *Neurol Clin N Am.* 2003;21:167–192.
22. Childhood Brain Tumor Consortium:The epidemiology of headache among children with brain tumor. *J Neurooncol.* 1991;10:31–46.
23. Wilne SH, Ferris RC, Nathwani A, et al. The presenting features of brain tumours: a review of 200 cases. *Arch Dis Child.* 2006;91:502–506.

24. Kaur A, Selwa L, Fromes G, et al. Persistent headache after supratentorial craniotomy. *Neurosurgery*. 2000;47:633–636.
25. de Gray LC, Matta BF. Acute and chronic pain following craniotomy: a review. *Anaesthesia*. 2005;60:693–704.
26. Purdy RA, Kirby S. Headaches and brain tumors. *Neurol Clin*. 2004;22:39–53.
27. Partap S, Walker M, Longstreth WT Jr, et al. Prolonged but reversible migraine-like episodes long after cranial irradiation. *Neurology*. 2006;66:1105–1107.
28. Pruitt A, Dalmau J, Detre J, et al. Episodic neurologic dysfunction with migraine and reversible imaging findings after radiation. *Neurology*. 2006;67:676–678.
29. Lewis D, Ashwal S, Hershey A, et al. (2004) Practice parameter: pharmacological treatment of migraine headache in children and adolescents: report of the American Academy of Neurology Quality Standards Subcommittee and the Practice Committee of the Child Neurology Society. *Neurology*. 2004;63:2215–2224.
30. Hershey AD, Powers SW, Bentti AL, et al. Effectiveness of amitriptyline in the prophylactic management of childhood headaches. *Headache*. 2000; 40:539–549.
31. Damen L, Bruijn J, Koes BW, et al. Prophylactic treatment of migraine in children. Part 1. A systematic review of non-pharmacological trials. *Cephalalgia*. 2006;26:373–383.
32. Lövblad K, Kelkar P, Ozdoba C, et al. Pure methotrexate encephalopathy presenting with seizures: CT and MRI features. *Pediatr Radiol*. 1998;28:86–91.
33. Riva D, Giorgi C, Nichelli F, et al. Intrathecal methotrexate affects cognitive function in children with medulloblastoma. *Neurology*. 2002;59:48–53.
34. Kishi T, Tanaka Y, Ueda K. Evidence for hypomethylation in two children with acute lymphoblastic leukemia and leukoencephalopathy. *Cancer*. 2000;89:925–931.
35. Matsumoto S, Nishizawa S, Murakami M, et al. Carmofur-induced leukoencephalopathy: MRI. *Neuroradiology*. 1995;37:649–652.
36. Wen PY, Schiff D, Kesari S, et al. Medical management of patients with brain tumors. *J Neurooncol*. 2006;80:313–332.
37. Rosen GM, Bendel AE, Neglia JP, et al. Sleep in children with neoplasms of the central nervous system: case review of 14 children. *Pediatrics*. 2003;112:e46–e54.
38. Anderson NE. Late complications in childhood central nervous system tumour survivors. *Curr Opin Neurol*. 2003;16:677–683.
39. Fearnley JM, Stevens JM, Rudge P. Superficial siderosis of the central nervous system. *Brain*. 1995;118:1051–1066.
40. McCarron MO, Flynn PA, Owens C, et al. Superficial siderosis of the central nervous system many years after neurosurgical procedures. *J Neurol Neurosurg Psychiatry*. 2003;74:1326–1328.
41. Koeppen AH, Dickson AC, Chu RC, et al. The pathogenesis of superficial siderosis of the central nervous system. *Ann Neurol*1993;34:646–653.
42. Anderson NE, Sheffield S, Hope JK. Superficial siderosis of the central nervous system: a late complication of cerebellar tumors. *Neurology*. 1999;52:163–169.
43. Pace A, Bove L, Nistico C, et al. Vinorelbine neurotoxicity: clinical and neurophysiological findings in 23 patients. *J Neurol Neurosurg Psychiatry*.1996;61:409–411.
44. Topp KS, Tanner KD, Levine JD. Damage to the cytoskeleton of large diameter sensory neurons and myelinated axons in vincristine-induced painful peripheral neuropathy in the rat. *J Comp Neurol*. 2000;424:563–576.
45. Nozaki-Taguchi N, Chaplan SR, Higuera ES, et al. Vincristine-induced allodynia in the rat. *Pain*. 2001;93:69–76.
46. Posner JB. *Neurologic Complications of Cancer*. Philadelphia: FA Davis; 1995.
47. London Z, Albers JW. Toxic neuropathies associated with pharmaceutic and industrial agents. *Neurol Clin*. 2007;25:257–276.
48. Antunes NL. Acute neurologic complications in children with systemic cancer. *J Child Neurol*.2000;15:705–16.
49. Reddy AT, Witek K. Neurologic complications of chemotherapy for children with cancer. *Curr Neurol Neurosci Rep*.2003;3:137–42.

50. Albers J, Chaudhry V, Cavaletti G, Donehower R. Interventions for preventing neuropathy caused by cisplatin and related compounds. *Cochrane Database Syst Rev*.2007;24: CD005228.
51. Hausheer FH, Schilsky RL, Bain S. Diagnosis, management, and evaluation of chemotherapy-induced peripheral neuropathy. *Semin Oncol*.2006;33:15–49.
52. Argyriou AA, Chroni E, Koutras A, et al. Vitamin E for prophylaxis against chemotherapy-induced neuropathy. *Neurology*.2005;64:26–31.

Chapter 10
Strokes Among Childhood Brain Tumor Survivors

Daniel C. Bowers

Introduction

Survivors of childhood brain tumors are at an increased risk of stroke. In contrast, strokes are exceptionally rare among children and young adults without brain tumors. Among children in the United States, the reported incidence of stroke is 2.7–3.3 per 100,000 children per year.[1–3] The most frequently reported risk factors for stroke during childhood include cardiac disorders, sickle cell disease, hypercoagulable states, and vascular disorders. Furthermore, risk factors for stroke in adulthood include hypertension, atherosclerotic cerebrovascular disease, diabetes, and dyslipidemia. Survivors of childhood brain tumors have multiple, often interrelated risk factors for stroke, including the history of a brain tumor and receiving anticancer therapy, as well as these evolving developmental risk factors for stroke.

Survivors of childhood brain tumors are at risk for late-occurring cerebrovascular accidents or strokes.[4–9] A report from the Childhood Cancer Survivors Study identified a rate of stroke of 267.6 per 100,000 person-years (95% CI: 206.8–339.2 per 100,000 person-years) among brain tumor patients who lived at least five years after diagnosis.[4] After adjusting for age, gender, and race, the relative risk of late-occurring stroke for brain tumor survivors compared with a sibling comparison group was 29.0% (95% CI: 13.8–60.7; $p < 0.0001$). The cumulative incidence of stroke among brain tumor survivors was 5.6% (95% CI: 3.8–7.4%) at 25 years. The mean interval from cancer diagnosis to late-occurring stroke was 13.9 years (SD: 6.3 years).

The objectives of this chapter are to review the pathophysiology of cerebrovascular disease among survivors of childhood brain tumors and to discuss therapeutic options for cancer survivors who experience a stroke. For the purposes of this chapter, etiology of strokes in childhood brain tumor survivors is subdivided into four groups: Strokes that result from the primary cancer;

D.C. Bowers (✉)
Division of Pediatric Hematology-Oncology, University of Texas Southwestern Medical School, 5323 Harry Hines Blvd, Dallas, TX 75390-9063, USA
e-mail: daniel.bowers@utsouthwestern.edu

S. Goldman, C.D. Turner (eds.), *Late Effects of Treatment for Brain Tumors*,
Cancer Treatment and Research 150, DOI 10.1007/b109924_10,
© Springer Science+Business Media, LLC 2009

strokes that result from cancer therapy and occur during therapy; strokes that result from cancer treatment and occur following completion of cancer therapy, and potential risk factors for cerebrovascular disease and stroke in childhood brain tumor survivors. Whereas few reports of cerebrovascular disease among childhood brain tumor survivors exist and the reports of cerebrovascular disease in children with cancer include small numbers of childhood brain tumor survivors, reports of cerebrovascular disease in adults with cancer are used to highlight etiology, pathophysiology, and treatment where appropriate. Likewise, there are no reports evaluating stroke prevention or treatment specifically for cancer survivors, and there are no prospective randomized studies of stroke prevention in young adults. Therefore, few reports justify the benefit of stroke prevention strategies for childhood brain tumor survivors. However, this chapter will propose which patients are most likely to benefit from stroke prevention therapies and review the available therapeutic options for clinicians caring for these patients.

Causes of Strokes in Brain Cancer Survivors

Mass Effect and Hemorrhage from Solid Tumors

A subarachnoid hemorrhage can be the presenting symptom of a CNS tumor.[10,11] Yokota and co-workers reported that six of 167 children less than 15-years-old with newly diagnosed brain tumors presented with subarachnoid hemorrhage.[10] Hemorrhages occurred in both benign and malignant CNS tumors, both in the posterior fossa and the hypothalamus in both neonates and older children. Although there was morbidity associated with the hemorrhage, subarachnoid hemorrhage did not cause perioperative or early patient death.

Although extra-CNS primary cancers among adults (e.g., lung cancer, breast cancer, etc.) often metastasize to the brain, pediatric solid tumors infrequently metastasize to the central nervous system. An exception is neuroblastoma, which has a propensity of metastasizing to the brain, skull, and dura. Metastatic tumor to the brain or surrounding structures can infiltrate or compress the superior sagittal sinus, resulting in venous stasis, thrombosis, and stroke. In a series by Packer and co-workers of children with cancer who experienced strokes, two of 78 children with neuroblastoma had direct tumor invasion of the torcular region and sagittal sinus thrombosis.[12] One child died of increased intracranial pressure; the other received emergency radiation therapy with clinical and radiographic improvement.

Strokes That Result from Cancer Therapy and Occur During Therapy

Stroke is a potential complication of any neurosurgical procedure, including brain tumor resection. The frequency of stroke associated with tumor resections is unknown, and the true incidence is likely underrepresented in the medical literature. A report by Sutton and co-workers of children with craniopharyngiomas who were treated with surgical resection identified nine of 31 (29%) patients as having fusiform dilatation of the supraclinoid carotid artery.[13] Dilatation of the carotid artery was identified at the time of surgery for recurrence for one patient and on routine surveillance by CT imaging for eight patients at 6–18 months postoperatively. Eight of the nine patients remain alive at a mean of 3.7 years after diagnosis. None have experienced hemorrhage or other symptoms referable to fusiform dilatation of the carotid artery, which was believed to result from surgical manipulation of the carotid artery.

Chemotherapy-Induced Thrombocytopenia

A common side effect and dose-limiting toxicity of most cytotoxic chemotherapeutic drugs is bone marrow suppression, including a decrease in platelet production. In fact, thrombocytopenia is among the most frequent dose-limiting toxicity of nearly all chemotherapeutic drugs.[14] The risk of life-threatening, spontaneous hemorrhage, including intracranial hemorrhage, increases as the platelet count drops below $20,000/mm^3$, and is especially a risk when the platelet count declines below $5,000/mm^3$.[15] Yet, despite the frequent occurrence of thrombocytopenia from cytotoxic chemotherapy, intracranial hemorrhages are rare. In the report from Packer and co-workers, only three of 700 patients with cancer experienced intracranial hemorrhages.[12] All had neuroblastoma and were refractory to platelet transfusions because of presumed alloimmunization.

Treatment of chemotherapy-induced thrombocytopenia consists of platelet transfusions. Prophylactic platelet transfusions are generally safe and can be effective in preventing spontaneous intracranial hemorrhage; however, platelet transfusions are expensive and are associated with side effects, including non-hemolytic febrile transfusion reactions; alloimmunization and, rarely, hemolysis, bacteremia, graft-versus-host disease, and acute pulmonary injury. Although there is considerable interest in therapies that stimulate bone marrow to produce more platelets, no therapy has yet been demonstrated as effective and safe and approved for use in children. Thrombopoietin receptor agonists include romiplostim, human interleukin-11, recombinant human thrombopoietin, and pegylated recombinant human megakaryocytic growth and development factor.

Strokes Occur Following Completion of Cancer Therapy

Radiation-Induced Vasculopathy and Thrombotic Strokes

Radiation therapy is an established component of therapy for many childhood malignancies, including primary brain tumors, sarcomas of the head and neck,

Hodgkin's disease, lymphomas, and CNS leukemia. Vasculopathy, including stroke, premature atherosclerosis, and carotid artery stenosis and thrombosis have been reported as late sequelae of radiation therapy.[16] In the report from the Childhood Cancer Survivors Study, the occurrence of late-occurring stroke among brain tumor survivors treated with cranial radiation therapy was significantly higher than those not treated with cranial radiation therapy ($p = 0.02$).[4] The rate of late-occurring stroke in brain tumor survivors who were treated with cranial RT was 339.5 per 100,000 person-years (95% CI: 249.7–448.5) compared with 117.9 per 100,000 person-years (95% CI: 53.9–219.5; $p = 0.02$). In another study, Bowers and co-workers reported symptomatic strokes among 13 of 807 consecutive patients with CNS tumors in the nonperioperative period.[17] The incidence of stroke among survivors of childhood CNS tumors was 4.03 strokes per 1,000 person-years. Risk factors for the subsequent development of a stroke were treatment with radiation therapy and a tumor type of an optic pathway glioma. Omura and co-workers reported cerebrovascular disease in six of 32 childhood brain tumor survivors at 2–13 years following cranial RT. All six patients had symptomatic cerebrovasular disease (stroke and transient ischemic attacks).[18] In all patients, stenotic or occlusive disease in the large cerebral arteries (internal carotid artery, anterior cerebral artery, and middle cerebral artery) was identified. Fouladi and co-workers reported 25 of 421 consecutive children with CNS tumors treated with radiation therapy (many also received chemotherapy) that developed clinically silent white matter lacunar lesions.[19] The lacunar lesions first appeared at an average of two years after radiation therapy, were more common in children less than five-years-old, and appeared to be progressive. Their clinical significance is not known.

In a report of adult patients treated with radiation therapy for head and neck cancer, stenosis of the internal carotid artery of greater than 70% was identified in 11.7% of patients.[20] Another study of adults with head and neck cancer identified a relative risk of 10.1 for carotid artery occlusive disease and stroke following treatment with radiation therapy.[21] Whereas the median interval from radiation therapy to stroke was 10.9 years in this report, radiation-induced vasculopathy is a disease that will likely affect childhood brain tumor survivors for many decades following completion of therapy.

Vascular Injury Induced by Chemotherapeutic Agents

In contrast to radiation therapy, the impact of chemotherapy on the risk of future stroke is poorly understood. In the report from the Childhood Cancer Survivors Study, treatment with an alkylating agent modified the risk of stroke in brain tumor survivors who had cranial radiation therapy.[4] Compared to the sibling cohort, the relative risk of late-occurring stroke among brain tumor survivors treated with cranial radiation therapy plus an alkylating agent was 78.3 (95% CI: 35.1–174.5; $P < 0.0001$).

Endothelial cell injury has been reported with many chemotherapeutic agents. Doxorubicin, vincristine, and bleomycin have been shown to cause endothelial cell retraction and increased platelet adhesion in vivo.[22] The clinical significance of this finding in children with cancer is not clear.

Mineralizing Microangiopathy

In 1978, Price and Birdwell reported distinctive vascular lesions within the brains of children with leukemia at autopsy.[23] They described noninflammatory, mineralizing microangiopathy that occurred within smaller arteries, arterioles, capillaries, and venules, usually accompanied by necrosis and calcification of adjacent neural tissue. The mineralizing process usually occluded the lumens of smaller vessels. The lesions always included the vessels of the putamen of the lenticular nucleus and, occasionally, other regions of the brain. Children most likely to have mineralizing microangiopathy had suffered multiple CNS leukemia relapses, been treated with CNS radiation therapy and methotrexate, and had survived for 10 months after CNS irradiation. They concluded that delayed-onset mineralizing microangiopathy in children with leukemia was the result of CNS radiation therapy, in doses as low as 1,500 cGy. Other authors report that the presence of CNS leukemia and treatment with either high-dose or intrathecal methotrexate is associated with the occurrence of mineralizing microangiopathy.[24,25]

Potential Risk Factors for Stroke in Childhood Brain Tumor Survivors

Hyperhomocysteinemia

Mild hyperhomocysteinemia is a strong, independent risk factor for stroke in otherwise healthy adults and children.[26–30] Through its inhibition of dihydrofolate reductase, methotrexate blocks normal intracellular folate cycling. The major methyl donor required by methionine synthase for the transmethylation of homocysteine to methionine is 5-methyltetrahydrofolate. Depletion of 5-methyltetrahydrofolate by methotrexate causes increased homocysteine and decreased methionine concentrations in plasma. Transient hyperhomocysteinemia and increased CSF concentrations of homocysteine have been reported after administering high-dose methotrexate in children with leukemia and osteosarcoma.[28–30] Atherosclerotic cerebrovascular disease as a result of hyperhomocysteinemia caused by treatment with methotrexate for brain tumors has not been studied.

Young adult survivors of childhood brain tumors are at increased risk of developing the combination of obesity, hyperinsulinemia, and dyslipidemia, which are strong risk factors for the development of atherosclerotic vascular disease and stroke.[31,32] Patients who are treated with cranial radiation therapy may be at particular risk for these conditions.[32] Although the absolute risk of stroke in these adult survivors of childhood leukemia is unknown, it is concerning that these patients frequently possess multiple risk factors for stroke in young adulthood.

Evaluation of Childhood Brain Tumor Survivors with Stroke

Whereas non-cancer-related causes may result in a stroke, childhood brain tumor survivors should be evaluated for an inherited predisposition to stroke. This includes a review of family history of thrombosis, including the occurrence of a stroke, deep vein thrombosis, and pulmonary embolus. A review of medications (e.g., oral contraceptive medications) and smoking history should also be performed. Finally, it is recommended that childhood brain tumor survivors who experience stroke should be evaluated for the presence of a hypercoaguable state by measuring activity of proteins C, S, and antithrombin, activated protein C resistance, Factor V Leiden, lipoprotein(a), lupus anticoagulant and anticardiolipin antibodies, and mutations of the MTHFR, FVL, prothrombin, and PAI genes.

The prognosis for stroke in childhood brain tumor survivors is highly variable, as a result of differences in patients' coagulation systems (both inherited and acquired), primary malignancy, cancer treatment (especially radiation therapy) and extent of neurological deficits. As a general rule, strokes that occur soon after diagnosis or during therapy are not likely to reoccur upon completion of therapy as long as patients' cancer remains in remission. However, strokes that occur after completion of therapy, such as a result of radiation-induced vasculopathy, may reoccur. Long-term stroke prophylaxis should be considered for childhood brain tumor survivors who have strokes after completing therapy.

Given their rarity and the multifactorial etiology of stroke in childhood brain tumor survivors, there have never been any studies to determine the best stroke prophylaxis in childhood brain tumor survivors. The following paragraphs on stroke prophylactic therapy are based on experience with adults with atherosclerotic cerebrovascular disease and should be interpreted with caution given the distinct differences in the disease processes.

There are no clinical trials evaluating the use of intravenous tissue plasminogen activator (t-PA) as urgent treatment of stroke among childhood brain tumor survivors. In studies of adults with acute stroke, the use of t-PA within three hours of symptoms was associated with improved patient outcomes.[33] The most common treatment-related side effect was intracranial hemorrhage. There is no experience with the use of t-PA in childhood brain tumor survivors who have had a stroke.

Aspirin is often the first drug for patients with cerebral ischemia.[34,35] However, there are no controlled trials on the use of aspirin or any other antiplatelet agents in children with ischemic cerebral infarction. Nevertheless, an antithrombotic dose of daily aspirin is frequently used for children with arterial ischemia stroke to prevent recurrent stroke. However, the clinical effectiveness of aspirin in preventing recurrent stroke in children and cancer survivors is unknown.

There have been no studies of the effectiveness of heparin or low-molecular weight heparin in childhood brain tumor survivors who have had a stroke. An initial study of adult patients with stroke who received low-molecular weight heparin for 10 days within 48 hours after diagnosis of stroke had a better outcome; however, subsequent larger studies have not confirmed these findings, and in fact have demonstrated that adult patients treated with aspirin therapy had superior outcome and less secondary hemorrhage than patients treated with heparin. Whether this observation is true in childhood cancer survivors is unknown. The use of heparin or low-molecular weight heparin for stroke may reduce the frequency of secondary infarction by an embolus, recurrence of an infarction, or extension of an infarction.[36] However, it should be used with caution because of the potential for secondary hemorrhage. In general, children can be treated along similar guidelines as adults with reasonably low frequency of secondary hemorrhage.

Note the use of heparin and low-molecular weight heparin may induce osteoporosis, which makes these agents unattractive for long-term anticoagulation in children and adults. Warfarin is the most effective method of long-term anticoagulation in children and adults. It is generally safe in children, with relatively low risks of hemorrhage. The dose of warfarin should be adjusted to achieve an internationalized normalized ratio (INR) of 2.0–3.0.

Conclusions

There are many cancer-specific and time-specific cerebrovascular insults among childhood brain tumor survivors. Familiarity with the clinical syndromes may lead to a better understanding of the etiology of strokes and their treatment in this patient population. Much additional research is needed to fully understand and prevent the many different causes of strokes among childhood brain tumor survivors.

References

1. Broderick J, Talbot GT, Prenger E, Leach A. Stroke in children within a major metropolitan area: the surprising importance of intracerebral hemorrhage. *J Child Neurol.* 1993;8: 250–255.
2. Schoenberg BS, Mellinger JF, Schoenberg DG. Cerebrovascular disease in infants and children: a study of incidence, clinical features, and survival. *Neurology.* 1978;28:763–768.

3. deVeber G, Roach ES, Riela AR, Wiznitzer M. Stroke in children: recognition, treatment, and future directions. *Semin Pediatr Neurol.* 2000;7:309–317.
4. Bowers DC, Liu Y, Leisenring W, et al. Late-occurring stroke among long-term survivors of childhood leukemia and brain tumors: a report from the Childhood Cancer Survivor Study. *J Clin Oncol.*2006;24: 5277–5282.
5. Grill J, Couanet D, Cappelli C, et al. Radiation-induced cerebral vasculopathy in children with neurofibromatosis and optic pathway glioma. *Ann Neurol.*1999;45:393–396.
6. Bowers DC, Mulne AF, Reisch JS, et al. Non-perioperative strokes in children with central nervous system tumors. *Cancer.*2002;94:1094–1101.
7. Omura M, Aida N, Sekido K, Kakehi M, Matsubara S. Large intracranial vessel occlusive vasculopathy after radiation therapy in children: clinical features and usefulness of magnetic resonance imaging.*Int J Radiat Oncol Biol Phys.*1997;38:241–249.
8. Poussaint TY, Siffert J, Barnes PD, et al. Hemorrhagic vasculopathy after central nervous system neoplasia in childhood: diagnosis and follow-up. *AJNR.*1995;16:693–699.
9. Epstein MA, Packer RJ, Rorke LB, Zimmerman RA, Goldwein JW, Sutton LN, Schut L. Vascular malformation with radiation vasculopathy after treatment of chiasmatic/hypothalamic glioma. *Cancer.*1992;70:887–893.
10. Yokota A, Kajiwara H, Matsuoka S, Kohchi M, Matsukado Y, Subarachnoid hemorrhage from brain tumors in childhood. *Child Nerv Sys.* 1987;3;65–69.
11. Scarfo GB, Piane R, Mencattini G, Tomaccini D. Stroke-like onset of pineal region tumors in two children. *Child's Brain.* 1982;9:274–279.
12. Packer RJ, Lange BJ, Rorke LB, Siegel KR, Evans AE. Cerebrovascular accidents in children with cancer. *Pediatrics.* 1985;76:194–201.
13. Sutton LN, Gusnard D, Bruce DA, Fried A, Packer RJ, Zimmerman RA. Fusiform dilatation of the carotid artery following radical surgery of childhood craniopharyngiomas. *J Neurosurg.*1991;74:695–700.
14. Cairo MS. Dose reductions and delays: limitations of myelosuppressive chemotherapy. *Oncology (Huntington).* 2000;14:21–31.
15. Schroeder ML. Principles and practice of transfusion medicine. In: Lee GR, Foerster J, Lukens J, eds. *Wintrobe's Clinical Hematology.* New York, NY: Thieme Medical, 1999:817–874.
16. Mitchell WG, Fishman LS, Miller JH, Nelson M, Zeltzer PM, Soni D. Stroke as a late sequela of cranial irradiation for childhood brain tumors. J Child Neurol. 1991;6:28–133.
17. Bowers DC, Mulne AF, Reisch JS, et al. Nonperioperative strokes in children with central nervous system tumors. *Cancer.* 2002;94:1094–1101.
18. Omura M, Aida N, Sekido K, Kakehi M, Matsubara S. Large intracranial vessel occlusive vasculopathy after radiation therapy in children: clinical features and usefulness of magnetic resonance imaging. *Int J Radiat Oncol Biol Phys.* 1997;38:241–249.
19. Fouladi M, Langston J, Mulhern R, et al. Silent lacunar lesions detected by magnetic resonance imaging of children with brain tumors: a late sequela of therapy. *J Clin Oncol.* 2000;18:824–831.
20. Murros KE, Toole JF. The effect of radiation on carotid arteries. *Arch Neurol.* 1989;46:449–455.
21. Dorresteijn LDA, Kappelle AC, Boogerd W, et al. Increased risk of ischemic stroke after radiotherapy on the neck in patients younger than 60 years. *J Clin Oncol.* 2002;20: 282–288.
22. Nicolson GL, Custead SE, Effects of chemotherapeutic drugs on platelet and metastatic tumor cell-endothelial cell interactions as a model for assessing vascular endothelial integrity. *Cancer Res.* 1985;45:331–336.
23. Price RA, Birdwell DA. The central nervous system in childhood leukemia. III. Mineralizing microangiopathy and dystrophic calcification. *Cancer.* 1978;42:717–728.
24. Phanthumchinda K, Intragumtornchai T, Kasantikul V. Stroke-like syndrome, mineralizing microangiopathy, and neuroaxonal dystrophy following intrathecal methotrexate therapy. *Neurology.* 1991;41(11):1847–1848.

25. Waber DP, Tarbell NJ, Fairclough D, Atmore K, Castro R, Isquith P. Cognitive sequelae of treatment in childhood acute lymphoblastic leukemia: cranial radiation requires an accomplice. *J Clin Oncol*. 1995;13:2490–2496.
26. Clarke R, Daly L, Robinson K, Naughten E, Cahalane S, Fowler B, et al. Hyperhomocysteinemia: an independent risk factor for vascular disease. *N Engl J Med*. 1991;324:1149–1155.
27. Bostom AG, Rosenberg IH, Silbershatz H, Jacques PF, Selhub J, D'Agostino RB. Nonfasting plasma total homocysteine levels and stroke incidence in elderly persons: the Framingham Study. *Ann Intern Med*. 1999;131(5):352–355.
28. Broxson EH Jr., Stork LC, Allen RH, Stabler SP, Kolhouse JF. Changes in plasma methionine and total homocysteine levels in patients receiving methotrexate infusions. *Cancer Res*. 1989;49:5879–5883.
29. Kishi S, Griener J, Cheng C, et al. Homocysteine, pharmacogenetics, and neurotoxicity in children with leukemia. *J Clin Oncol*. 2003;21:3084–3091.
30. Quinn CT, Griener JC, Bottiglieri T, Hyland K, Farrow A, Kamen BA. Elevation of homocysteine and excitatory amino acid neurotransmitters in the CSF of children who receive methotrexate for the treatment of cancer. *J Clin Oncol*. 1997;15:2800–2806.
31. Talvensaari KK, Lanning M, Tapanainen P, Knip M. Long-term survivors of childhood cancer have an increased risk of manifesting the metabolic syndrome. *J Clin Endocrinol Metab*. 1996;81:3051–3055.
32. Oeffinger KC, Buchanan GR. Eshelman DA, et al. Cardiovascular risk factors in young adult survivors of childhood acute lymphoblastic leukemia. *J Pediatr Hematol Oncol*. 2001 23:424–430.
33. Brott T, Bogousslavsky J. Treatment of acute ischemic stroke. *N Eng J Med*.2000; 343:710–722.
34. Antiplatelet Trialists' Collaboration. Collaborative overview of randomised trials of antiplatelet therapy. I. Prevention of death, myocardial infarction, and stroke by prolonged antiplatelet therapy in various categories of patients. *Brit Med J*. 1994;308:81–106.
35. Barnett HJM, Eliasziw M. Meldrum HE. Drugs and surgery in the prevention of ischemic stroke. *N Engl J Med*. 1995;332:238–248.
36. Dix D, Andrew M, Marzinotto V, et al. The use of low molecular weight heparin in pediatric patients: a prospective cohort study. *J Pediatr*. 2000;136:439–445.

Chapter 11
Endocrine Late Effects: Manifestations and Treatments

Jason R. Fangusaro and Elizabeth Eaumann Littlejohn

Introduction

Central nervous system (CNS) tumors are the most common solid tumors encountered in pediatrics and are a significant cause of morbidity in adults. The Central Brain Tumor Registry of the United States (CBTRUS) reports that the incidence rate of all primary CNS tumors is 14.8 per 100,000 person-years for adults and 4.3 cases per person-years for children.[1] Overall, CNS tumors are second only to acute lymphoblastic leukemia (ALL) as the most common malignancy among children, and brain tumors account for approximately 25% of all cancer deaths among children in addition to the significant morbidities associated with treatment.

The range of endocrine abnormalities that arise in survivors of brain tumors is wide. Dysfunction can arise from numerous abnormalities including direct endocrine organ damage and/or abnormalities of the hypothalamic-pituitary axis. Many patients will develop growth hormone deficiency as a direct consequence of radiation damage to the hypothalamic-pituitary axis.[2] A common late effect of radiotherapy in children is the development of precocious puberty. This is thought be a consequence of disinhibition of cortical control upon the hypothalamus.[3] One of the endocrine organs with the most prevalent and common late effects is the thyroid gland. Late effects upon the thyroid can include thyroid stimulating hormone (TSH) deficiency or central hypothyroidism, primary hypothyroidism, the development of thyroid nodules and thyroid malignancy, as well as hyperthyroidism.[4] Radiotherapy to the hypothalamic-pituitary axis can also lead to hyperprolactinemia in addition to the more well-recognized central hypothyroidism.[5] Gonadotropin deficiency is also a common finding among adult survivors who received high

J.R. Fangusaro (✉)
Department of Pediatric Hematology/Oncology and Stem Cell Transplantation, Children's Memorial Hospital, 2300 Children's Plaza, Box #30, Chicago, IL, USA
e-mail: jfangusaro@childrensmemorial.org

S. Goldman, C.D. Turner (eds.), *Late Effects of Treatment for Brain Tumors*, Cancer Treatment and Research 150, DOI 10.1007/b109924_11, © Springer Science+Business Media, LLC 2009

155

doses of radiation as part of their brain tumor therapy.[6,7] Many patients will also develop gonadal failure and infertility, often secondary to chemotherapy, in addition to radiotherapy.[7–9]

As suggested by the abnormalities mentioned above, many patients will develop panhypopituitarism with dysfunction of the entire anterior pituitary axis.[6,10] As is common among many survivors of childhood acute lympho-blastic leukemia (ALL), patients with a history of pediatric brain tumors have an increased risk of developing obesity.[11,12] This obesity can be multifactorial; causes include hypothyroidism and hypothalamic obesity. There is also a risk of osteopenia, particularly after craniospinal irradiation (CSI).[13–16] Manage-ment strategies for osteopenia remain poorly defined in children due to the risk of fertility problems associated with the use of bisphosphonates. Finally, many patients are at risk for developing spinal radiation syndrome which leads to short stature. Each of these endocrinologic abnormalities will be addressed individually within the context of this chapter. We will focus upon the pathophysiology, detection, evaluation and treatment of each endocrine abnormality.

Hypothalamic-Pituitary and Growth Hormone Axes

A broad overview of the hypothalamic-pituitary axis and function of this system is required in order to understand the implications of damage to this area. The hypothalamus can be considered the coordinating center of the pituitary endocrine system. It consolidates signals derived from upper cortical inputs, autonomic function, environmental cues such as light and tempera-ture, as well as peripheral endocrine feedback. In turn, the hypothalamus delivers precise signals to the pituitary gland which then releases hormones that influence most endocrine organs in the body. Specifically, the hypotha-lamic-pituitary (HP) axis directly affects the functions of the thyroid gland, the adrenal gland or stress system and the reproductive system, as well as influencing growth, milk production and water balance

The pituitary secretes seven sets of hormones. Those manufactured and secreted from the anterior pituitary are growth hormone (GH), adrenocortico-tropin hormone (ACTH), luteinizing hormone (LH)/follicle stimulating hormone (FSH), thyroid stimulating hormone (TSH) and Prolactin (PRL).[17] The hormones that are manufactured and secreted from the posterior pituitary are Arginine vasopressin (AVP) or antidiuretic hormone (ADH) and Oxytocin. (Please refer to the Table 11.1 and Fig. 11.1). The major pituitary hormones are stimulated or inhibited by a number of factors (Table 11.1).

Some general statements that can be made about the effects of cancer therapies on the HP axis are as follows. There is correlation between the total radiation dose and the development of pituitary hormone deficits.[18] For instance, after lower radiation as used in the treatment of some brain tumors,

Table 11.1 Major hypothalamic hormones and their effect on anterior pituitary hormones

Hypothalamic stimulatory hormones	Pituitary hormones
Corticotropin-releasing hormone – 41 amino acids; released from paraventricular neurons as well as supraoptic and arcuate nuclei and limbic system	Adrenocorticotropic hormone – basophilic corticotrophs represent 20% of cells in anterior pituitary; ACTH is product of proopiomelanocortin (POMC) gene Melanocyte-stimulating hormone – alternate product of POMC gene Endorphins – also products of POMC gene
Growth hormone-releasing hormone – two forms, 40 and 44 amino acids	Growth hormone – acidophilic somatotrophs represent 50% of cells in anterior pituitary
Gonadotropin-releasing hormone – 10 amino acids; mostly released from preoptic neurons	Luteinizing hormone and follicle-stimulating hormone – gonadotrophs represent about 15% of anterior pituitary cells
Thyrotropin-releasing hormone – three amino acids; released from anterior hypothalamic area	Thyroid-stimulating hormone – thyrotropes represent about 5% of anterior pituitary cells
Prolactin-releasing factors – include serotonin, acetylcholine, opiates, and estrogens	Prolactin – lactotrophs represent 10 to 30% of anterior pituitary cells
Hypothalamic inhibitory hormones	
Somatostatin – 14 amino acids	Inhibits the release of growth hormone

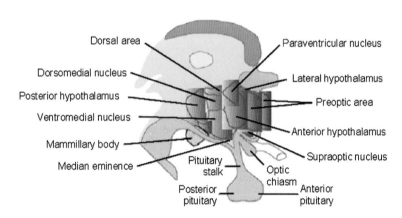

Fig. 11.1 Anatomy of the hypothalamic-pituitary axis
Anatomic relationships of the hypothalamic-pituitary axis. Hormones released from the hypothalamus are released into the median eminence and then move down the pituitary stalk to the pituitary gland. Antidiuretic hormone and corticotropin-releasing hormone are secreted by the paraventricular and supraoptic nuclei, gonadotropin-releasing hormone by the preoptic area, and thyrotropin-releasing hormone by the anterior hypothalamus.
Adapted from Krieger, DT, in: Neuroendocrinology, Krieger, DT, Hughes, JC (Eds), Sinauer Associates, Sunderland, MA, 1980, Chapter 2

one may develop GH deficiency in isolation. However, after higher doses of radiation (>60 Gy), panhypopituitarism may develop. Interestingly, diabetes insipidus is not likely to develop following irradiation to the HP axis. Also, the same dose given in fewer fractions over a short period of time is likely to cause greater damage and severity of pituitary hormone deficiencies than the same dose given over a longer time interval with a greater number of fractions.[19] More specifically, the degree of anterior pituitary hormone deficiency has been correlated with the biological effective dose of radiation affecting the HP axis. The hypothalamus is more radiosensitive and is damaged by lower doses of cranial radiation than the pituitary gland. Thus, after lower doses of radiation (<50 Gy) the hypothalamus is affected and leads to isolated GH deficiency, whereas higher doses cause direct anterior pituitary damage as well and, thus, contribute to early and multiple pituitary hormone deficiencies.[20] HP dysfunction is also time-dependent. There is an increase in the frequency and severity of hormonal deficits with increasing time after radiotherapy. This phenomenon can be attributed to atrophy of the pituitary gland following previous hypothalamic damage.[21] The damaging effects of radiation on HP axis function is increased when the HP axis is already affected by an additional pathology (e.g., such as interference by a central nervous system malignancy itself and/ or surgery). GH producing cells appear to be the most radiosensitive followed by ACTH producing cells. TSH producing cells are least likely to be affected. Children seem more radiosensitive than adults, and older children are less vulnerable than younger children.[19] Chemotherapy may potentiate the damaging effects of radiation.[22]

Given the fact that children affected by pituitary hormone deficiencies post-therapy often present with short stature, it is prudent to understand some basics with regard to the assessment of the short child. The differential diagnosis of short stature in cancer survivors is the same as that considered for all children undergoing an evaluation for statural growth. A general paradigm is as follows: understanding the basic concept that normal children enter puberty at a pubertal somatic maturational age (bone age). Intrinsic short stature (ISS) is commonly a normal variant that has a polygenic and characteristically non-pathologic basis. It is characterized by a normal bone age (age for which the bone maturation is average) that is equal to the chronologic age (calendar age) with both being greater than height age (age for which the height is average) in the presence of a normal growth velocity. However, this growth pattern can also result from a variety of congenital disorders with or without intrauterine growth retardation (IUGR). Although most infants with IUGR catch up to their normal peers in the first 6–12 months postnatally, the remainder follow a pattern consistent with that of ISS or a delayed pattern of growth (see below). Occasionally, IUGR is associated with severe postnatal growth failure (primordial growth failure). Multiple congenital anomalies or dysmorphisms may suggest chromosomal or genetic disorders. Bone dysplasia may be indicated by disproportionate growth, achondroplasia being the most common. The most common primordial dysmorphic syndrome is Russell-Silver syndrome. Patients exhibit normal head circumference in the presence of short stature, small and triangular facies, clinodactyly, bony asymmetry and poor weight gain in infancy. Turner's syndrome is the most common pathologic cause of short stature in girls. Pseudohypoparathyroidism and hypocalcemia is associated with ISS.[23] Radiation damage to the spinal cord would also be placed into the category of ISS.

An extreme variation of normal or "constitutional delay" (CGD) is the most common cause of a delayed pattern of growth defined as height age (HA) equaling bone age (BA) with both less than the chronologic age (CA) in the presence of a normal growth velocity. Frequently there is familial precedence. Birth size is generally normal; however, length then crosses growth channels by 2–3 years of age with BA and weight age retarded, then HA and BA advance at a normal rate. There is delay of puberty until the child reaches a pubertal BA. A normal pubertal growth spurt culminates in a normal adult height, albeit late, thus allowing a catch up of growth. This pattern of growth may also be detected in cancer survivors and is a normal variant. It may confound the evaluation of short stature due to hormone deficits. Alternatively, a delayed pattern of growth has other causes that may also be pertinent to post-cancer treatment patients. Other causes include undernutrition, rickets, tissue hypoxia, chronic anemia, heart disease and chronic diseases of any variety of organ systems. Since CGD is a diagnosis of exclusion and is difficult to distinguish from subtle deficits of GH or gonadotropins, which can occur in cancer survivors,[23] one must follow and evaluate further if indicated.

An attenuated growth pattern is clearly abnormal and is the result of endocrine, metabolic, severe systemic disease or a combination of these. The pattern is characterized by HA = BA or HA < BA with both less than CA in the presence of a subnormal growth velocity for BA. It is usually the result of hormonal deficiencies due to HP axis abnormalities and/or primary endocrinopathies, severe medical illnesses and/or extra HP-axial abnormalities that seriously alter the functioning of the HP axis.[23] Deficiency of GH is the most common and occurs in post-cancer survivors. Functional GH deficiency can also occur in emotional deprivation (or extreme stress) and resistance to GH occurs rarely. Attenuation of growth is experienced in glucocorticoid excess and primary or secondary/tertiary hypothyroidism (pituitary or hypothalamic dysfunction, respectively). Severe chronic disease of any organ system and/or severe malnutrition can attenuate linear growth if sustained long enough.[23]

Supra-normal height occurs as the result of inherent genetic endowment or an excessive stimulation of rate of bone growth. The diagnostic approach is similar to that used for the patient who is short. In the cancer patient it may be encountered as a growth pattern that is familial or the result of hormone excesses (sex steroids or GH) that might occur after HP axis disturbance due to surgery or irradiation,[23] but is rare in comparison to stunting of growth post-therapy.

Specific and commonly encountered diagnoses in post-brain cancer treatment that are related to the HP axis must include GH deficiency as the most commonly encountered pituitary hormone deficiency. GH deficiency is a known consequence of brain tumors themselves, and/or central nervous system (CNS) irradiation as treatment for primary brain tumors, or total body irradiation (TBI) in preparation for hematopoietic stem cell transplantation in brain tumors or other cancers. We will concentrate on the GH deficiency encountered in the former. GH deficiency is diagnosed by documenting an abnormal GH secretion in response to two stimulatory events of the growth axis (stimulation testing, sleep-related GH secretion or physiologic stimuli such as exercise or hypoglycemia), in the presence of a delayed BA and subnormal growth velocity. Once the diagnosis is made, GH replacement is provided to the patient to administer subcutaneously using either the pediatric or adult recommended dosages while monitoring for adverse effects and serum levels of insulin-like growth factor-1 (IGF-1).

The pituitary or the hypothalamic area that communicates to the somatotroph in the pituitary is often directly affected by radiation. The relationship between the radiation dose to the hypothalamus and the time to onset of clinically significant GH deficiency is unknown. A study correlating the dosimetry of radiation to the hypothalamus and the peak GH value after cranial-spinal radiotherapy (CRT) in children with localized primary brain tumors, demonstrated that peak GH responses within 12 months after CRT depends on hypothalamic dose-volume effects and may be predicted on the basis of a linear model that sums the effects of the entire distribution of the dose. The modeled effects may be used to optimize radiotherapy while minimizing and treating GH deficienc.[24] Recent evidence suggests that 100% of pediatric patients treated with radiation doses in excess of 30 Gy have blunted responses to GH stimulation tests and that those with less than 30 Gy will have normal responses to GH stimulation testing even after 2–5 years post-therapy.[25]

Radiation-induced GH neurosecretory dysfunction (or hypothalamic dysfunction) is a known clinical entity that is poorly described, following radiation to the HP axis, and is not easy to diagnose using standard criteria. It is characterized by preserved response to GH provocative testing with diminished physiological GH secretion in the presence of slowed linear growth. The reported frequency may thus be low and the prevalence may be underestimated. However, the discrepancy between stimulated and physiological spontaneous GH secretion disappears with time, suggesting that those who develop impaired GH provocative responses might have had a neurosecretory deficit at an earlier stage.[26]

It has been suggested that radiation-induced GH neurosecretory dysfunction exists more commonly in childhood cancer survivors than in adults. The pathophysiology is poorly understood and has mostly been studied in adults. One study looked at 24-hour spontaneous GH secretion in adult cancer survivors with normal GH status defined by two GH provocative tests, 13.1 +/- 1.6 (range, 3–28) years after cranial irradiation (18–40 Gy) for nonpituitary brain tumors or leukemia in comparison with age and body mass index matched normal controls. Using previously published diagnostic thresholds, all patients had stimulated peak GH responses in the normal range in response to both an insulin tolerance test and the combined growth hormone-releasing hormone (GHRH) plus arginine stimulation test, as well as normal individual mean profile GH levels during the fed and fasting states. However, despite gender-specific comparisons that revealed marked reduction (by 40%) in the overall peak GH responses to both provocative tests, but similar GH secretory profiles, no differences were seen in the pulsatile attributes of GH secretion (cluster analysis) or the profile absolute and mean GH levels in the fed state or when the hypothalamic-pituitary axis was stimulated by fasting. Thus, it was concluded that radiation-induced GH neurosecretory dysfunction either does not exist or is a very rare phenomenon in irradiated adult cancer survivors. Yet the phenomenon is known to exist in children using the end points of growth, e.g., poor growth in the presence of normal stimulatory release of GH post-pituitary stimulation, and response to GH after replacement. Whether hypothalamic control of the somatotrophs is important after childhood is, therefore, controversial. Regardless, neurosecretory dysfunction remains poorly defined in childhood, yet we believe it to be an entity that requires evaluation and treatment.

Alternatively, normality of physiological GH secretion in the context of reduced maximum somatotroph reserve might suggest compensatory overdrive of the partially damaged somatotroph axis. This may constitute a relative argument against somatotroph dysfunction being explained purely by hypothalamic damage with secondary atrophy due to GHRH deficiency. It is therefore possible that radiation in doses less than 40 Gy may actually cause dual damage to both the pituitary and the hypothalamus.[27] It appears that this phenomenon may be more relevant and affect children more so than adults due to the demands of growth. For instance, perhaps for adults with these minor deficits, the overall GH status may be compensated, whereas in children they are not well compensated for due to the rigors of growth. In other words, neurosecretory defect or minor somatotroph abnormality with compensation may be clinically unapparent in adults, yet apparent in children via poor growth velocity. These controversies require acknowledgement due to the fact that neurosecretory defect remains an entity that is poorly understood in childhood survivors of cancer.

As in vitro and in vivo studies, epidemiologic observations provide some evidence that the GH-IGF-1 axis is associated with tumorigenesis, and it is important to assess, in practice, the incidence of tumors related to GH treatment as this remains a concern as endocrine replacement therapy of the cancer survivors ensue. Reassuringly, surveillance studies in large cohorts of children and in smaller cohorts of adults indicate that GH is not associated with an increased incidence of tumor occurrence or recurrence. Nevertheless, all children who have received GH, in particular cancer survivors and those receiving GH in adulthood, should be in surveillance programs to assess whether an increased rate of late-onset and rare tumors may occur.[28] Tumor recurrence rates in surviving patients with brain tumors receiving GH treatment do not appear to be increased compared with published reports. However, longer follow-up regarding recurrences and secondary neoplasms is essential.[29]

The Hypothalamic-Pituitary-Gonadal and Adrenal Axes

The effect of cranial irradiation on the hypothalamic-pituitary-gonadal axis is dose-dependent; specifically doses of radiation >50 Gy are likely to result in gonadotropin deficiency whereas doses <50 Gy often result in sexual precocity.[3] Early puberty may occur as the result of loss of inhibition at the hypothalamic level. The mechanism for early puberty following irradiation is thought to be due to the disinhibition of cortical influences on the hypothalamus.[30,31] In contrast to lower doses associated with sexual precocity in girls, higher doses in boys with brain tumors are associated with sexual precocity as well.[32] Thus, there appears to be a disappearance of sexual dichotomy with higher doses.

As the dose of radiation exceeds 50 Gy in the treatment of brain tumors, there is a progressive increase in the incidence of gonadotropin deficiency. The prevalence also increases with time post-irradiation; a cumulative incidence of 20–50% has been reported in patients followed long-term. Thus, it is the second most common hormone deficit in many serie[18] after GH deficiency. Gonadotropin deficiency exists in a range of severity from subtle or subclinical abnormalities with low normal sex hormone levels to severe impairment associated with subnormal circulating estrogen and/or testosterone levels.

Cranial irradiation for brain tumors not involving the HP axis demonstrated that only 19% of individuals developed ACTH deficiency, even after 15 years of follow-up.[33] It is possible that the hypothalamic-pituitary-adrenal (HPA) axis is affected late by radiation and adequate follow-up data is lacking. Dose of radiation is important as little damage to this axis is encountered in lower doses whereas subtle problems are noticed with higher doses as used in brain tumor treatments over a similar follow-up time. A dose-response relationship was confirmed by a recent follow-up study done in brain tumor survivors.[33] Although an insulin tolerance test is the gold standard for diagnosing ACTH deficiency, it is dangerous as hypoglycemia is induced. The authors use a very low-dose ACTH test (0.6 mcg/1.0 m^2, intravenous push over 30 seconds),[34] to detect a blunted response (serum cortisol of < 17 mcg/dl) in the presence of a normal ACTH level and low dehypdroepiandrosterone-sulphate level, indicative of adrenal atrophy, in the presence of clinical symptomotolgy to make a diagnosis of ACTH deficiency. Stimulation of the HPA axis with corticotrophin-releasing factor (or CRF) is novel and currently under study for detecting ACTH deficiency in children.

The Hypothalamic-Pituitary-Thyroid Axis

The hypothalamic-pituitary-thyroid (HPT) axis is the least vulnerable to radiation damage. The frequency of radiation-induced TSH deficiency is dose-dependen[18] and related to time since irradiation.[35] Making the diagnosis of central hypothyroidism, however, is very difficult. Most clinicians compare baseline thyroid function tests (TFTs) to those after CNS manipulation and make the diagnosis when there is low-normal free T4 level or declining T4 levels in the presence of a low-normal or slightly raised TSH level with or without frank symptoms of hypothyroidism. This concept, along with a free T4 level by dialysis, can be used instead of total T4 levels, as the former is more accurate and less confounded by binding proteins and other environmental disturbances.[36] Some claim that baseline TFTs are insensitive and thyrotropin-releasing hormone (TRH) tests along with the presence or absence of a nocturnal TSH surge are more diagnostically useful.[37] Yet there are problems with the specificity of the TRH test and determining the "absence" of a nocturnal TSH surge in the presence of a normal T4 level, such that these criteria likely are less helpful in making the diagnosis.

The Hypothalamic-Neurohypophyseal System

Central diabetes insipidus is the end result of a number of different insults affecting the hypothalamic-neurohypophyseal system. In many patients, especially children and young adults, it is caused by the destruction or degeneration of neurons that originate in the supraoptic and paraventricular nuclei of the hypothalamus. The broad differential that incorporates all known causes of these lesions include germinoma or craniopharyngioma; Langerhans cell histiocytosis; local inflammatory, autoimmune or vascular diseases; trauma resulting from surgery or an accident; sarcoidosis; metastases, and midline cerebral and cranial malformations. In rare cases, genetic defects in AVP synthesis that are inherited as autosomal dominant, autosomal recessive or X-linked recessive traits are the underlying cause.[38] Most cases of diabetes insipidus that are related to brain tumors arise as a result of surgery in the location of the pituitary or growth of the lesion itself causing interruption of the neurons that supply the posterior pituitary.[39] Rarely has diabetes insipidus been reported following cranial irradiation. There is one case report of a woman who underwent surgical removal of a frontal capillary hemangioblastoma and received cranial irradiation. She presented 10 months later with features of diabetes insipidus that were confirmed to be of central origin. She responded well to desmopressin nasal spray.[40] Radiation-induced damage to the HP axis presents usually with anterior pituitary hormone deficiencies, most commonly that of growth hormone as noted above; thus presentation with central diabetes insipidus is very uncommon.

Hypothalamic Obesity

Obesity is a late effect of cancer survivors and is a risk factor for morbidity in the general population. In brain tumor survivors, radiation in doses of 50 Gy or higher were associated with abnormal 10-year post-therapy body mass index

(BMI) increases and, therefore, is a primary risk factor for obesity as well as young age at diagnosis.[41] BMI weight category at diagnosis, rather than type of CNS treatment received, predicted adult weight in long-term survivors of childhood hematologic malignancies.[42]

Damage to the hypothalamus, particularly to the ventromedial hypothalamus (VMH), is postulated to be responsible for obesity. The VMH theoretically integrates blood-borne information from leptin, ghrelin and insulin, translating the information into regulation of energy balance. Thus, dysregulation of the VMH results in excessive caloric intake and decreased caloric expenditure which results in weight gain.[43] It is hypothesized that VMH damage causes either hyperphagia that results in obesity and compensatory hyperinsulinemia, or dis-inhibition of efferent output of the vagus nerve which acts on the pancreatic β cell to promote excessive insulin secretion. Lustig et al. demonstrated that reducing hyperinsulinemia in 18 cancer survivors with hypothalamic damage using octreo-tide, a long-acting somatostatin analogue that binds to the somatostatin receptor 5 (SSTR5) on the β cell, resulted in inhibition of intracellular calcium influx and attenuated insulin release.[44]

Other factors that induce obesity in patients with brain tumors include the use of high-dose glucocorticoids which promotes obesity by affecting appetite, regulation of energy intake, alteration in substrate oxidation and/or alteration in energy expenditure.[45] Hypopituitarism and resultant GH deficiency has numerous metabolic effects placing the individual at risk for obesity; GH therapy has been shown to reverse these effects.[46] More specifically, an elevated systolic blood pressure, increased waist-hip ratio and an adverse lipid profile were commonly seen in brain tumor survivors more so than in normal controls. These abnormalities were particularly pronounced in those with untreated GH deficiency.[47]

Additionally, neurological complications associated with intracranial tumors and their treatment may have adverse effects on motor function which may reduce physical activity and predispose to obesity. Lifestyle advice on diet and exercise must be employed early, yet hypothalamic obesity may be resistant to these measures. More focal irradiation schedules for tumors in the posterior fossa and temporal lobes may reduce incidental hypothalamic irradiation. A role for controlling hyperinsulinemia by octreotide for severe cases may be present, yet randomized control trials of efficacy are required.[48]

Hyperinsulinism (HI) and its associated metabolic abnormalities, including diabetes mellitus (DM), have been reported in long-term survivors of childhood cancer, mainly after bone marrow transplant (BMT); however, the predisposing factors are unclear, and early markers have not been identified. Overweight/obesity was not increased when comparing subjects with controls; however, the prevalence of abdominal adiposity in prepubertal and pubertal subjects was roughly doubled ($P \leq 0.04$). Fasting insulin concentrations were higher in prepubertal and pubertal subjects compared with their controls ($P < 0.001$) and were similar in adult and pubertal subjects. HI, impaired glucose tolerance (IGT) or DM was detected in 39 of 212 (18%) pubertal or adult subjects (23 of

67 with BMT). Ten of 88 (11%) pubertal and 14 of 124 (11%) adult subjects had IGT/DM (vs. 0 and 4.9% controls, respectively; P < 0.001). Total body irradiation, untreated hypogonadism, and abdominal adiposity emerged as independent risk factors for the development of HI, IGT, or DM in a multivariate regression analysis. The risk factors identified suggest a need to reconsider BMT protocols and regular screening of survivors. The increased prevalence of abdominal adiposity among prepubertal subjects, none of whom had developed HI/IGT/DM, suggests that a waist–to–height ratio greater than 0.5 has potential as a clinical screening tool.[49]

Direct Endocrine Organ Damage

Many of the endocrinologic pathologies encountered in adult survivors of brain tumors are the result of a direct toxicity upon one of the many endocrine organs either from surgical trauma, chemotherapy, radiotherapy or a combination of the three. This damage often renders the specific organ as non-functional or dysfunctional, leading to a variety of endocrinopathies.

Gonadal Function

Many brain tumor survivors sustain gonadal damage and failure both from dysregulation and damage to the hypothalamic-pituitary axis as well as secondary to a direct toxic effect upon the gonads. This direct gonad toxicity arises almost exclusively as a result of the gonado-toxic effects of adjuvant chemotherapy. The toxicity sustained by the gonads is often dose–dependent, and it is most often seen after the use of alkylating agents such as ifosfamide, cyclophosphamide and lomustine. Other chemotherapeutic agents known to be associated with direct gonadal toxicity include procarbazine, cisplatin, busulfan and vinblastine.[9,50,51] Scattered radiation from spinal irradiation is also known to contribute to gonadal toxicity, particularly in females.[52]

In males, spermatogenesis is more sensitive to the toxic effects of chemotherapy compared to Leydig cell function. Therefore, it is possible for a male to have normal levels of testosterone and still be infertile. It is believed that adjuvant chemotherapy causes direct damage to the Sertoli cells and germ cells leading to decreased spermatogenesis and a reduction in testicular volume.[7] Chemotherapy also significantly impacts semen quality causing decreased sperm concentration and motility.[53] Spinal radiation does not appear to significantly contribute to the development of primary gonadal failure in males.[50] In a study evaluating the gonadal status of male survivors of childhood brain tumors, there was evidence of increased primary gonadal failure in the group of patients treated with chemotherapy and radiation versus the group that received radiation alone.The adverse effects upon the hypothalamic-pituitary regulation of the gonads seemed similarly effected in the two groups. This suggests that spinal radiation may contribute more to a secondary or central gonadal failure while chemotherapy has more direct gonadal toxicity.[7]

Chemotherapy-induced primary gonadal dysfunction is seen more commonly in males compared to females. However, females are by no means spared from this late effect. In fact, in a study evaluating patients with ALL treated with a combination of spinal irradiation and chemotherapy, 60% of female patients developed ovarian dysfunction.[54] Again, the alkylating agents appear to be associated with the highest risk of ovarian failure and are known to cause ovarian fibrosis as well as follicular and oocyte depletion.[55] Contrary to the male population, the damage sustained to the female gonads often results in a decline in sex steroid production and a concomitant destruction of germ cells. Therefore, this can result in failure to progress through puberty or premature menopause, depending upon the patient's age. In addition, the damage also leads to infertility. There is also evidence to suggest that spinal radiation alone in females will contribute to primary ovarian failure. In a study evaluating brain tumor survivors, 65% of females who received craniospinal irradiation (CSI) alone exhibited signs of primary ovarian failure as assessed by elevated gonadotrophin levels.[56]

Postpubertal patients are at a much higher risk of developing gonadal failure as a consequence of chemotherapy and spinal radiation, whereas prepubertal patients seem less susceptible to this late effect.[6,57] In prepubertal males, there appears to be less of a toxic effect upon the germinal epithelium; however, prepubertal males may still experience long-term gonadal damage and infertility.[58] Since females possess their lifetime supply of oocytes at birth, even prepubertal females can have gonadal toxicity and develop infertility from chemotherapy and radiation therapy; however, the risks of menstrual irregularity, primary ovarian failure and infertility clearly increases with age at treatment.[59]

Since infertility is a common and anticipated side effect in many cancer patients who receive specific chemotherapeutic agents and spinal radiation, there has been great interest in developing reproductive alternatives for these patients. For male patients, there is the option of cryopreservation of spermatozoa before initiating treatment in an effort to preserve viable sperm for future use.[59] Viable sperm can be collected from males newly diagnosed with cancer pretreatment and successfully utilized for future fertility.[53,60] There are also newer techniques available for those males unable to bank sperm, such as testis sperm extraction. This method has been utilized successfully in male survivors of germ cell tumors.[61] In females who are postpubertal, gonadotrophins can be utilized in an attempt to stimulate the ovaries and retrieve mature oocytes for cryopreservation.[62] In vitro fertilization and embryo cryopreservation has proven successful. A more recent modality is the cryopreservation of ovarian cortical strips. This technique has been suggested as an acceptable way of preserving fertility in prepubertal female patients.[63] Live births have been successfully achieved utilizing this technique after orthotopically transplanted ovaries.[64,65] Other protective maneuvers are described later in this chapter.

Thyroid Gland

The thyroid gland is one of the most commonly effected endocrine organs in survivors of brain tumors. Most of the damage to the thyroid is the result of radiation therapy either directly upon the gland itself or secondarily by causing damage to the hypothalamic-pituitary axis as described previously. The effects of chemotherapy alone on thyroid function are less clearly understood. The late effects to the thyroid seen in brain tumor survivors include hypothyroidism, thyroid nodules, thyroid malignancy and, rarely, hyperthyroidism.[4]

Hypothyroidism

Hypothyroidism is one of the most commonly encountered thyroid late effects to the neuroaxis seen after radiation therapy. Hypothyroidism is the state in which there is insufficient thyroid hormone production by the thyroid gland. Inadequate stimulation of cells and organs in the body due to low levels of thyroid hormone can result in a general slowing of the body's metabolism and cell processes. Patients can develop bradycardia, tiredness, cold intolerance, constipation and poor growth. Frank primary hypothyroidism can be diagnosed by both an elevated TSH and decreased free T4 level. Compensated primary hypothyroidism can also develop whereby a patient has an elevated TSH with a low to normal and somewhat compensated T4 level.[66] Since hypothyroidism can result in poor growth, poor energy and declining work or school performance, early diagnosis of patients at increased risk is important so that appropriate treatment can begin. Ideally, routine screening should begin at the time of brain tumor diagnosis. In this way, a patient's baseline thyroid function can be documented. TSH and free T4 levels can be monitored routinely each year following treatment and as needed for new suspicious symptoms.

The most common malignant pediatric brain tumor is medulloblastoma. This patient population has helped us to more completely understand the toxic effects of radiation upon the thyroid, especially since there is some uniformity of treatment over time. Most up-front treatment strategies in children diagnosed at an age greater than three years includes surgical resection followed by CSI with a radiation boost to the tumor bed or entire posterior fossa, followed by chemotherapy. The radiation volume most often includes the entire neuroaxis. Because of its midline location near the cervical spine, the thyroid is invariably affected by CSI. The risk that medulloblastoma patients who receive CSI will develop primary hypothyroidism is between 20–30%, while their risk of central hypothyroidism is much lower.[67] Also, it appears that those patients who receive CSI at a younger age are at an increased risk of direct thyroid toxicity and the development of hypothyroidism.[68] The majority of patients who develop hypothyroidism secondary to radiation therapy do so within 2–5 years posttreatment; however, delayed presentations beyond five years have been reported.[69,70]

The degree of thyroid dysfunction depends upon numerous contributing factors including radiation dose, technique, patient age at treatment, length of patient follow-up and the diagnostic criteria used to make the diagnosis.[71] Hyperfractionated radiotherapy decreases the risk of hypothyroidism as compared to conventional radiotherapy. Studies evaluating thyroid dysfunction in survivors of pediatric medulloblastoma and primitive neuroectodermal tumors (PNET) have found that patients who received hyperfractionated radiation are statistically less likely to develop hypothyrodism as compared to those who received conventional radiotherapy.[72,73] It was anticipated that lower CSI doses would also decrease a patient's risk of developing hypothyroidism; however, the addition of adjuvant chemotherapy utilized to balance the reduction of CSI doses has contributed significantly to the development of hypothyroidism.[68] The exact mechanism whereby chemotherapy contributes to thyroid dysfunction is not yet understood, but it clearly increases the risk of hypothyroidism in those patients who are also receiving radiation therapy. In a study evaluating patients treated for medulloblastoma with either 3,600 cGY CSI versus 2,340 cGY CSI, those patients who received lower doses of radiation with adjuvant chemotherapy had an increased risk of hypothyroidism compared to those who received higher radiation doses without adjuvant chemotherapy.[68] A clear pattern has been recognized whereby chemotherapy plus radiotherapy is more damaging to the thyroid than radiation alone.[74] The mainstay of treatment in patients with hypothyroidism, regardless of the cause, is usually thyroid hormone replacement therapy.

Hyperthyroidism

Less commonly, hyperthyroidism has also been documented in survivors of brain tumors who have received radiation therapy.[4,69,75] Hyperthyroidism is often characterized by an enlarged thyroid gland, elevated T4, depressed TSH, increased uptake of radioactive iodine and the development of thyroid autoantibodies. As opposed to hypothyroidism, there is an overproduction of thyroid hormone leading to a hypermetabolic state. Patients may develop symptoms including tachycardia, tremors, weight loss and heat intolerance. In a study evaluating survivors of Hodgkin's disease, the risk of developing hyperthyroidism was statistically increased significantly compared to sibling controls.[4] Interestingly, hyperthyroidism developed later than is typical for hypothyroidism and was seen at a mean of eight years from radiation treatment. Higher doses of radiation were also associated with an increased risk of developing hyperthyroidism.[4] Patients can also develop acute hyperthyroidism during or shortly thereafter radiation therapy secondary to a thyroiditis leading to destruction and leakage of thyroid hormone, but this is typically a transient process and often does not require intervention.[76] Depending upon the degree of dysfunction, patients with hyperthyroidism can be treated with observation alone, antithyroid medications and/or surgical removal of the thyroid or radioactive iodine. The use to the latter treatment modality remains controversial in children.

Thyroid Nodules

Cancer survivors who have received radiation therapy are also at risk of developing thyroid nodules which may or may not be malignant. Sklar et al. found an increased risk of thyroid nodules in Hodgkin's survivors as compared to sibling controls, and an increased risk of thyroid malignancy as compared to the general population.[4] The patients in this study were diagnosed with a thyroid nodule at a mean of 14 years after initial diagnosis of Hodgkin's disease, and there was an increased risk of developing a nodule at higher radiation doses, greater time since diagnosis and among females compared to males.[4] The Hodgkin's experience emphasizes the need for thorough physical exams throughout a survivor's lifetime, including a routine thyroid exam on an annual basis.

Thyroid Screening

The key to primary thyroid pathologies in survivors of pediatric malignancies is routine surveillance, education/awareness and early detection. Patients who are known to be at risk for these late effects (for example, any brain tumor patient who received CSI with or without chemotherapy) must be routinely monitored with thorough physical examinations and routine thyroid hormone testing (TSH and free T4). The Children's Oncology Group (COG) has established long-term follow-up guidelines for survivors of childhood and adolescent cancers. The recommendations for those survivors who have received radiation therapy involving the thyroid, including CSI, is yearly thyroid examinations and yearly evaluation of TSH and free T4 levels.[77] It is recommended that this annual interval be decreased during periods of rapid growth, such as puberty. It is important to remember that some thyroid dysfunction typically occurs earlier, like hypothyroidism, whereas thyroid nodules and malignancy can occur 10–20 years after therapy.

Craniopharyngioma and CNS Germ Cell Tumors

Craniopharyngiomas and CNS germ cell tumors (GCT) are two specific pediatric brain tumors that are more consistently associated with specific endocrinopathies, both in the acute setting at diagnosis and as a continued long-term consequence. Often these endocrinopathies arise as a consequence of the tumor's location in addition to late effects of surgery and/or adjuvant treatments. Since these tumors are often intimately associated with the endocrine control system within the brain including the HP axis, it is understandable that they cause dysfunction to this system. The endocrinopathies can arise from tumor compression upon adjacent endocrine structures, surgical intervention causing damage to the HP axis and as a consequence of chemotherapy and radiation therapy.[78–82]

Craniopharyngioma

Craniopharyngiomas are rare epithelial tumors that are thought to be of mal-developmental origin. One hypothesis is that they develop from embryonic remnants of Rathke's pouch.[83] Although these tumors are considered histologically "benign," they can often be very aggressive and difficult to manage. Craniopharyngiomas represent approximately 6–10% of all pediatric brain tumors and are most commonly seen in children ages 5–14 years.[84] They often originate within a midline location either within the pituitary stalk or arising from the floor of the third ventricle. Despite their midline origin, they can often expand superiorly, inferiorly and laterally, causing local compression and damage. Due to the tumor's proximity to the hypothalamus and pituitary gland, patients often sustain significant endocrine dysfunction.

Patients with craniopharyngiomas most commonly present with headaches, emesis, visual field deficits and endocrinopathies. Overall, between 80–90% of patients display some type of HP dysfunction at presentation when they are evaluated thoroughly, even though it may not be their chief complaint.[85,86] Primary treatment strategies for craniopharyngioma usually consist of a complete surgical resection when possible, with or without adjuvant radiation therapy.[83,87] The endocrinologic abnormalities common to patients with craniopharyngioma include growth hormone deficiency, gonadotropin deficiency, central hypothyroidism, ACTH deficiency, ADH dysfunction or central diabetes insipidus and hypothalamic obesity.[84,85,88]

Growth Hormone Deficiency

The most common endocrine abnormality observed in children with craniopharyngioma is growth hormone deficiency leading to growth failure or growth deceleration. It is often observed pre-diagnosis and continues after surgical excision.[85,89] It is recommended that patients be followed at regular intervals following diagnosis and treatment, including evaluation of serum IGF-1, insulin-like growth factor binding protein-3 (IGBP-3) and radiographs to evaluate bone age. Interestingly, some patients who have laboratory evidence of growth hormone deficiency do not always exhibit growth failure. This was originally documented by Matson in 1964 and later became known as the "growth without growth hormone" phenomenon.[90] Matson suggested that either there was enough pituitary tissue left behind post-surgically to function or, perhaps, some secretion of growth hormone is independent of the hypothalamus.[90] Most endocrinologists agree that these patients do not need growth hormone replacement.

In those patients with growth failure or decline who are clearly diagnosed with growth hormone deficiency as evaluated by an endocrinologist, growth hormone replacement is a treatment alternative. There is still significant controversy over its use, however, especially in patients who may have residual tumor. It is yet unclear what the consequence of growth hormone may be upon patients with residual tumor and, therefore, most clinicians will not utilize it in this setting. However, in patients who are free from disease and exhibit symptomatic growth hormone deficiency, growth hormone replacement has been shown to improve growth without increasing the risk of tumor recurrence.[91,92]

Gonadotropin Deficiency

LH and FSH deficiency and subsequent delays in puberty are present in a significant number of adolescents who develop craniopharyngioma.[93] It is not completely clear what percentage of younger children also have gonadotropin deficiency because the measurements of these hormones in prepubertal children are often less sensitive and inconclusive. In patients with gonadotropin deficiency, it is important to begin replacement at an appropriate age in order to induce pubertal development. Initiating replacement hormones needs to be individualized for each patient and conducted under the supervision and guidance of an experienced endocrinologist in order to ensure appropriate maturation and pubertal development.[85]

Hypothyroidism

Up to 25% of patients with craniopharyngioma will present with symptoms or laboratory evidence of hypothyroidism.[93] Postoperatively, the incidence of hypothyroidism significantly increases.[94] Therefore, it is important to test the thyroid function routinely, even in those patients who exhibited normal function at diagnosis and pretreatment. The hypothyroidism experienced in these patients is most commonly a central hypothyroidism, whereby there is a decrease in TSH production and lack of stimulation of the thyroid gland. There are patients, however, who display a low level of thyroxine with a normal or mildly elevated level of TSH. This has subsequently been shown to result from abnormally glycated TSH which has decreased biologic activity.[95] As is typical for most patients with hypothyroidism, either central or primary, thyroid hormone replacement is effective in maintaining normal thyroid hormone levels and minimizing symptoms.

ACTH Deficiency

Although the signs and symptoms of ACTH deficiency may be subtle, a significant number of craniopharyngioma patients will be deficient upon presentation.[86,93] Post-surgery, ACTH deficiency is also a common finding among these patients.[96] The common signs and symptoms of ACTH deficiency include anorexia, poor weight gain, hypoglycemia, decreased energy and nausea. These symptoms are exacerbated in times of stress upon the body and, in an extreme setting, can lead to hypotension and even death. Survivors who are ACTH deficient should receive replacement hydrocortisone. The exact maintenance dosage utilized is based upon the body surface area, patient's age and symptomotolgy.[97,98] Higher doses or "stress" doses are necessary during times of stress upon the body, for example during surgical procedures, febrile illnesses and/or infection.

Diabetes Insipidus

ADH deficiency or diabetes insipidus can be seen in up to 38% of patients newly diagnosed with craniopharyngioma.[86,99] Postoperative diabetes insipidus has been seen in as many as 94% of craniopharyngioma patients.[96] Hypothalamic diabetes insipidus usually presents acutely with symptoms of thirst and excessive urination. Laboratory evaluation includes evaluation of serum osmolality, urine osmolality, urine specific gravity, and serum electrolytes. Patients present with dilute urine in the presence of a serum osmolality that is elevated due to a lack of ADH. ADH is secreted by the posterior pituitary gland. Its effect in the kidney is mediated via the vasopressin V2 receptor on the cells on the basolateral surface of the collecting duct. The key action of ADH in the kidney is to increase permeability of water and allow free water to be reabsorbed from the collecting duct within the renal medulla. A more definitive test of diabetes insipidus is a water deprivation test in which the patient is unable to concentrate his urine despite elevation of plasma osmolality. Treatment for both acute and chronic diabetes insipidus is DDAVP, a synthetic agonist of the AVP V2 receptor.[85]

Interestingly, glucocorticoids have an inhibitory effect on ADH secretion. Therefore, in patients that have both ADH and ACTH deficiency, the ACTH deficiency may actually mask the ADH deficiency. Also, concomitant TSH deficiency may also mask diabetes insipidus by assisting the kidney's ability to concentrate urine.[85] Replacement of glucocorticoids in ACTH deficiency and thyroid hormone in TSH deficiency, therefore, may unmask significant diabetes insipidus.

Syndrome of Inappropriate Secretion of Antidiuretic Hormone

Another postoperative complication seen in craniopharyngioma patients is the syndrome of inappropriate secretion of antidiuretic hormone (SIADH) in which the patient has a low serum sodium and osmolality in the presence of highly concentrated urine. In SIADH, the abnormally elevated vasopressin levels enhance the reabsorption of water leading to concentrated urine, an inability to excrete water and hyponatremia. Often patients who initially develop SIADH postoperatively may go on to develop diabetes insipidus. These patients must be monitored very carefully and consistently as the treatment strategies for these two entities differ.

Hypothalamic Obesity

Finally, many patients treated for craniopharyngioma are at risk of developing hypothalamic obesity as discussed above. Neural damage to the ventromedial hypothalamus leads to excessive eating, rapid weight gain and hyperinsulinemia. This obesity is often associated with other hypothalamic endocrinopa- thies.[12,100,101] Unfortunately, in hypothalamic obesity, the weight gain is often intractable and does not respond to diet or exercise. There have been some beneficial effects of octreotide therapy in pediatric patients with hypothalamic obesity. Octreotide suppresses insulin and can stabilize weight providing patients with an improved quality of life.[44]

CNS Germ Cell Tumors (GCT)

CNS GCT represent approximately 2–3% of all childhood CNS tumors in the Western World; however, incidences vary with geography. For example, in Japan, CNS GCT can account for up to 18% of all pediatric CNS tumors.[102,103] CNS GCTs are thought to arise from pluripotent primordial germ cells. They most commonly arise in midline locations such as the pituitary gland and the pineal region and, less commonly, they arise in other areas of the brain such as the thalamus and basal ganglia. Historically, these tumors have been classified based upon their histologic components and their varying degrees of differen- tiation. Most commonly, they have been divided into either pure germinomas or nongerminomatous germ cell tumors (NGGCT). The NGGCT group includes choriocarcinoma, endodermal sinus or yolk sac tumor, embryonal carcinoma and mixed tumors. Outcomes vary among the differing tumors, but in general, those patients with pure germinomas have much better outcomes compared to the NGGCT group.[102,104]

Most CNS GCT patients are evaluated and treated with a combination of tumor marker evaluation in serum and cerebrospinal fluid (CSF), biopsy, chemotherapy and radiation therapy. Patients with CNS GCT tumors may develop a variety of endocrine abnormalities secondary to tumor location, surgery and adjuvant therapy. Many patients do not exhibit endocrinopathies at diagnosis or post-surgical resection, but they may develop endocrine dysfunction after adjuvant radiotherapy.[80] The endocrine dysfunctions encountered in these patients include the following: panhypopituitarism, growth hormone deficiency, gonadotrophin deficiency, thyroid hormone abnormalities, cortisol deficiency and diabetes insipidus.[78,82]

Diabetes Insipidus

In a prospective evaluation and long-term follow-up of nine pediatric patients diagnosed with CNS GCT, the only endocrine abnormality that caused sig- nificant symptoms at the time of diagnosis was diabetes insipidus; however, all nine patients eventually developed endocrine abnormalities that required some type of prolonged hormone replacement.[78] In this study, patients with tumors centered within the sella developed more significant and complex endocrinopathies compared to patients with tumors in other locations.[78] This same pattern has been observed in other series as well.[80] Diabetes insipidus has been documented as a common finding at presentation among many patients with CNS GCT.[79,81,82] For most patients, this is a lifelong complication requiring continued management with DDAVP therapy.[78]

Growth Hormone Deficiency

Growth hormone deficiency is also commonly seen among patients with CNS GCT. As has been seen in craniopharyngioma patients, growth hormone deficiency does not always equate with poor growth. In a study evaluating endocrine status in children with CNS GCT, among the seven patients diagnosed with growth hormone deficiency, only three patients actually exhibited poor growth and required growth hormone replacement. All three of these patients also received adjuvant radiation therapy as part of their treatment course.[82] In another study, among 23 patients evaluated with CNS GCT, 20 (87%) exhibited impaired growth hormone secretion at the time of diagnosis.[81]

Hyperprolactinemia and Hypothyroidism

Another commonly seen endocrine abnormality seen among patients with CNS GCTs is hyperprolactinemia.[79,82] This complication is often seen in patients who have other endocrinological disturbances such as gonadotrophin deficiency and growth failure.[79,82] Although some patients will have elevated prolactin levels, few patients develop frank galactorrhea.[79] As has been seen in other patients who receive radiation to the pituitary, sellar and pineal region, these patients can also sustain thyroid dysfunction either from radiation splay directly affecting the thyroid or from damage to the HP axis causing a central hypothyroidism.[78] Routine laboratory monitoring is recommended, including TSH and free T4. Those patients with documented hypothyroidism are treated with thyroid hormone replacement therapy.

Hematopoietic Cell Rescue and Endocrine Late Effects

In an effort to avoid and delay radiation therapy in very young children with newly diagnosed brain tumors, some treatment strategies have employed high-dose chemotherapy with autologous hematopoietic cell rescue (AuHCR).[105–108] Those patients who have undergone AuHCR may be at additional risk for developing endocrinopathies.[109–111]

In a study evaluating the endocrine function of 29 patients who had undergone AuHCR for a variety of hematologic and solid malignancies, a variety of endocrine abnormalities were observed.[112] Nine out of 10 females reported secondary amenorrhea and required hormonal replacement for a minimum of two years following transplantation. In the male patients, Leydig cell function remained intact; however, many male patients exhibited elevated FSH levels suggesting germinal aplasia.[112] Since many of the patients received gonado-toxic chemotherapy and/or radiation therapy, it was difficult to decipher the specific contribution of the AuHCR to endocrine dysfunction. Interestingly, in this study the thyroid and adrenocortical system were both grossly within normal limits in the majority of patients tested.[112]

In another larger study evaluating early and late post-AuHCR endocrine function among patients undergoing 95 consecutive autologous transplants, numerous endocrine abnormalities were again documented.[109] One year following AuHCR, many patients had low IGF-1 levels, ovarian failure and subclinical hypothyroidism. Interestingly, a portion of the endocrine abnormalities documented within the first three months following AuHCR improved or resolved by the time the patient was re-evaluated one year post-AuHCR.[109]

Of the patients who undergo AuHCR as part of the treatment for their brain tumor, many have already received gonado-toxic chemotherapies or will eventually receive radiation therapy to the neuroaxis. For this reason, it is often difficult to distinguish what degree each treatment modality is contributing to late endocrine toxicity. However, these patients are best served by following their endocrine function closely on a yearly basis post-AuHCR in order to identify any endocrine dysfunction and begin appropriate therapy, whatever the underlying cause.

Endocrine Evaluation/Assessment and Treatment

The endocrine assessment and treatment must be done in a thorough fashion. The essentials are the same as for the routine endocrine consultation and include a complete history and physical examination with an appropriate laboratory evaluation. In general, it is recommended that the initial evaluation begin with a comprehensive metabolic panel including a glucose level, free thyroxine and TSH level, ACTH and cortisol levels, renin and aldosterone levels (if needed), IGF-1 and IGFBP-3 levels, LH, FSH, testosterone and estradiol levels (as indicated based upon gender), prolactin level and a bone age (for pediatric patients). Depending upon the results of the initial evaluation one can proceed with specific stimulation tests for GH and/or GnRH and ACTH stimulation testing as indicated. A free thyroxine level by dialysis or sleep study for LH, FSH and sex steroids may be obtained, depending upon clinical suspicions.[23] Brain or other organ imaging would ensue after dysfunction of the endocrine system is confirmed.

Specific therapies should then be applied, depending upon which system(s) require replacement or inhibition. It is important to consider quality of life issues such as attempting to maximize statural growth at a critical age prior to epiphyseal closure, improving general psychological well-being, improving lipid metabolism, ensuring bone health and/or initiating or restoring sexual development or functioning. Additionally, clinical interventions involve trying to maximize or preserve fertility both at the time of diagnosis and post-cancer therapy, as well as evaluation and treatment of ostepenia.

Advances in the field of assisted reproductive technology (ART) provide hope that the reproductive impact of cancer therapy can be reduced. The technologies that may be applicable prior to gonadotoxic therapy are pretreatment ovarian protection with oral contraceptives or gonadotropin releasing hormone agonist (GnRHa) therapy; ART using pretreatment cryopreservation of embryos or gametes; posttreatment ART with donor gametes or embryos, or adoption. Ovarian protection is not of proven benefit and oocyte/ovary cryopreservation has had only limited success to date. Regardless, information on cancer treatment's effects on fertility and ways to circumvent these should be part of routine counseling so the patient can make decisions before treatment commences.[113] In a study of adolescent female cancer patients receiving polychemotherapy (PCT), a study of GnRHa treatment before and during was instrumental in enhancing ovarian function and preserving adolescent fertility. Results require confirmation in larger studies.

Conclusion

Brain tumor survivors are often left with significant lifelong late effects and morbidities secondary to the tumor itself, surgical intervention, chemotherapy and radiotherapy. One of the most common and anticipated late effects seen in many survivors is endocrine dysfunction. Endocrine dysfunction can manifest early at the time of diagnosis, acutely after a surgical procedure and/or as a complication of tumor compression and damage to adjacent brain tissue. It can also develop years later as a consequence of chemotherapy and radiotherapy. The endocrine abnormalities seen in brain tumor survivors are significant and can involve multiple endocrine processes.

If left undiagnosed and untreated, many of these endocrine abnormalities can lead to quality of life concerns, severe illness and/or death. However, by anticipating dysfunction and monitoring patients with routine evaluations and physical exams, many of these abnormalities can be easily treated with hormonal replacement. Patient education about the signs and symptoms of endocrine dysfunction, routine laboratory monitoring and physical exams are key in diagnosing endocrinopathies early and initiating treatment when necessary. Most of these dysfunctions can be treated without significant morbidity, especially when diagnosed early and monitored carefully.

References

1. Miller B. *SEER Cancer Statistics Review*. Maryland: NIH Publication; 1993:93.
2. Spoudeas HA, Hindmarsh PC, Matthews DR, et al. Evolution of growth hormone neurosecretory disturbance after cranial irradiation for childhood brain tumours: a prospective study. *J Endocrinol*. 1996;150(2):329–342.
3. Gleeson HK, Shalet SM. The impact of cancer therapy on the endocrine system in survivors of childhood brain tumours. *Endocr Relat Cancer*. 2004;11(4):589–602.
4. Sklar C, Whitton J, Mertens A, et al. Abnormalities of the thyroid in survivors of Hodgkin's disease: data from the Childhood Cancer Survivor Study. *J Clin Endocrinol Metab*. 2000;85(9):3227–3232.
5. Constine LS, Rubin P, Woolf PD, et al. Hyperprolactinemia and hypothyroidism following cytotoxic therapy for central nervous system malignancies. *J Clin Oncol*. 1987;5(11): 1841–1851.
6. Constine LS, Woolf PD, Cann D, et al. Hypothalamic-pituitary dysfunction after radiation for brain tumors. *N Eng J Med*. 1993;328(2):87–94.
7. Schmiegelow M, Lassen S, Poulsen HS, et al. Gonadal status in male survivors following childhood brain tumors. *J Clin Endocrinol Metab*. 2001;86(6):2446–2452.
8. Clayton PE, Shalet SM, Price DA. Gonadal function after chemotherapy and irradiation for childhood malignancies. *Horm Res*. 1988;30(2–3):104–110.
9. Clayton PE, Shalet SM, Price DA, et al. Ovarian function following chemotherapy for childhood brain tumours. *Med Pediatr Oncol*. 1989;17(2):92–96.
10. Clayton PE, Shalet SM. Dose dependency of time of onset of radiation-induced growth hormone deficiency. *J Pediatr*. 1991;118(2):226–228.
11. Didi M, Didcock E, Davies HA, et al. High incidence of obesity in young adults after treatment of acute lymphoblastic leukemia in childhood. *J Pediatr*. 1995;127(1):63–67.
12. Lustig RH, Post SR, Srivannaboon K, et al. Risk factors for the development of obesity in children surviving brain tumors. *J Clin Endocrinol Metab*. 2003;88(2):611–616.
13. Barr RD, Simpson T, Webber CE, et al. Osteopenia in children surviving brain tumours. *Eur J Cancer*. 1998;34(6):873–877.
14. Krishnamoorthy P, Freeman C, Bernstein ML, et al. Osteopenia in children who have undergone posterior fossa or craniospinal irradiation for brain tumors. *Arch Pediatr Adolesc Med*. 2004;158(5):491–496.
15. Odame I, Duckworth J, Talsma D, et al. Osteopenia, physical activity and health-related quality of life in survivors of brain tumors treated in childhood. *Pediatr Blood Cancer*. 2006;46(3):357–362.
16. Pietila S, Sievanen H, Ala-Houhala M, et al. Bone mineral density is reduced in brain tumour patients treated in childhood. *Acta Paediatr*. 2006;95(10):1291–1297.
17. Chrousos G. Seminars in Medicine of the Beth Israel Hospital, Boston. The hypothalamic-pituitary axis and immune mediated inflammation. *N Engl J Med*. 1995;332:1351.
18. Constine L, Woolf P, Cann D, et al. Hypothalamic-pituitary dysfunction after radiation for brain tumors. *N Engl J Med*. 1993;328:87–94.
19. Shalet S, Breadwell C, Pearson D, et al. The effect of varying doses of cerebral irradiation on growth hormone production in childhood. *Clin Endocrinol*. 1976;5:287–290.
20. Samaan N, Vieto R, Schultz P, et al. Hypothalamic; ituitary and thryroid dysfunction after radiotherapy to the head and neck. *Int J Radiat Oncol Biol Phys*. 1982;8:1857–1867.
21. Schmiegelow M, Lassen S, Poulsen H, et al. Cranial radiotherapy of childhood brain tumors: growth hormone deficiency and its relation to the biological effective dose of irradiation in a large populaiton based study. *Clin Endocrinol*. 2000;53: 191–197.
22. Gleeson H, Gattamaneni H, Smethhurst L, et al. Reassessment of growth hormone status is required at final height in children treated with growth hormone replacement after radiation therapy. *J Clin Endocrinol Metab*. 2004;89:662–666.

23. Rosenfield RL. Essentials of growth diagnosis. *Endocrinol Metab Clin North Am.* 1996;25 (3):743–758.
24. Merchant T, Goloubeva O, Pritchard DL, et al. Radiation dose-volume effects on growth hormone secretion. *Int J Radiat Oncol Biol Phys.* 2002 Apr 1;52(5):1264–1270.
25. Clayton P, Shalet S. Dose dependency of time of onset of radiation-induced growth hormone deficiency. *J Pediatr.* 1991;118:226–228.
26. Darzy K, Aimaretti G, Wieringa G, et al. The usefulness of the combined growth hormone (GH)-releasing hormone secretion and arginine stimulation test int ehdignosis of radiation-induced Gh deficiency is dependent on the post-irradiation time interval. *J Clin Endocrinol Metab.* 2003;88:95–102.
27. Darzy K, Pezzoli SS, Thorner MO, Shalet SM. Cranial irradiation and growth hormone neurosecretory dysfunction: a critical appraisal. *J Clin Endocrinol Metab.* 2007 May;92 (5):1666–1672.
28. Banerjee I, Clayton PE. Growth hormone treatment and cancer risk. *Endocrinol Metab Clin North Am.* 2007 Mar;36(1):247–263.
29. Darendeliler F, Karagiannis G, Wilton P, et al. Recurrence of brain tumours in patients treated with growth hormone: Analysis of KIGS (Pfizer International Growth Database). *Acta Paediatr.* 2006;95(10):1284–1290.
30. Roth C, Lakomek M, Lakomek M, Schmidberger H, Jarry H. Cranila irradiation inducespremature activation of the gonadotropin-releasing hormone. *Klin Padiatr.* 2001;213:239–243.
31. Roth C, Schmidberger H, Schaper O, et al. Cranial irradiation of female rats causes dose-dependent and age-dependent activation or inhibition of pu bertal development. *Pediatr Res.* 2000;47:586–591.
32. Ogilvy-Stuart A, Clayton P, Shalet MS. Cranial irradiation and early puberty. *J Clin Endocrinol Metab.* 1994;78:1282–1286.
33. Schmiegelow M, Feldt-Rasmussen U, Rasmussen AK, Lange M, Poulsen HS, Müller J. Assessment of the hypothalamic-pituitary-adrenal axis in patients treated with radio-therapy and chemotherapy for childhood brain tumor. *J Clin Endocrinol Metab.* 2003;88: 3149–3154.
34. Crowley S, Hindmarsh PC, Holownia P, et al. The use of low doses of ACTH in the investigation of adrenal function in man. *J Endocrinol.* 1991;130(3):475–479.
35. Schmiegelow M, Feldt-Rasmussen U, Rasmussen AK, Poulsen HS, Müller J. A population-based study of thyroid function alfter radiotherapy and chemotherapy for a childhood brain tumor. *J Clin Endocrinol Metab.* 2003;88:136–140.
36. Sapin R, Thyroxine SJ (T4) and tri-iodothyronine (T3) determinations: techniques and value in the assessment of thyroid function. [Article in French]. *Ann Biol Clin*(Paris). 2003 Jul–Aug;61(4):411–420.
37. Rose S, Lustig RH, Pitukcheewanont P, et al. Diagnosis of hidden central hypothyroidism in survivors of childhood cancer. *J Clin Endocrinol Metab.* 1999;84:4472–4479.
38. Ghirardello S, Garrè ML, Rossi A, Maghnie M. The diagnosis of children with central diabetes insipidus. *J Pediatr Endocrinol Metab.* 2007 Mar;20(3):359–375.
39. De Buyst J, Massa G, Christophe C, Tenoutasse S, Hein-richs C. Clinical, hormonal and imaging findings in 27 children with central diabetes insipidus. *Eur J Pediatr.* 2007 Jan;166(1):43–49.
40. Jyotsna V, Singh SK, Chaturvedi R et al. Cranial irradiation – an unusual cause for diabetes insipidus. *J Assoc Physicians India.* 2000 Nov;48(11):1107–1108.
41. Lustig R, Post SR, Srivannaboon K, et al. Risk factors for the development of obesity in children surviving brain tumors. *J Clin Endocrinol Metab.* 2003;88:611–616.
42. Razzouk B, Rose SR, Hongeng S, et al. Obesity in survivors of childhood acute lympho-blastic leukemia and lymphoma. *J Clin Oncol.* 2007 Apr1;25(10):1183–1189.
43. Schwartz M, Woods SC, Porte D Jr, Seeley RJ, Baskin DG. Central nervous system control of food intake. *Nature.* 2000;404:661–671.

44. Lustig RH, Hinds PS, Ringwald-Smith K, et al. Octreotide therapy of pediatric hypothalamic obesity: a double-blind, placebo-controlled trial. *J Clin Endocrinol Metab.* 2003;88 (6):2586–2592.
45. Tataranni PA, Larson DE, Snitker S, et al. Effects of glucocorticoids on energy metabolism and food intake in humans. *Am J Physiol.* 1996;271(2 Pt 1):E317–325.
46. Salomon F, Cuneo RC, Hesp R, et al. The effects of treatment with recombinant human growth hormone on body composition and metabolism in adults with growth hormone deficiency. *N Engl J Med.* 1989;321(26):1797–1803.
47. Heikens J, Ubbink MC, van der Pal HP, et al. Long term survivors of childhood brain cancer have an increased risk for cardiovascular disease. *Cancer.* 2000;88(9):2116–2121.
48. Gregory J, Reilly J. *Body Composition and Obesity.* London: Arnold; 2004;155–158.
49. Neville K, Cohn RJ, Steinbeck KS, Johnston K, and Walker JL. Hyperinsulinemia, impaired glucose tolerance, and diabetes mellitus in survivors of childhood cancer: prevalence and risk factors. *J Clin Endocrinol Metab.* 2006 Nov;91(11):4401–4407.
50. Ahmed SR, Shalet SM, Campbell RH, et al. Primary gonadal damage following treatment of brain tumors in childhood. *J Pediatr.* 1983;103(4):562–565.
51. Duffner PK. Long-term effects of radiation therapy on cognitive and endocrine function in children with leukemia and brain tumors. *The Neurologist.* 2004;10(6):293–310.
52. Livesey EA, Hindmarsh PC, Brook CG, et al. Endocrine disorders following treatment of childhood brain tumours. *Br J Cancer.* 1990;61(4):622–625.
53. Ginsberg JP, Ogle SK, Tuchman LK, et al. Sperm Banking for Adolescent and Young Adult Cancer Patients: Sperm Quality, Patient, and Parent Perspectives. *Pediatr Blood Cancer.* 2008;50(3):594–598.
54. Pasqualini T, McCalla J, Berg S, et al. Subtle primary hypothyroidism in patients treated for acute lymphoblastic leukemia. *Acta Endocrinol.* 1991;124(4):375–380.
55. Familiari G, Caggiati A, Nottola SA, et al. Ultrastructure of human ovarian primordial follicles after combination chemotherapy for Hodgkin's disease. *Hum Reprod.* 1993;8 (12):2080–2087.
56. Livesey EA, Brook CG. Gonadal dysfunction after treatment of intracranial tumours. *Arch Dis Child.* 1988;63(5):495–500.
57. Moshang T, Jr., Grimberg A. The effects of irradiation and chemotherapy on growth. *Endocrinol Metab Clin North Am.* 1996;25(3):731–741.
58. Dhabhar BN, Malhotra H, Joseph R, et al. Gonadal function in prepubertal boys following treatment for Hodgkin's disease. *Am J Pediatr Hematol Oncol.* 1993;15(3):306–310.
59. Thomson AB, Critchley HO, Kelnar CJ, et al. Late reproductive sequelae following treatment of childhood cancer and options for fertility preservation. *Best Pract Res.* 2002;16(2):311–334.
60. Edge B, Holmes D, Makin G. Sperm banking in adolescent cancer patients. *Arch Dis Child.* 2006;91(2):149–152.
61. Damani MN, Master V, Meng MV, et al. Postchemotherapy ejaculatory azoospermia: fatherhood with sperm from testis tissue with intracytoplasmic sperm injection. *J Clin Oncol.* 2002;20(4):930–936.
62. Donnez J, Godin PA, Qu J, et al. Gonadal cryopreservation in the young patient with gynaecological malignancy. *Curr Opin Obstet Gynecol.* 2000;12(1):1–9.
63. Simon B, Lee SJ, Partridge AH, et al. Preserving fertility after cancer. *CA Cancer J Clin.* 2005;55(4):211–228; quiz 263–214.
64. Donnez J, Dolmans MM, Demylle D, et al. Livebirth after orthotopic transplantation of cryopreserved ovarian tissue. *Lancet.* 2004;364(9443):1405–1410.
65. Meirow D, Levron J, Eldar-Geva T, et al. Pregnancy after transplantation of cryopreserved ovarian tissue in a patient with ovarian failure after chemotherapy. *N Engl J Med.* 2005;353(3):318–321.
66. Hancock SL, McDougall IR, Constine LS. Thyroid abnormalities after therapeutic external radiation. *Int J Radiat Oncol Biol Phys.* 1995;31(5):1165–1170.

67. Duffner PK, Cohen ME. Long-term consequences of CNS treatment for childhood cancer, Part II: Clinical consequences. *Pediatr Neurol.* 1991;7(4):237–242.
68. Paulino AC. Hypothyroidism in children with medulloblastoma: a comparison of 3600 and 2340 cGy craniospinal radiotherapy. *Int J Radiat Oncol Biol Phys.* 2002;53(3):543–547.
69. Hancock SL, Cox RS, McDougall IR. Thyroid diseases after treatment of Hodgkin's disease. *N Engl J Med.* 1991;325(9):599–605.
70. Constine LS, Donaldson SS, McDougall IR, et al. Thyroid dysfunction after radiotherapy in children with Hodgkin's disease. *Cancer.* 1984;53(4):878–883.
71. Gleeson HK, Darzy K, Shalet SM. Late endocrine, metabolic and skeletal sequelae following treatment of childhood cancer. *Best Pract Res.* 2002;16(2):335–348.
72. Chin D, Sklar C, Donahue B, et al. Thyroid dysfunction as a late effect in survivors of pediatric medulloblastoma/primitive neuroectodermal tumors: a comparison of hyperfractionated versus conventional radiotherapy. *Cancer.* 1997;80(4):798–804.
73. Ricardi U, Corrias A, Einaudi S, et al. Thyroid dysfunction as a late effect in childhood medulloblastoma: a comparison of hyperfractionated versus conventionally fractionated craniospinal radiotherapy. *Int J Rad Oncol Biol Phys.* 2001;50(5):1287–1294.
74. Ogilvy-Stuart AL, Shalet SM, Gattamaneni HR. Thyroid function after treatment of brain tumors in children. *J Pediatr.* 1991;119(5):733–737.
75. Loeffler JS, Tarbell NJ, Garber JR, et al. The development of Graves' disease following radiation therapy in Hodgkin's disease. *Int J Radiat Oncol Biol Phys.* 1988;14(1):175–178.
76. Nishiyama K, Kozuka T, Higashihara T, et al. Acute radiation thyroiditis. *Int J Radiat Oncol Biol Phys.* 1996;36(5):1221–1224.
77. Group CsO. *Long-Term Follow-up Guidelines for Survivors of Childhood, Adolescent and Young Adult Cancers.* Volume Version 2.0. 2006.
78. Benesch M, Lackner H, Schagerl S, et al. Tumor- and treatment-related side effects after multimodal therapy of childhood intracranial germ cell tumors. *Acta Paediatr.* 2001;90 (3):264–270.
79. Janmohamed S, Grossman AB, Metcalfe K, et al. Suprasellar germ cell tumours: specific problems and the evolution of optimal management with a combined chemoradiotherapy regimen. *Clin Endocrinol.* 2002;57(4):487–500.
80. Merchant TE, Sherwood SH, Mulhern RK, et al. CNS germinoma: disease control and long-term functional outcome for 12 children treated with craniospinal irradiation. *Int J Radiat Oncol Biol Phys.* 2000;46(5):1171–1176.
81. Ono N, Kohga H, Zama A, et al. A comparison of children with suprasellar germ cell tumors and craniopharyngiomas: final height, weight, endocrine, and visual sequelae after treatment. *Surg Neurol.* 1996;46(4):370–377.
82. Schmugge M, Boltshauser E, Pluss HJ, et al. Long-term follow-up and residual sequelae after treatment for intracerebral germ-cell tumour in children and adolescents. *Ann Oncol.* 2000;11(5):527–533.
83. Jane JA, Jr., Laws ER. Craniopharyngioma. *Pituitary.* 2006;9(4):323–326.
84. Kendall-Taylor P, Jonsson PJ, Abs R, et al. The clinical, metabolic and endocrine features and the quality of life in adults with childhood-onset craniopharyngioma compared with adult-onset craniopharyngioma. *Eur J Endocrinol.* 2005;152(4):557–567.
85. Halac I, Zimmerman D. Endocrine manifestations of craniopharyngioma. *Childs Nerv Syst.* 2005;21(8–9):640–648.
86. Sklar CA. Craniopharyngioma: endocrine abnormalities at presentation. *Pediatr Neurosurg.* 1994;21(Suppl 1):18–20.
87. Stripp DC, Maity A, Janss AJ, et al. Surgery with or without radiation therapy in the management of craniopharyngiomas in children and young adults. *Int J Radiat Oncol Biol Phys.* 2004;58(3):714–720.
88. Gonc EN, Yordam N, Ozon A, et al. Endocrinological outcome of different treatment options in children with craniopharyngioma: a retrospective analysis of 66 cases. *Pediatr Neurosurg.* 2004;40(3):112–119.

89. Blethen SL, Weldon VV. Outcome in children with normal growth following removal of a craniopharyngioma. *Am J Med Sci.* 1986;292(1):21–24.

90. Matson DD. Craniopharyngioma. *Clin Neurosurg.* 1964;10:116–129.

91. Moshang T, Jr., Rundle AC, Graves DA, et al. Brain tumor recurrence in children treated with growth hormone: the National Cooperative Growth Study experience. *J Pediatr.* 1996;128(5 Pt 2):S4–7.

92. Jostel A, Mukherjee A, Hulse PA, et al. Adult growth hormone replacement therapy and neuroimaging surveillance in brain tumour survivors. *Clin Endocrinol.* 2005;62(6): 698–705.

93. de Vries L, Lazar L, Phillip M. Craniopharyngioma: presentation and endocrine sequelae in 36 children. *J Pediatr Endocrinol Metab.* 2003;16(5):703–710.

94. Bin-Abbas B, Mawlawi H, Sakati N, et al. Endocrine sequelae of childhood craniopharyngioma. *J Pediatr Endocrinol Metab.* 2001;14(7):869–874.

95. Persani L, Ferretti E, Borgato S, et al. Circulating thyrotropin bioactivity in sporadic central hypothyroidism. *J Clin Endocrinol Metab.* 2000;85(10):3631–3635.

96. Lyen KR, Grant DB. Endocrine function, morbidity, and mortality after surgery for craniopharyngioma. *Arch Dis Child.* 1982;57(11):837–841.

97. Kerrigan JR, Veldhuis JD, Leyo SA, et al. Estimation of daily cortisol production and clearance rates in normal pubertal males by deconvolution analysis. *J Clin Endocrinol Metab.* 1993;76(6):1505–1510.

98. Linder BL, Esteban NV, Yergey AL, et al. Cortisol production rate in childhood and adolescence. *J Pediatr.* 1990;117(6):892–896.

99. Paja M, Lucas T, Garcia-Uria J, et al. Hypothalamic-pituitary dysfunction in patients with craniopharyngioma. *Clin Endocrinol.* 1995;42(5):467–473.

100. Bray GA, Inoue S, Nishizawa Y. Hypothalamic obesity. The autonomic hypothesis and the lateral hypothalamus. *Diabetologia.* 1981:20 Suppl:366–377.

101. Ullrich NJ, Scott RM, Pomeroy SL. Craniopharyngioma therapy: long-term effects on hypothalamic function. *The Neurologist.* 2005;11(1):55–60.

102. Diez B, Balmaceda C, Matsutani M, et al. Germ cell tumors of the CNS in children: recent advances in therapy. *Childs Nerv Syst.* 1999;15(10):578–585.

103. Matsutani M, Sano K, Takakura K, et al. Primary intracranial germ cell tumors: a clinical analysis of 153 histologically verified cases. *J Neurosurg.* 1997;86(3): 446–455.

104. Jubran RF, Finlay J. Central nervous system germ cell tumors: controversies in diagnosis and treatment. *Oncology*(Williston Park, NY). 2005;19(6):705–711; discussion 711–702, 715–707, 721.

105. Chi SN, Gardner SL, Levy AS, et al. Feasibility and response to induction chemotherapy intensified with high-dose methotrexate for young children with newly diagnosed high-risk disseminated medulloblastoma. *J Clin Oncol.* 2004;22(24): 4881–4887.

106. Gururangan S, McLaughlin C, Quinn J, et al. High-dose chemotherapy with autologous stem-cell rescue in children and adults with newly diagnosed pineoblastomas. *J Clin Oncol.* 2003;21(11):2187–2191.

107. Mason WP, Goldman S, Yates AJ, et al. Survival following intensive chemotherapy with bone marrow reconstitution for children with recurrent intracranial ependymoma – a report of the Children's Cancer Group. *J Neuro Oncol.* 1998;37(2):135–143.

108. Mason WP, Grovas A, Halpern S, et al. Intensive chemotherapy and bone marrow rescue for young children with newly diagnosed malignant brain tumors. *J Clin Oncol.* 1998;16(1):210–221.

109. Tauchmanova L, Selleri C, De Rosa G, et al. Endocrine disorders during the first year after autologous stem-cell transplant. *Am J Med.* 2005;118(6):664–670.

110. Schimmer AD, Ali V, Stewart AK, et al. Male sexual function after autologous blood or marrow transplantation. *Biol Blood Marrow Trans.* 2001;7(5):279–283.

111. Schimmer AD, Quatermain M, Imrie K, et al. Ovarian function after autologous bone marrow transplantation. *J Clin Oncol*. 1998;16(7):2359–2363.
112. Keilholz U, Max R, Scheibenbogen C, et al. Endocrine function and bone metabolism 5 years after autologous bone marrow/blood-derived progenitor cell transplantation. *Cancer*. 1997;79(8):1617–1622.
113. Davis VJ. Female gamete preservation. *Cancer*. 2006;107(7 Suppl):1690–1694.

Chapter 12
Ocular Consequences and Late Effects of Brain Tumor Treatments

María E. Echevarría and Joanna L. Weinstein

Introduction

A wide variety of ocular complications may occur in pediatric and adult patients treated for brain tumors and other cancers. These conditions, which may present at diagnosis and during treatment or may develop more insidiously, vary in their severity and their impact on the patient's quality of life. Because vision can have a significant impact on the patient's daily living, it is essential to identify which patients are at highest risk for developing these complications in order to establish regular evaluations by trained ophthalmologists, to make prompt diagnoses and to start the appropriate treatment when indicated.

Risk factors for ophthalmic complications in cancer patients include ocular or visual dysfunction related to tumor location, surgical intervention and associated morbidity, radiation therapy (RT), chemotherapy, other medications such as corticosteroids, and medical comorbidities. At diagnosis, patients with primary brain tumors may present with decreased visual acuity, nystagmus, diplopia, abnormal visual fields or cranial nerve palsies. Surgical interventions with or without tumor resection may lead to additional cranial nerve or other deficits which may affect vision, ocular motility and ocular function. Some of the resulting symptoms and signs may persist beyond treatment and contribute to additional ocular pathology.[1]

Long-term ophthalmologic complications can also affect any portion of the eye, including the lacrimal glands, eyelids, conjunctiva, sclera, cornea, lens, iris, retina and optic nerve (See Table 12.1). Accordingly, patients may experience a range of symptoms not limited to decreased tear production, lacrimal duct atrophy, eyelid or corneal ulceration, telangiectases, conjunctival neovascularization, keratinization, cataracts, glaucoma, retinopathy and optic neuropathy.[2]

M.E. Echevarría (✉)
San Jorge Children's Hospital, Division of Hematology/Oncology and Stem Cell Transplant, San Juan, PR, USA
e-mail: mechevarria@sjcms.com

S. Goldman, C.D. Turner (eds.), *Late Effects of Treatment for Brain Tumors*,
Cancer Treatment and Research 150, DOI 10.1007/b109924_12,
© Springer Science+Business Media, LLC 2009

Table 12.1 Ophthalmologic effects of cancer therapies

Structure	Pathology	Contributing factors	Treatment	Reference
Periocular skin, eyelid, lashes	Dermatitis Skin atrophy Lymphedema Ectropion Entropion Lid notching Madarosis	RT	Topical	[6–8, 10, 11, 25, 80]
Lacrimal glands, meibomian glands	Dry Eye (KCS)	RT CT	Punctual occlusion Topicals	[7, 8, 12–31, 80]
Iris, anterior chamber	Iridocyclitis Atrophy Neovascularization Neovascular glaucoma	RT	Topical IOP-lowering agents Surgery Enucleation	[7, 32, 33, 38]
Conjunctiva	Dry Eye (KCS) Conjunctivitis Pseudomembranous conjunctivitis Chemosis	RT SCT/GVHD	Topicals Topical IS Systemic IS Surgery	[6, 8, 30, 34–37, 80, 81]
Sclera	Scleritis Atrophy Necrosis	RT SCT/GVHD		[7, 32, 33]
Lens	Cataract	Corticosteroids RT SCT Comorbidity*	surgery	[7, 18, 32, 37, 39–56]
Cornea	Keratitis Ulceration Vascularization	SCT Endocrinopathy	Topicals Surgery	[6, 80]
Retina, choroid	Retinopathy Chorioretinopathy Choroiditis	RT SCT/GVHD Endocrinopathy Comorbidity*	surgery	[48, 57–69, 82]
Optic nerve	Optic neuropathy	RT	Unclear, ?HBO	[4, 5, 7, 70–78]

Abbreviations: RT = radiotherapy; SCT = stem cell transplantation; GVHD = graft-versus-host disease; CT = chemotherapy; CS = corticosteroids; S = surgical; T = tumor-related; HBO = hyperbaric oxygen therapy, IOP = intraocular pressure, IS = immunosuppression

For the purposes of this review we will describe the most commonly seen ophthalmic complications, symptoms and risk factors. Finally, we will focus upon current evaluation, treatment and outcomes in patients with long-term ocular complications after being treated for a brain tumor.

Radiation therapy is the therapeutic modality most commonly associated with ophthalmologic late effects. The different tissues of the eye vary greatly in their radiosensitivity.[3] Even though the goals of RT are to maximize the dose delivered to the target tissue and to minimize dose to neighboring normal tissue, ocular damage can result from the direct use of irradiation for intraocular tumors, or from indirect effects when irradiating nearby structures, such as the brain, nasopharynx or paranasal sinuses. In general, radiation damage to the anterior visual pathway is not usually seen until the RT dose exceeds 50 Gy,[4] but other morbidities and concurrent treatment may lead to damage at lower cumulative doses.[5] Post-irradiation complications may develop at the time of treatment or months to years following treatment. Acute lesions usually affect the most rapidly dividing cells, such as the cornea and skin, and may be prevented or reversed with appropriate management. Examples of acute lesions include blepharitis, conjunctivitis and keratitis. Later RT-induced effects can occur secondary to ischemia caused by vascular changes and may include cataracts, retinopathy, optic neuropathy and keratoconjunctivitis sicca. Current fractionated and conformal radiation modalities such as intensity-modulated radiotherapy (IMRT), proton beam radiotherapy, and stereotactic radiosurgery, may minimize the possible associated long-term effects.[6]

Periocular Skin, Eyelids, Lacrimal Glands and Lacrimal Ducts

The periocular skin and eyelids may undergo acute and late reactions after irradiation to the orbital or paranasal areas. Complications, which may appear during radiation, are typically dose-dependent and include dermatitis, madarosis (loss of eyelashes) and palpebral conjunctivitis.[6,7] These conditions may progress to atrophy, telangiectasia, hyperpigmentation, permanent madarosis, or lymphedema. Telangiectasia, which may result from RT-induced activation of angiogenic factors, and lymphedema may occur one to five years after treatment.[6-9] Moist dermatitis with ulceration can occur as a late finding when radiation doses exceed 40 Gy.[8,10] Such eyelid changes may lead to ectropion or entropion, skin atrophy, keratinization and lid notching, especially when doses exceed 50 Gy.[11] The resulting incomplete eyelid closure can compromise normal lid and tear function, leading to corneal damage in the form of an exposure keratopathy. The skin may be treated with skin balms and topical and/or oral corticosteroids, and the associated pathology must be treated as well (see below). It is controversial whether use of prophylactic topical steroid reduces this risk of developing these late dermatologic complications.[7]

Therapeutic ionizing radiation can also cause atrophy of the lacrimal glands and of the meibomian glands,[12] causing dose-dependent dysfunction.[7,13-17] This glandular atrophy leads to a combined lacrimal insufficiency-evaporative dry state; xerophthalmia occurs with doses greater than 40–50 Gy,[18] while doses greater than 60 Gy may cause permanent loss of secretion.[8,17,19] Such dry eye syndrome or keratoconjuntivitis sicca (KCS) is likely after the cumulative radiation dose exceeds 50–60 G[15,19]. Affected patients may report symptoms of dry, irritated red eyes and foreign body sensation and, with progression, excessive tearing secondary to reflex secretion by the accessory and major lacrimal glands.[20] When severe, this condition can produce rapid visual loss secondary to corneal opacification, ulceration or neovascularizatio.[8,19] which sometimes can become unresponsive to treatment.[21] Parsons et al. reported that of 33 patients with extracranial head and neck tumors treated with orbital radiation, 20 developed KCS. The greatest risk of this complication occurred in those who received a total radiation dose of 57 Gy or greater, though severe KCS was seen in some patients following lower doses (30–45 Gy).[15] At the higher doses, presented within a year of therapy, but at lower doses years after treatment.[15]

Radiotherapy can also affect the lacrimal ducts, punctae and canaliculi, causing inflammation and fibrosis leading to stenosis of the lacrimal drainage system.[22] Concurrent chemotherapy with such agents as 5-fluoroucil or docetaxel may cause punctual-canalicular stenosis as well.[7,23,24] Patients experience excessive tearing, and dilation of the lacrimal duct is often therapeutic.

Treatment of KSC consists of tear replacement, topical lubricants and punctual occlusion. The use of proton-beam and intensity-modulated radiotherapy (IMRT) and shielding, if appropriate, may minimize these effects to the lacrimal glands.[7]

Following stem cell transplantation, KCS can accompany graft-versus-host disease, most typically in the chronic form. This condition, which can affect up to 57% of patients,[25] can be treated with tear drops. More severe cases that do not improve with local or surgical care may require different treatment approaches such as autologous serum eye drops, tacrolimus, topical retinoic acid, topical cyclosporine, systemic steroids or other immunomodulatory agents.[26–31]

Cornea, Sclera and Conjunctiva

Effects on the cornea can be secondary to direct radiation damage,KCS or epithelial toxicity.[6] Temporary keratopathy, usually seen after radiation doses of 30–50 Gy, manifests as epithelial erosions or corneal scarring. At higher radiation doses, a keratopathy caused by the loss of the corneal stem cells which maintain the integrity of the cornea can present months after treatment.[6,7] Corneal dystrophy and necrosis can cause corneal anesthesia that may progress to occult corneal ulceration.[6–8] Additionally, dysfunction of the fifth cranial nerve can cause corneal disease, due to epithelial damage, while seventh nerve dysfunction leading to impaired blinking can lead to corneal exposure keratopathy.[6]

The characteristic symptoms of keratopathy including irritation, tearing and photophobia, may be alleviated by topical steroids and antibiotics and usually improve weeks to months after radiation.[7] Patients with ulceration often experience pain, foreign body sensation, decreased visual acuity and photosensitivity. Diagnosis is made by slit lamp examination. Treatment options include tear replacement, antibiotics, soft bandages and surgery.

The avascularity of the sclera makes it more radioresistant than other ocular structures. Nonetheless, complications such as scleral atrophy and necrosis have been described, independent of radiation doses, type of fractionation or patient's age.[32,33] These conditions may be seen with any form of radiotherapy, but commonly follow brachytherapy.[7]

Changes in the conjunctiva may be secondary to radiation therapy or associated with other ophthalmic pathology.[6,34] Varying doses of radiation affect the goblet cells of the conjunctiva and epithelium causing patients to experience dryness, irritation, and foreign body sensation. Acute conjunctival changes include hyperemia and inflammation, and following higher doses of radiation, may progress to telangiectasia, vascular engorgement and epithelial keratinization.[6,8] Conjunctival necrosis, lid deformities, limited ocular motility and subconjunctival hemorrhage may also develop as a result.[6] Necrosis requires steroids and antibiotic drops. Scarring usually resolves spontaneously with artificial drops, while lid deformities usually require surgical correction.[6,8]

Graft-versus-host disease can cause pseudomembranous conjunctivitis or sloughing of the corneal epithelium. The former can be treated in severe cases with excision, and the latter is treated with lubricants, anti-inflammatory agents and artificial tears.[30,35–37]

Iris and Anterior Chamber

Complications affecting the iris and the anterior chamber, such as iridocyclitis, iris atrophy and neovascularization, and secondary neovascular glaucoma (NVG), have become less common due to reduced radiation doses and conformal and sparing techniques.[7] Radiation may cause direct damage to the iris vessels, as well as ischemic changes to the retina. Both events drive neovascularization of the iris, which is usually asymptomatic, but can lead to a potentially severe complication, neovascular glaucoma (NVG).

NVG may arise in up to 35% of eyes treated with radiotherapy, either from direct toxicity or secondary to radiation retinopathy.[7,32,33,38] The risk of NVG appears to be dependent on radiation factors, medical comorbidities such as diabetes, and other factors. Patients with glaucoma may experience eye pain, headache, nausea and vomiting, decreased peripheral vision and increased intraocular pressure. Treatments to decrease intraocular pressure include beta-blocker drops, atropine or acetazolamide, but in some cases, enucleation may be required.[7]

Lens

Cancer therapies can lead to the development of cataracts, which are the result of disorganized healing of the normally transparent lens following damage, compensatory mitosis and proliferation of the lens epithelium.[18,39–43] Patients with cataracts may experience decreased visual acuity or, on examination, show an abnormal red reflex and an opaque lens. Chemotherapy agents, such as busulfan, used as part of preparatory regimes for high-dose chemotherapy regimens with autologous hematopoietic cell rescue can lead to cataract formation. Corticosteroids, widely used to treat edema caused by brain tumors, in treatment regimens for various cancers, including hematological malignancies, and for graft-versus-host disease following stem cell transplantation, can as well. The incidence of steroid-associated and treatment-associated cataracts varies with cumulative exposure and other, less well-defined cofactors.[44–46]

Radiation-induced cataracts are a well-characterized adverse effect of radiation therapy. They most commonly develop 2–3 years after radiotherapy; however, they can develop from six months to 35 years after treatment.[7,47] Even though most of the cases reported developed after RT doses greater than 8–10 Gy,[7,48] damage to the lens can occur even with low-dose irradiation (i.e., 2 Gy).[49,50] The risk of developing cataracts may be dependent on the mode of RT delivery and fractionation factors.[7,32] Cataracts appear more commonly in patients treated with higher penetrating electrons and brachytherapy.[7,48,50,51] In one large study of patients with choroidal melanoma treated with iodine-125 brachytherapy, 83% of eyes developed cataracts by five years posttreatment;[52] those patients who had received doses of at least 24 Gy to the lens were more likely to undergo subsequent cataract surgery.[52]

Patients treated with total body irradiation (TBI), such as that used in stem cell transplant conditioning regimens, are also at substantial risk of cataract development; occurrence in this setting ranges from 10% to 60% at 10 years.[51,53–56] Risk depends on cumulative radiation dosage and fractionation parameters,[51,53–56] as well as other cofactors. The report by Belkacemi et al. of 494 patients undergoing TBI identified high instantaneous dose rate (greater than 8 Gy) as the main risk factor for cataractogenesis;[53,54] in this study heparin used to treat transplant-associated veno-occlusive disease may have been protective again cataract development. The risk for developing cataracts appears to increase in patients concomitantly treated with corticosteroids, or patients with graft-versus-host disease (GVHD).

Preventive measures include the use of shielding or lens sparing positioning during treatment and protection from UV light. Cataracts are no longer considered a severe complication because vision can be successfully restored by surgical extraction. However, ultimate visual acuity may depend on other cofactors and underlying comorbidities, such as the presence of other ocular radiation-induced effects, including radiation retinopathy.[52]

Retina

Retinopathy can result from radiation therapy and concurrent therapies, underlying medical conditions, and as well as other factors.[48,57–66] RT-induced retinopathy has been reported following external beam RT (EBRT) or brachytherapy.[57] The posterior retina is more sensitive to radiation than the peripheral retina.[58,61,62] Radiation retinopathy is characterized by progressive degenerative and proliferative vascular changes characterized by capillary occlusion, macular edema, telangiectasia, microaneurysm formation, neovascularization, microangiopathy and retinal pigmental changes or hemorrhage. Though radiation retinopathy does not tend to occur at cumulative RT doses less than 45 Gy, concomitant chemotherapeutic agents and vascular diseases such as diabetes and hypertension have been shown to increase the likelihood of this complication, even at lower RT doses, and tend to increase the severity.[58–60] The most predictive factors of retinopathy are patient's age, total dose to the retina, and fractionation parameters.[60] Radiation-induced changes typically appear six months to three years after treatment with irradiation, but can present earlier or much later.[7] A study of patients with head and neck cancer treated with irradiation demonstrated that the incidence of retinopathy can be reduced with hyperfractionation, especially at doses greater than 50 Gy.[60] Intensity-modulated techniques may provide targeted distribution of dose so that the retina can be spared from these high dose.[60] and may decrease the risk of this complication.

Patients with retinopathy may experience blurred or distorted vision or abnormal color vision. This retinopathy can progress to permanent visual loss. When neovascularization is present, patients may be treated with photocoagulation in an attempt to prevent further visual loss. Hyperbaric oxygen and systemic corticosteroids have not consistently shown efficacy in the treatment of radiation retinopathy.[60] Some studies report vision improvement with intravitreal triamcinolone or focal laser therapy.[58,67–69] Intravitreal or systemic bevacizumab, a monoclonal antibody to vascular endothelial growth factor (VEGF) that inhibits the formation of abnormal blood vessels and decreases vascular permeability, may have a role in the treatment of radiation retinopathy, but further investigation is needed before definitive recommendations can be made.[70,71]

Acute occlusion of the central retinal artery is a rare complication following high doses of radiation and can cause permanent visual impairment.[48,64]

Optic Nerve

Radiation optic neuropathy (RON) is a rare, but potentially serious complication of radiotherapy.[72] RON occurs more commonly following radiation of primary extracranial head and neck tumors, but it may present after treatment for tumors of the eye and orbit, or any periorbital or nasopharyngeal structures.[7,73] Though not usually seen until RT doses exceed 50 Gy,[73,74] this condition may also be affected by radiation variables such as volume of irradiated tissue and fraction size. Additionally, concomitant chemotherapy or other comorbidities, including hypertension, diabetes, and endocrinopathies, may potentiate the effects of RT leading to pathology at lower RT doses.[5,75]

The pathogenesis of radiation-induced optic neuropathy appears to involve primarily vascular, but also neuropathic factors,[4,7,76] that affect both vascular endothelial and neuroglial cells. Affected patients present an average of 18 months from radiation, but symptoms may develop from three months to years following treatment.[4,7] Many patients experience an irreversible, fulminant course, characterized by painless and potentially rapid, progressive vision loss over weeks to months; affected eyes can become completely blind.

The optimal management for radiation-induced optic neuropathy remains unclear.[76] Corticosteroids and anticoagulation have not been effective.[72,73,76,77] A few reports have demonstrated potential benefit of hyperbaric oxygen therapy if initiated soon after the onset of symptoms.[72,75–77] A recent case report demonstrated visual improvement following intravitreal bevacizumab in one patient treated for RON.[78]

Ophthalmologic Screening Recommendations

At this time, cancer survivor surveillance guidelines would recommend annual ophthalmologic exams by an experienced ophthalmologist for the patients at highest risk. These apply to patients with a tumor involving the eye or orbit, with history of radiation to the brain, orbit, or eye (or surrounding structures), and with current or previous evidence of graft-versus-host disease following stem cell transplantation.[79] Relatively lower-dose radiation exposure may permit less frequent ophthalmologic screening every three years. It is critical that the ophthalmologic practitioner be aware of the patient's cancer history, prior therapy and other present or past medical conditions. This annual screening should include vision screening, examination for cataracts, and full dilated ophthalmoscopy examining the internal structures of the eye. Recommendations should be made regarding the protection of vision, including the use of sunglasses with UV protection, and protective eyewear during sports and use of power equipment.

References

1. Punt J. Cinical syndromes In: Walker D, Periolongo G, Punt J, Taylor R, eds. *Brain and Spinal Tumors of Childhood*. London: Arnold; 2004:99–106.
2. Schwartz C HW, Constine L. *Survivors of Childhood Cancer: Assessment and Management*. St. Louis, Mo: Mosby; 1994.

3. Friedman DL CL. *Late Effects on Cancer Treatment*. Fourth Edition: Lippincott Williams and Wilkins; 2005.
4. Lessell S. Friendly fire: neurogenic visual loss from radiation therapy. *J Neuroophthalmol*. 2004;24:243–250.
5. Fishman ML, Bean SC, Cogan DG. Optic atrophy following prophylactic chemotherapy and cranial radiation for acute lymphocytic leukemia. *Am J Ophthalmol*. 1976;82:571–6.
6. Barabino S, Raghavan A, Loeffler J, et al. Radiotherapy-induced ocular surface disease. *Cornea*. 2005;24:909–914.
7. Durkin SR, Roos D, Higgs B, et al. Ophthalmic and adnexal complications of radiotherapy. *Acta Ophthalmol Scand*. 2007;85:240–250.
8. Brady LW, Shields J, Augusburger J, et al. Complications from radiation therapy to the eye. *Front Radiat Ther Oncol*. 1989;23:238–250; discussion 51–4.
9. Riekki R, Jukkola A, Oikarinen A, et al. Radiation therapy induces tenascin expression and angiogenesis in human skin. *Acta Derm Venereol*. 2001;81:329–333.
10. Pilapil F, Studva KV, Dietz KA. Programmed instruction: cancer care. Radiation therapy: external radiation. *Cancer Nurs*. 1979;2:129–138.
11. Roth J, Brown N, Catterall M, et al. Effects of fast neutrons on the eye. *Br J Ophthalmol*. 1976;60:236–244.
12. Karp LA, Streeten BW, Cogan DG. Radiation-induced atrophy of the Meibomian gland. *Arch Ophthalmol*. 1979;97:303–305.
13. Bessell EM, Henk JM, Whitelocke RA, et al. Ocular morbidity after radiotherapy of orbital and conjunctival lymphoma. *Eye*. 1987;1(Pt 1):90–96.
14. Kennerdell JS, Flores NE, Hartsock RJ. Low-dose radiotherapy for lymphoid lesions of the orbit and ocular adnexa. *Ophthal Plast Reconstr Surg*. 1999;15:129–133.
15. Parsons JT, Bova FJ, Fitzgerald CR, et al. Severe dry-eye syndrome following external beam irradiation. *Int J Radiat Oncol Biol Phys*. 1994;30:775–780.
16. Stafford SL, Kozelsky TF, Garrity JA, et al. Orbital lymphoma: radiotherapy outcome and complications. *Radiother Oncol*. 2001;59:139–144.
17. Parsons JT, Fitzgerald CR, Hood CI, et al. The effects of irradiation on the eye and optic nerve. *Int J Radiat Oncol Biol Phys*. 1983;9:609–622.
18. Parsons JT, Bova FJ, Mendenhall WM, et al. Response of the normal eye to high dose radiotherapy. *Oncology* (Williston Park). 1996;10:837–847; discussion 47–8, 51–52.
19. Kwok SK, Ho PC, Leung SF, et al. An analysis of the incidence and risk factors of developing severe keratopathy in eyes after megavoltage external beam irradiation. *Ophthalmology*. 1998;105:2051–2055.
20. Weber DC, Chan AW, Lessell S, et al. Visual outcome of accelerated fractionated radiation for advanced sinonasal malignancies employing photons/protons. *Radiother Oncol*. 2006;81:243–249.
21. Nakissa N, Rubin P, Strohl R, et al. Ocular and orbital complications following radiation therapy of paranasal sinus malignancies and review of literature. *Cancer*. 1983;51:980–986.
22. Buatois F, Coquard R, Pica A, et al. [Treatment of eyelid carcinomas of 2 cmm or less by contact radiotherapy]. *J Fr Ophtalmol*. 1996;19:405–409.
23. Eiseman AS, Flanagan JC, Brooks AB, et al. Ocular surface, ocular adnexal, and lacrimal complications associated with the use of systemic 5-fluorouracil. *Ophthal Plast Reconstr Surg*. 2003;19:216–224.
24. Esmaeli B, Hidaji L, Adinin RB, et al. Blockage of the lacrimal drainage apparatus as a side effect of docetaxel therapy. *Cancer*. 2003;98:504–507.
25. Sanders JE. Chronic graft-versus-host disease and late effects after hematopoietic stem cell transplantation. *Int J Hematol*. 2002;76(Suppl 2):15–28.
26. Ahmad SM, Stegman Z, Fructhman S, et al. Successful treatment of acute ocular graft-versus-host disease with tacrolimus (FK506). *Cornea*. 2002;21:432–433.
27. Kiang E, Tesavibul N, Yee R, et al. The use of topical cyclosporin A in ocular graft-versus-host-disease. *Bone Marrow Transplant*. 1998;22:147–151.

28. Murphy PT, Sivakumaran M, Fahy G, et al. Successful use of topical retinoic acid in severe dry eye due to chronic graft-versus-host disease. *Bone Marrow Transplant.* 1996;18:641–642.
29. Ogawa Y, Okamoto S, Mori T, et al. Autologous serum eye drops for the treatment of severe dry eye in patients with chronic graft-versus-host disease. *Bone Marrow Transplant.* 2003;31:579–583.
30. Robinson MR, Lee SS, Rubin BI, et al. Topical corticosteroid therapy for cicatricial conjunctivitis associated with chronic graft-versus-host disease. *Bone Marrow Transplant.* 2004;33:1031–1035.
31. Rocha V, Wagner JE, Jr., Sobocinski KA, et al. Graft-versus-host disease in children who have received a cord-blood or bone marrow transplant from an HLA-identical sibling. Eurocord and international bone marrow transplant registry working committee on alternative donor and stem cell sources. *N Engl J Med.* 2000;342:1846–1854.
32. Shields CL, Naseripour M, Shields JA, et al. Custom-designed plaque radiotherapy for nonresectable iris melanoma in 38 patients: tumor control and ocular complications. *Am J Ophthalmol.* 2003;135:648–656.
33. Shields CL, Shields JA, Cater J, et al. Plaque radiotherapy for retinoblastoma: long-term tumor control and treatment complications in 208 tumors. *Ophthalmology.* 2001;108: 2116–2121.
34. Morita K, Kawabe Y. Late effects on the eye of conformation radiotherapy for carcinoma of the paranasal sinuses and nasal cavity. *Radiology.* 1979;130:227–232.
35. Jabs DA, Wingard J, Green WR, et al. The eye in bone marrow transplantation. III. Conjunctival graft-vs-host disease. *Arch Ophthalmol.* 1989;107:1343–1348.
36. Przepiorka D, Weisdorf D, Martin P, et al. 1994 Consensus Conference on Acute GVHD Grading. *Bone Marrow Transplant.* 1995;15:825–828.
37. Saito T, Shinagawa K, Takenaka K, et al. Ocular manifestation of acute graft-versus-host disease after allogeneic peripheral blood stem cell transplantation. *Int J Hematol.* 2002;75:332–334.
38. Bacin F, Kwiatkowski F, Dalens H, et al. [Long-term results of cobalt 60 curietherapy for uveal melanoma]. *J Fr Ophtalmol.* 1998;21:333–344.
39. Worgul BV, Merriam GR, Szechter A, et al. Lens epithelium and radiation cataract. I. Preliminary studies. *Arch Ophthalmol.* 1976;94:996–999.
40. Worgul BV, Rothstein H. On the mechanism of thyroid mediated mitogenesis in adult anura. I. Preliminary analysis of growth kinetics and macromolecular syntheses, in lens epithelium, under the influence of exogenous triiodothyronine. *Cell Tissue Kinet.* 1974;7: 415–424.
41. Paulino AC. Role of radiation therapy in parameningeal rhabdomyosarcoma. *Cancer Invest.* 1999;17:223–230.
42. Alter AJ, Leinfelder PJ. Roentgen-ray cataract; effects of shielding of the lens and ciliary body. *AMA Arch Ophthalmol.* 1953;49:257–260.
43. Macfaul PA, Bedford MA. Ocular complications after therapeutic irradiation. *Br J Ophthalmol.* 1970;54: 237–247.
44. Livingston PM, Carson CA, Taylor HR. The epidemiology of cataract: a review of the literature. *Ophthal Epidemiol.* 1995;2:151–164.
45. West SK, Valmadrid CT. Epidemiology of risk factors for age-related cataract. *Sur Ophthalmol.* 1995;39:323–334.
46. Dai E, et al. In: Yanoff M, Duker JS eds. *Ophthalmology.* C. V. Mosby. 2nd edition.
47. Anteby I, Ramu N, Gradstein L, et al. Ocular and orbital complications following the treatment of retinoblastoma. *Eur J Ophthalmol.* 1998;8:106–111.
48. Takeda A, Shigematsu N, Suzuki S, et al. Late retinal complications of radiation therapy for nasal and paranasal malignancies: relationship between irradiated-dose area and severity. *Int J Radiat Oncol Biol Phys.* 1999;44:599–605.
49. Wilde G, Sjostrand J. A clinical study of radiation cataract formation in adult life following gamma irradiation of the lens in early childhood. *Br J Ophthalmol.* 1997;81: 261–266.

50. Schipper J, Tan KE, van Peperzeel HA. Treatment of retinoblastoma by precision megavoltage radiation therapy. *Radiother Oncol.* 1985;3:117–132.
51. Deeg HJ, Flournoy N, Sullivan KM, et al. Cataracts after total body irradiation and marrow transplantation: a sparing effect of dose fractionation. *Int J Radiat Oncol Biol Phys.* 1984;10:957–964.
52. Group COMS. Incidence of cataract and outcomes after cataract surgery in the first 5 years afetr iodine 125 bracgytherapy in the Collaborative Ocular Melanoma Study: COMS Report No. 27. *Ophthalmology.* 2007;114(7):1363–1371.
53. Belkacemi Y, Labopin M, Vernant JP, et al. Cataracts after total body irradiation and bone marrow transplantation in patients with acute leukemia in complete remission: a study of the European Group for Blood and Marrow Transplantation. *Int J Radiat Oncol Biol Phys.* 1998;41:659–668.
54. Belkacemi Y, Ozsahin M, Pene F, et al. Cataractogenesis after total body irradiation. *Int J Radiat Oncol Biol Phys.* 1996;35:53–60.
55. Zierhut D, Lohr F, Schraube P, et al. Cataract incidence after total-body irradiation. *Int J Radiat Oncol Biol Phys.* 2000;46:131–135.
56. Beyzadeoglu M, Dirican B, Oysul K, et al. Evaluation of fractionated total body irradiation and dose rate on cataractogenesis in bone marrow transplantation. *Haematologia (Budap).* 2002;32:25–30.
57. Parsons JT, Bova FJ, Fitzgerald CR, et al. Radiation retinopathy after external-beam irradiation: analysis of time-dose factors. *Int J Radiat Oncol Biol Phys.* 1994;30:765–773.
58. Gupta A, Dhawahir-Scala F, Smith A, et al. Radiation retinopathy: case report and review. *BMC Ophthalmol.* 2007;7:6.
59. Subramanian PS, Bressler NM, Miller NR. Radiation retinopathy after fractionated stereotactic radiotherapy for optic nerve sheath meningioma. *Ophthalmology.* 2004;111:565–567.
60. Monroe AT, Bhandare N, Morris CG, et al. Preventing radiation retinopathy with hyperfractionation. *Int J Radiat Oncol Biol Phys.* 2005;61:856–864.
61. Zamber RW, Kinyoun JL. Radiation retinopathy. *West J Med.* 1992;157:530–533.
62. Brown GC, Shields JA, Sanborn G, et al. Radiation retinopathy. *Ophthalmology.* 1982;89:1494–1501.
63. Anderson NG, Regillo C. Ocular manifestations of graft versus host disease. *Curr Opin Ophthalmol.* 2004;15:503–507.
64. Shukovsky LJ, Fletcher GH. Retinal and optic nerve complications in a high dose irradiation technique of ethmoid sinus and nasal cavity. *Radiology.* 1972;104:629–634.
65. Kim RY, Anderlini P, Naderi AA, et al. Scleritis as the initial clinical manifestation of graft-versus-host disease after allogenic bone marrow transplantation. *Am J Ophthalmol.* 2002;133:843–845.
66. Alvarez MT, Hernaez JM, Ciancas E, et al. Multifocal choroiditis after allogenic bone marrow transplantation. *Eur J Ophthalmol.* 2002;12:135–137.
67. Hykin PG, Shields CL, Shields JA, et al. The efficacy of focal laser therapy in radiation-induced macular edema. *Ophthalmology.* 1998;105:1425–1429.
68. Shields CL, Demirci H, Dai V, et al. Intravitreal triamcinolone acetonide for radiation maculopathy after plaque radiotherapy for choroidal melanoma. *Retina.* 2005;25:868–874.
69. Sutter FK, Gillies MC. Intravitreal triamcinolone for radiation-induced macular edema. *Arch Ophthalmol.* 2003;121:1491–1493.
70. Finger PT, Chin K. Anti-vascular endothelial growth factor bevacizumab (avastin) for radiation retinopathy. *Arch Ophthalmol.* 2007;125:751–756.
71. Solano JM, Bakri SJ, Pulido JS. Regression of radiation-induced macular edema after systemic bevacizumab. *Can J Ophthalmol.* 2007;42:748–749.
72. Boschetti M, De Lucchi M, Giusti M, et al. Partial visual recovery from radiation-induced optic neuropathy after hyperbaric oxygen therapy in a patient with Cushing disease. *Eur J Endocrinol.* 2006;154:813–818.

73. Parsons JT, Bova FJ, Fitzgerald CR, et al. Radiation optic neuropathy after megavoltage external-beam irradiation: analysis of time-dose factors. *Int J Radiat Oncol Biol Phys.* 1994;30:755–763.
74. Hopewell JW, van der Kogel AJ. Pathophysiological mechanisms leading to the development of late radiation-induced damage to the central nervous system. *Front Radiat Ther Oncol.* 1999;33:265–275.
75. Guy J, Schatz NJ. Hyperbaric oxygen in the treatment of radiation-induced optic neuropathy. *Ophthalmology.* 1986;93:1083–1088.
76. Miller NR. Radiation-induced optic neuropathy: still no treatment. *Clin Experiment Ophthalmol.* 2004;32:233–235.
77. Levy RL, Miller NR. Hyperbaric oxygen therapy for radiation-induced optic neuropathy. *Ann Acad Med Singapore.* 2006;35:151–157.
78. Finger PT. Anti-VEGF bevacizumab (Avastin) for radiation optic neuropathy. *Am J Ophthalmol* 2007;143:335–338.
79. Landier W, Bhatia S, Eshelman DA, et al. Development of risk-based guidelines for pediatric cancer survivors: the Children's Oncology Group Long-Term Follow-Up Guidelines from the Children's Oncology Group Late Effects Committee and Nursing Discipline. *J Clin Oncol.* 2004;22:4979–4990.
80. Mohammadpour M, Javadi MA. Keratitis associated with multiple endocrine deficiency. *Cornea.* 2006;25:112–114.
81. Franklin RM, Kenyon KR, Tutschka PJ, et al. Ocular manifestations of graft-vs-host disease. *Ophthalmology.* 1983;90:4–13.
82. Cheng LL, Kwok AK, Wat NM, et al. Graft-vs-host-disease-associated conjunctival chemosis and central serous chorioretinopathy after bone marrow transplant. *Am J Ophthalmol.* 2002;134:293–295.

Chapter 13
Auditory Late Effects of Chemotherapy

Anna K. Meyer and Nancy M. Young

Introduction

Sensorineural hearing loss is the primary ototoxicity of chemotherapy in pediatric CNS tumors. The majority of toxicity is secondary to the platinums, in particular cisplatin and to a lesser degree, carboplatin. Multiple risk factors have been investigated that contribute to this loss including age, cumulative dose, method of dosing, pretreatment hearing loss, renal function, cranial radiation, and individual sensitivity. A large number of chemoprotectant treatments have been studied, with varying results. In addition, recent attention has emphasized the need for early detection of hearing loss and new methodologies besides the standard audiometry that is currently being utilized. Children who are found to have speech range hearing loss will need early intervention by audiology and speech pathology in order to maximize their hearing and language development.

Specific Agents with Ototoxicity

Cisplatin

Cisplatin is the most commonly implicated ototoxic chemotherapeutic agent used to treat pediatric CNS tumors. Traditionally, the dose limiting effect has been nephrotoxicity. The incidence of ototoxicity at conventional doses ranges from 4% to 91%, with most studies in the range of 35–50%.[1-6] This wide range is due to considerable variability in inclusion criteria, mode of hearing assessment, platinum therapy dosage and schedule, and follow-up. Cisplatin ototoxicity

A.K. Meyer (✉)
Division of Pediatric Otolaryngology, Department of Otolaryngology – Head & Neck Surgery, University of California, San Francisco, 400 Parnassus Avenue, Suite A730, San Francisco, CA 94143-0342, USA
e-mail: annakatrinemeyer@gmail.com

S. Goldman, C.D. Turner (eds.), *Late Effects of Treatment for Brain Tumors*,
Cancer Treatment and Research 150, DOI 10.1007/b109924_13,
© Springer Science+Business Media, LLC 2009

predominates in the high frequency with an overall high frequency sensorineural hearing loss (HFSNHL) incidence of 26 to >90%.[5–10] Transient and permanent tinnitus is a less common complaint.[6,11] Vestibular toxicity has not been evaluated in children. The hearing loss can have progressive involvement that eventually includes the speech frequencies in 15–54% of patients.[4,7,12,13] The loss is almost exclusively irreversible, with rare case reports of recovery, most commonly in adults.[11,14–16]

The population of patients who have pediatric CNS tumors may be the most vulnerable to ototoxicity due to their young age and exposure to cranial radiation. Several studies of cisplatin toxicity have focused on children with CNS tumors. Study sizes have been small (range $n = 11–39$) and have confirmed date seen in larger trials of young children. In five studies pediatric CNS tumors treated with cisplatin and/or carboplatin,[3,9,17–19] 20–33% had hearing loss in the speech range (250–4,000 Hz) and 20–64% had losses in the high frequency range. Younger age (<5 years old), high cumulative dose, and deteriorating renal function posed a greater than 50% risk for severe loss.[9]

A number of larger studies have been performed to evaluate cisplatin ototoxicity. Schell et al.[20] studied 177 children and young adults who received cisplatin, cranial radiation or both with exclusion of patients who had received previous ototoxic drugs or who had inadequate renal function. Eleven percent had >50 dB loss in the speech range (500–3,000 Hz); whereas over 50% had high frequency loss (4,000–8,000 Hz). Risk factors for ototoxicity, especially in the speech range, were higher cumulative dose, cranial radiation, presence of a CNS tumor, and younger age. A review of 153 children treated with cisplatin for a variety of tumors[5] identified young age and individual and cumulative doses as significant risks for moderate to severe high frequency loss. Another large study of 173 patients treated for neuroblastoma (median age 3-years-old) with cisplatin with/without carboplatin[4] showed severe loss (greater than 40 dB in the speech range) in 25% of patients treated with the standard dose (SD) of cisplatin (400 mg/m^2), 54% of patients treated with high-dose (HD) cisplatin (600 mg/m^2), and 50% of patients treated with standard dose cisplatin followed by carboplatin. This data is supported by Simon et al.'s [21] large study of 1,170 neuroblastoma patients in which post-cisplatin carboplatin and higher stage disease, but not age, were risks for ototoxicity.

Carboplatin

Historically the dose limiting toxicity of carboplatin has been myelosuppression. Carboplatin was initially used as a substitute for cisplatin due to its similiar antineoplastic activity and diminished nephrotoxicity. At standard doses in adults, clinical ototoxicity was believed to be minimal. Subclinical ototoxicity was observed at a rate as high as 15%.[22,23] Children were also found to have very low levels of severe hearing loss.[24–26]

Dose limiting myelotoxicity in carboplatin therapy has been mitigated by the advent of autologous stem cell rescue. High-dose carboplatin in conjunction with autologous stem cell rescue is now an essential aspect of the treatment of high risk solid tumors. Higher doses of carboplatin, especially following previous cisplatin therapy, have resulted in higher rates of ototoxicity. Kennedy et al.[27] conducted an early study of large cumulative carboplatin dosing in adults and found a 19% incidence of high frequency sensorineural hearing loss (HFSNHL) of 30 dB or greater. Escalating doses, without previous cisplatin treatment, have also shown a high rate of ototoxicity, though some idiosyncratic or first-dose ototoxicity has also been observed.[28,29] In a small study of high-dose carboplatin (total dose 2 g/m^2) for pre-bone marrow transplant neuroblastoma,[12] all patients ($n = 11$) had worsening hearing loss and 82% had loss in the speech frequency range for which hearing aids were recommended. The majority had previous exposure to cisplatin, as well as additional risk factors for hearing loss including aminoglycosides, diuretics, and noise exposure (Fig. 13.1). As noted previously, other large studies have confirmed a high risk of loss (40–50%) with carboplatin following cisplatin treatment.[4,21] Carboplatin has also been linked to ototoxicity in patients with osmotic opening of the blood-brain barrier, especially in cases of intravertebral artery infusion.[30,31]

In general, hearing loss from carboplatin is likely to be considerably larger than previously estimated, especially when given at a high dose or after cisplatin. Children who are older, treated with standard dose, and who did not sustain previous cisplatin treatment are at less risk for hearing loss.

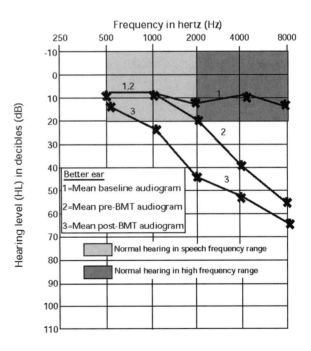

Fig. 13.1 Better ear mean audiograms. Hearing loss was symmetrical. None of the patients had greater than a 15 dB difference between better and worse ear at any frequency.[12] BMT = Bone Marrow Transplant

Vincristine

Peripheral neuropathy is the most well-documented toxicity of vincristine. A few case reports have identified patients in whom high-dose vincristine (2–2.5 mg/m^2) has caused bilateral sensorineural hearing loss.[32] In at least one report the effect was transient.[33] A study of the distortion product otoacoustic emissions (DPOAEs) and medial olivocochlear bundle (MOCB) function in 36 children treated with vincristine (and gentamycin) showed a transient effect on the DPOAEs that can last weeks, and an effect on the MOCB that can last years.[34] Further clinical investigation of this effect and its long-term outcomes is necessary.

Pathophysiology

The platinums destroy the outer hair cells (OHCs) in the organ of Corti of the cochlea.[35-37] The basal turn of the cochlea contains the OHCs for the highest frequencies and is the most common site for loss. Cumulative damage to the OHCs ascends the cochlea resulting in loss in the lower frequencies, including the speech range.[35] Additionally, atrophy of the stria vascularis and damage to the spiral ganglion cells has been documented with cisplatin treatment.[38]

The pathogenesis of the specific damage to OHCs has been linked to the overproduction of reactive oxygen species and iron-induced free radicals which deplete cellular antioxidant protection.[39,40] Damage to the organ of Corti from carboplatin has also been observed.[41] Free radicals are created by platinum-generated depletion of antioxidants by a multitude of mechanisms (see Chapter 4). The use of antioxidants and the elimination of free radicals has been the subject of intense focus for treatment and prevention of ototoxicity (See Adjuvant Therapy).

Risk Factors

Multiple risk factors for cisplatin ototoxicity have been investigated, including cumulative dose, mode of administration, cranial radiation, age, treatment with other ototoxic medications, previous hearing loss, renal dysfunction, and individual susceptibility.

Cranial Radiation

Cranial radiation alone can cause conductive hearing loss (CHL) secondary to middle and external ear alterations, including middle ear effusion and eustachian tube dysfunction. Sensorineural hearing loss (SNHL) is uncommon, but more likely to be permanent than CHL.[42] A synergistic effect between cranial radiation and post-radiation cisplatin has been documented in children.[19,20,43] Temporal bone evaluation of patients undergoing cisplatin and radiation have shown extensive loss of OHCs.[38] Knight et al.[44] found that 70% of patients with cranial radiation and cisplatin had hearing loss; however, there was no significant difference in ototoxicity from patients who received chemotherapy alone. Other studies support the increased risk of ototoxicity with both radiation and platinum therapy as compared to platinum therapy alone. Schell et al.[20] observed a high probability of moderate hearing loss in patients with cranial radiation followed by cisplatin therapy even at cumulative doses as low as 270 mg/m^2. A study of 31 patients with intracranial tumors treated postsurgically in three arms (radiation alone, cisplatin alone, combined therapy),[19] found significantly worse hearing in those receiving combined therapy. Conversely, pre-radiation treatment does not seem to be a risk factor for additional ototoxicity.[3] In addition, ototoxicity incurred from cranial radiation may be delayed for up to a year.[43] Recent advances in radiation therapy, particularly intensity-modulated radiation therapy, are promising auditory system sparing modalities that limit ototoxicity even at higher doses of cisplatin.[45]

Cumulative Dose

Increasing cumulative dose has been implicated as a risk for increased ototoxicity from platinums, particularly cisplatin.[6,46,47] Clinically significant ototoxicity has been observed in children at cumulative cisplatin doses of 400 mg/m^2, and the maximum dose is considered 600 mg/m^2.[8] In adults, the threshold for cisplatin is as high as 600 mg/m^2.[11] A wide range of cumulative doses is used in children (300–450 mg/m^2), and the severity of ototoxicity correlates to this range. Li et al.[5] showed a three-fold increased risk for hearing loss between cisplatin doses at 100–300 versus 700–1,300 mg/m^2. Incidences of HFSNHL at doses above 450 mg/m^2 have been found to be as high as 88%.[47] Simon et al.[21] found no statistical difference in ototoxicity between children treated with 401–600 mg/m^2 (26%) and those treated with greater than 600 mg/m^2 (22%); whereas Bertolini et al.[2] found a small, but significant difference between doses less than 400 mg/m^2 (37%) and doses above 400 mg/m^2 (44%), and Kushner et al.[4] found the most significant difference with 25% severe loss at 400 mg/m^2 and 54% severe loss at 600 mg/m^2. Caution should be exercised, with diligent monitoring, in doses over 400 mg/m^2. However, an absolute cut-off for dosage is less useful than the clinician's awareness that a relatively linear relationship between cumulative dose and ototoxicity exists, with a plateau at higher doses.[20]

The addition of carboplatin to patients previously treated with cisplatin has also been linked to an increased risk of ototoxicity. In a large study[4] ($n = 173$), 50% of children treated with carboplatin 1,500–1,700 mg/m^2 after 400 mg/m^2 of cisplatin had severe ototoxicity, while only 25% of those treated with

400 mg/m^2 of cisplatin alone had such ototoxicity levels. In 67 patients, Knight et al.[44] found that 84% of children treated with variable doses of cisplatin followed by carboplatin had ototoxicity, whereas 38 and 55% of children treated with carboplatin therapy followed by cisplatin, respectively, suffered ototoxicity.

Pretreatment Hearing Loss

The majority of data for risk of ototoxicity in patients with pre-cisplatin exposure hearing loss is within the adult literature[13] and is due to the much higher frequency of hearing loss in the adult cancer population. Parsons et al.[12] have identified that children with pre-bone marrow transplant (BMT) HFSNHL were at risk for speech frequency hearing loss post-BMT.

Age

In most studies, an inverse relationship between age and severity of ototoxicity has been observed.[2,6,48] Kushner et al.'s [4] large study of 173 clearly showed increased ototoxicity from high-dose cisplatin in children less than five-years-old, and Li et al.[5] showed a 21 times higher incidence of moderate to severe hearing loss in children less than five-years–old, compared to patients aged 15–20-years-old. Studies in which higher rates of ototoxicity have been observed in children over 36 months, versus those that were younger, are attributed to a higher cumulative dose in the older patients and use of standard dose carboplatin and low-dose cisplatin in the younger patients.[2,6,48] The elderly are also more likely to be at risk, which is confounded by the much higher incidence of pretreatment hearing loss.[49] In general, children with CNS tumors are quite young and, thus, fall into a higher risk category for ototoxicity.

Renal Function

Ototoxicity in platinum therapy may be affected by creatinine clearance (CrCl) and some advocate dose reduction based upon CrCl.[50] Individual variation in maximum plasma concentration and platinum clearance may account for variations in ototoxicity.[51,52]

Mode of Administration

While the evidence for reduced nephrotoxicity from continuous infusion instead of bolus dosage has been well characterized,[53,54] the evidence in the case of ototoxicity is equivocal. Humes et al.[55] identified increased ototoxicity with bolus infusion in both adults and children. Several studies have shown increased overall tissue toxicity from pulsed platinum infusions.[56,57] Gupta et al.[58] in a study of only continuous cisplatin infusion, had only one patient ($n = 39$) with ototoxicity, an individual who also had a high dose of 500 mg/m^2. However, other researchers have found that continuous cisplatin infusion versus bolus infusion showed diminished nephrotoxicity, but not ototoxicity in children.[59]

Genetic Polymorphism

Individual sensitivity to platinum therapy has generated exploration of genetic susceptibilities. Glutathione S-transferase genotype variation in patients with testicular cancer confers a four-fold increased risk of ototoxicity in certain genotypes.[60,61] Further study of these and other genotype variations will perhaps offer insight into the pediatric population.

Ototoxic Medications

The use of other ototoxic medications, particularly aminoglycosides and diuretics, is difficult to study. The majority of patients undergoing cisplatin therapy are exposed to aminoglycosides and/or diuretics. Animal models have shown interaction between cisplatin, aminoglycoside antibiotics, and loop diuretics.[37,62] Coradini et al.[63] found no difference in exposure to other ototoxic agents between patients who developed hearing loss and those that did not. Skinner et al.[6] found that the number of days of exposure to other ototoxic drugs did not influence the severity of hearing loss. In summary, data regarding the effect of additional ototoxic medication on platinum ototoxicity is difficult to obtain and worthy of further investigation.[64,65]

Counseling

A necessary component of initiating chemotherapy is extensive discussion of toxicities and the cost/benefit of therapy versus toxicity. All patients who will be treated with platinums, and their parents, should be advised about the risk of hearing loss, the need for frequent and prolonged monitoring, and rehabilitative options including hearing aids, speech therapy, and cochlear implantation.

Screening for Loss

Cisplatin ototoxicity typically has an onset within hours to days.[66] Most studies confirm that this rapid onset is permanent and neither improves or worsens over time.[4,8,12] However, a few studies have shown continued loss up to 11 years after platinum therapy.[2,44,67] In a study of 123 children, Brock grade 2 ototoxicity incidence increased from 11% within two years of treatment, to 44% after two years (see "Assessment of Hearing Loss" section for Brock criteria).[2] Two cases of recovery in children after ototoxicity have been reported.[6]

Because it is unclear if pretreatment loss is a risk factor for ototoxicity from chemotherapy, it is recommended that patients undergo pretreatment audiometry. All children who undergo cisplatin or high-dose carboplatin should be evaluated at the completion of treatment.[68] Though many cisplatin protocols ask for audiologic screening during treatment, there is no consensus among practitioners on how to proceed when early subclinical ototoxicity has been detected. No clear data has surfaced to indicate that chemotherapy doses should be limited in this setting and whether an unacceptable effect on survival rates would be justified for an undetermined effect on ototoxicity progression. Most current treatment protocols with platinums recommend dose modification to limit ongoing ototoxicity in the setting of clinical ototoxicity. This generally includes a 50% dose reduction for Brock Grade 2 and discontinuation of the drug for Grades 3 and 4. The potential for less chemotherapeutic effect should be considered and discussed with the family.

The frequency and duration of posttreatment interval screening has not been established. Given the small risk of ongoing or delayed loss months to years following treatment, a conservative approach would be to screen children every six months for greater than two years.

Assessment of Hearing Loss

Multiple criteria exist for evaluating and reporting hearing loss from ototoxicity. The variation in hearing loss that is included in the grading accounts for some of the wide variability in reported chemotherapy-induced ototoxicity.[44]

Chemotherapeutic ototoxicity papers most frequently utilize the Brock criteria[8] (Table 13.1). This criteria grades hearing loss based on pure tone thresholds in a range from 0 to 4. Grade 0 represents thresholds less than 40 dB; Grade 1 (minimal hearing loss) is greater than 40 dB threshold above 8,000 Hz; Grade 2

Table 13.1 Brock grading

Bilateral hearing loss	Grade	Designation
< 40 dB at all frequencies	0	Minimal
≥ 40 dB at 8,000 Hz only	1	Mild
≥ 40 dB at 4,000 Hz and above	2	Moderate
≥ 40 dB at 2,000 Hz and above	3	Marked
≥ 40 dB at 1,000 Hz and above	4	Severe

Grading system for cisplatin-induced bilateral high frequency hearing loss (Brock et al.[112–115]).

(moderate hearing loss) is greater than 40 dB at or above 4,000 Hz; Grade 3 (severe hearing loss) is greater than 40 dB between 2,000 and 8,000 Hz, and Grade 4 (severe hearing loss) is greater than 40 dB between 1,000 and 8,000 Hz. This scale is useful in that it emphasizes the increased risk of hearing loss in the high frequencies and specifically reflects the risk of speech or learning difficulties.[58] However, it should be noted that Grade 0 does not discriminate between normal hearing and mild hearing loss (>15 to 40 dB) according to standard audiometric measurement.[69] In addition, it may miss early signs of hearing loss in the highest frequencies that portend further loss with continued platinum treatment. In addition, the Brock criteria assumes normal hearing at baseline.

Other criteria account for baseline hearing loss by assessing change in hearing thresholds. The American Speech-Language-Hearing Association (ASHA) criteria[70] (Table 13.2) was specifically designed to detect ototoxicity early in

Table 13.2 Degree of hearing loss: Severe degree of hearing loss refers to the severity of the loss. The numbers are representative of the patient's thresholds, or the softest intensity at which sound is perceived. The following is one of the more commonly used classification systems[70]

Degree of hearing loss	Hearing loss range (dB HL)
Normal	–10 to 15
Slight	16 to 25
Mild	26 to 40
Moderate	41 to 55
Moderately severe	56 to 70
Severe	71 to 90
Severe Profound	91 +

Source: Clark JG. Uses and abuses of hearing loss classification *Asha*. 1981;23:493–500.

order to prevent or minimize loss. The criteria include: (A) 20 dB or greater decrease in pure tone threshold at one test frequency; (B) 10 dB or greater decrease in pure tone threshold at two adjacent frequencies, and (C) loss of response at three consecutive test frequencies where responses were previously obtained. The National Cancer Institute Common Terminology Criteria for Adverse Events (NCI CTCAE) ototoxicity grades include: Grade 1, threshold shift or loss of 15–25 dB relative to baseline, averaged at two or more contiguous frequencies in at least one ear; Grade 2, threshold shift or loss of >25–90 dB, averaged at two contiguous test frequencies in at least one ear; Grade 3, hearing loss sufficient to indicate therapeutic intervention, including hearing aids (e.g., > 20 dB bilateral HL in the speech frequencies; >30 dB unilateral HL, and requiring additional speech-language related services), and Grade 4, indication for cochlear implant and requiring additional speech-language related services. The NCI CTCAE criteria are used widely in clinical trials and are criticized for not specifically identifying high frequency hearing loss.[8]

Additionally, many clinical trials report only Grade 3 and 4, and both fail to emphasize the importance of milder loss and adequately report the magnitude of ototoxicity. In Knight's series of 82 patients, use of CTCAE Grades 3 and 4 only would have missed reporting 36% of patients with hearing loss.[44] This milder hearing loss may not only be a harbinger of further loss, but also may have a significant impact on academic and socio-emotional development.[71] ASHA and NCI CTCAE grades correlate well, but both poorly correlate with the Brock criteria.[44]

The Muenster classification attempts to specifically assess the ototoxicity of cisplatin therapy[59,72] (Table 13.3). It is an effective tool for cisplatin-specific loss, identifying early high frequency loss and offering the user a guideline for intervention with hearing aids or possible cochlear implantation. Its limitations are that it only assesses bilateral loss and that it is new and has not been thoroughly compared to the other criteria.

Table 13.3 Muenster classification for early detection of cisplatin-induced bilateral high frequency hearing loss[59,72]

Bilateral hearing loss	Pediatric audiological valuation according to WHO classification	Grade
10 dB at all frequencies	No considerable damage	0
>10 to 20 dB at all frequencies or tinnitus	Questionable, commencing damage	1
Hearing loss 4 kHz; >20 dB	Moderate damage	
>20 to 40 dB		2a
>40 to 60 dB		2b
>60 dB		2c
Hearing loss <4 kHz; >20 dB	Impairment compensable with hearing aid	
>20 to 40 dB		3a
>40 to 60 dB		3b
>60 dB		3c
Mean hearing loss <4 kHz; 80 dB	Loss of function, compensable by cochlear implantation	4

The emphasis on detecting early loss has resulted in investigation of the use of alternatives to pure tone audiometry. While pure tone audiometry remains the gold standard, it is often not reliable in children younger than three-years-old[73] and may be limited in the assessment of ill children who are unwilling to participate.[58,74] Otoacoustic emissions (OAEs) have been found to be very helpful in assessing children.[75-77] OAEs test outer hair cell function specifically and are uniquely suited to detect early change that may represent subclinical damage. Clinical forms of OAEs are distortion product OAEs (DPOAEs) and transient-evoked OAEs (TEOAEs), both of which are induced with a stimulus. OAEs have high test-retest reliability, do not require active patient participation, and are rapid, objective and noninvasive. They provide ear-specific information. This is often limited in small children in which audiometry is performed in the sound field and only provides information about the best hearing ear.

OAEs are an excellent screening tool; however, they do not establish a hearing threshold and thus are nondiagnostic for degree of loss. If abnormal OAEs are obtained, a follow-up audiogram or auditory brainstem response testing (ABR) should be pursued. OAEs are limited by the inability to measure loss in patients with middle ear pathology or to be obtainable in a crying or moving child.

The criteria for ototoxic change has not been established in OAEs in children. DPOAEs have been established as a sensitive measure of hearing loss in aminoglycoside and noise-induced hearing loss.[78,79] A study comparing pure tone average (PTA) to DPOAEs after the first dose of cisplatin showed a more pronounced effect on DPOAEs than PTA and suggested that DPOAEs are an easy and reliable test to monitor hearing as the patients underwent treatment.[73] Toral-Martinon et al.[77] have confirmed their reliability for monitoring in cisplatin treatment.

The emphasis on early detection has resulted in the investigation of combining evaluation methods. Extended high frequency audiometry (EHF) (8–20 kHz), in conjunction with DPOAEs, has been shown to be a more sensitive evaluation of initial ototoxic change than PTA.[12,80–83] In a study of 32 children, 63% showed bilateral ototoxicity by conventional PTA (0.5–8 kHz), 81.3% had bilateral decreased DPOAEs and dynamic range, and 94% had bilateral ototoxicity on extended high frequency audiometry (EHF) (9–16 kHz).[83]

Auditory brain stem response (ABR) testing is also a reliable, objective test of bilateral hearing that can be utilized in the uncooperative or young child. ABR is more costly, time-consuming, and requires sedation; thus, it should be reserved to assess thresholds in children with altered DPOAEs who cannot undergo audiometry.

As more emphasis has been placed on detecting early signs of ototoxicity, a pertinent question is whether high frequency loss, even that outside the usual speech range, has any effect on learning or communication. High frequency sound has the least acoustic power, yet it has been shown to make a major contribution to speech intelligibility.[84] High frequency loss reduces recognition of some speech sounds above 2,000 Hz, including: s, f, th, sh, h, k, and t. Some estimates show that 50% of consonants in the English language can be aided by the perception of high frequency sound.[85] In children, hearing loss above 4,000 Hz may impede the hearing of plurals, especially from women and children.[86] Adults are much more capable of tolerating high frequency loss, both due to their full language competence and their ability to use semantic and syntactic clues.[87] Diminished or absent high frequency hearing may also affect comprehension of speech in noise or overheard and indirect conversation.[85,88] A study of 1,218 children with minimal hearing loss showed that 37% failed at least one grade.[71] Children in this group also showed greater dysfunction in behavior energy, stress, self-esteem, and social support.

In assessing the pediatric population, several different testing modalities may need to be used. The oncologist should be familiar with age-related audiometric testing and the possible use of ototoxicity-specific testing, such as EHF audiometry, DPOAEs, and ABR. Table 13.4 provides age-specific testing recommendations.

Table 13.4 Recommended audiologic testing by age

Age (or approximate developmental age)	Testing
6 to 10 months	Behavior Observation Audiometry (BOA)
	DPOAEs
	ABR (if DPOAEs fail)
10 months to 2 ½ years	Visual Reinforcement Audiometry (VRA)
	DPOAEs
	ABR (if DPOAEs fail)
2 1/2 to 5 years	Conditioned Play Audiometry (CPA)
	High frequency threshold audiometry
	Speech audiometry
	DPOAEs
	ABR (if DPOAEs fail)
Greater than 5-years-old	Threshold audiometry
	High frequency threshold audiometry
	Speech audiometry

Adapted from Dhooge et al.[80]

Adjuvant Treatment

A multitude of adjuvant treatments to mitigate the effects of platinums have been investigated. Nearly all are sulfur or sulfhydryl compounds (thio compounds) that act as antioxidants and heavy metal chelators.

Amifostine

Amifostine (WR-2721, Ethylol) has been approved for treatment of toxicities from chemotherapy and radiation such as myelosuppression and radiation-induced xerostomia, and has had efficacy in the prevention of nephrotoxicity.[89–91] Amifostine is a prodrug that, when phosphorylated to its active form, acts to protect tissues by increasing vascularity, pH and the level of activity of alkaline phosphatase.[92] Significant toxicities, including hypocalcemia, hypersensitivity reactions and hypotension have been associated with amifostine.[93] In guinea pigs, it has been shown to reduce cisplatin-induced hearing loss.[94] Amifostine, given in conjunction with high-dose cisplatin in adults with melanoma, had poor results. Three out of 15 patients had a dose limiting ototoxicity and went on to wear hearing aids; all patients had audiometric changes at one or more frequencies.[95] In one study, amifostine given with high-dose cisplatin for pediatric germ cell tumors had no effect on ototoxicity.[96] This lack of effect may be due to the blood-brain barrier impeding the effect of amifostine in the inner ear.[97]

Sodium Thiosulfate

Animal models have shown a chemoprotective effect by sodium thiosulfate (STS).[98] Sodium thiosulfate reduces ototoxicity in adults treated with high-dose carboplatin.[30,99] However, concern about the reduction of efficacy of carboplatin by STS has been raised.[100,101] Attempts at circumventing this in CNS tumors have involved making the blood-brain barrier more permeable to carboplatin, but then diminishing its permeability to STS (the two-compartment theory).[30] Rat models in which STS was delayed after cisplatin infusion were effective for ototoxity prevention, and were thought not to affect cisplatin antineoplastic activity.[102] The efficacy of delayed STS treatment in platinum therapy needs to be studied in pediatric CNS tumors.

D-Methionine

D-Methionine given systemically or to the round window has been shown to be chemoprotective for cisplatin-induced OHC loss.[103–105] It has also shown a protective effect on the stria vascularis.[106] Administration to rats has also shown protection against cisplatin-induced ABR threshold shifts and DPOAE decreases.[103,104,107,108] As with STS, concern exists about limiting the cytotoxic effect of platinums, and trials of D-Methionine in humans have not yet occurred.

Other

Lipoic acid, methylthiobenzoic acid (MBTA), histone deacetylase inhibitors, fosfomycin, and diethyldihydrothiocarbamate (DDTC) are additional otoprotectants that have been studied. Several comparison studies in animals have indicated that STS and DDTC are the most promising otoprotectants.[109,110]

Treatment of Hearing Loss

The result of diligent screening for early ototoxicity and continued surveillance should be appropriate treatment of hearing loss. Children who have any hearing loss, delayed or decreased speech and language development, compromised communication, or decreased educational performance should be referred for further audiologic evaluation. Children with mild loss or unilateral loss may benefit from preferential seating in the classroom or use of an FM system. The latter is designed to minimize the deleterious effects of background noise on the child's ability to understand spoken language by having the teacher use a wireless microphone so the student may listen to instruction through headphones, classroom or personal desktop speakers. Moderate to severe hearing loss will necessitate hearing aids. The clinician should also have a low threshold for referral to speech therapy.

Cochlear implantation should be strongly considered in patients with severe to profound loss. The minimum FDA-approved age for implantation is one year, though children younger than this have been implanted on a selective basis. For children with congenital hearing loss, a hearing aid trial of 4–6 months in which no benefit is observed precedes approval for cochlear implantation.[111] However, in the setting of acute losses of hearing, particularly meningitis, the trial period is eliminated. Given that postlingually deaf children and adults have better outcomes with a shorter time period between the onset of deafness and implantation, children with ototoxicity-induced hearing loss should be expedited in the cochlear implantation process.

Summary

Ototoxicity secondary to platinum treatment is a serious effect that should be closely watched for and treated appropriately when detected. Good understanding of audiologic testing and intervention on the part of the oncologist will facilitate both prevention or limitation of hearing loss and rehabilitation of patients with ototoxicity. In addition, as the search for therapies that will limit or eliminate otoxicity continues, the physician should stay abreast of studies in this area.

References

1. Fausti SA, Schechter MA, Rappaport BZ, et al. Early detection of cisplatin ototoxicity. Selected case reports. *Cancer*. 1984;53:224–231.
2. Bertolini P, Lassalle M, Mercier G, et al. Platinum compound-related ototoxicity in children: long-term follow-up reveals continuous worsening of hearing loss. *J Pediatr Hematol Oncol*. 2004;26:649–655.
3. Kretschmar CS, Warren MP, Lavally BL, et al. Ototoxicity of preradiation cisplatin for children with central nervous system tumors. *J Clin Oncol*. 1990;8:1191–1198.
4. Kushner BH, Budnick A, Kramer K, et al. Ototoxicity from high-dose use of platinum compounds in patients with neuroblastoma. *Cancer*. 2006;107:417–422.
5. Li Y, Womer RB, Silber JH. Predicting cisplatin ototoxicity in children: the influence of age and the cumulative dose. *Eur J Cancer*. 2004;40:2445–2451.
6. Skinner R, Pearson AD, Amineddine HA, et al. Ototoxicity of cisplatinum in children and adolescents. *Br J Cancer*. 1990;61:927–931.
7. Blakley BW, Myers SF. Patterns of hearing loss resulting from cis-platinum therapy. *Otolaryngol Head Neck Surg*. 1993;109:385–391.
8. Brock PR, Bellman SC, Yeomans EC, et al. Cisplatin ototoxicity in children: a practical grading system. *Med Pediatr Oncol*. 1991;19:295–300.
9. Ilveskoski I, Saarinen UM, Wiklund T, et al. Ototoxicity in children with malignant brain tumors treated with the "8 in 1" chemotherapy protocol. *Med Pediatr Oncol*. 1996;27:26–31.
10. Montaguti M, Brandolini C, Ferri GG, et al.[Cisplatin and carboplatin-induced ototoxicity in children: clinical aspects and perspectives for prevention]. *Acta Otorhinolaryngol Ital*. 2002;22:14–18.

11. Bokemeyer C, Berger CC, Hartmann JT, et al. Analysis of risk factors for cisplatin-induced ototoxicity in patients with testicular cancer. *Br J Cancer*. 1998;77:1355–1362.

12. Parsons SK, Neault MW, Lehmann LE, et al. Severe ototoxicity following carboplatin-containing conditioning regimen for autologous marrow transplantation for neuroblastoma. *Bone Marrow Transplant*. 1998;22:669–674.

13. Brown RL, Nuss RC, Patterson R, et al. Audiometric monitoring of cis-platinum ototoxicity. *Gynecol Oncol*. 1983;16:254–262.

14. Schaefer SD, Post JD, Close LG, et al. Ototoxicity of low- and moderate-dose cisplatin. *Cancer*. 1985;56:1934–1939.

15. Aguilar-Markulis NV, Beckley S, Priore R, et al. Auditory toxicity effects of long-term cis-dichlorodiammineplatinum II therapy in genitourinary cancer patients. *J Surg Oncol*. 1981;16:111–123.

16. Truong MT, Winzelberg J, Chang KW. Recovery from cisplatin-induced ototoxicity: a case report and review. *Int J Pediatr Otorhinolaryngol*. 2007;71:1631–1638.

17. Cohen BH, Zweidler P, Goldwein JW, et al. Ototoxic effect of cisplatin in children with brain tumors. *Pediatr Neurosurg*. 1990;16:292–296.

18. Freilich RJ, Kraus DH, Budnick AS, et al. Hearing loss in children with brain tumors treated with cisplatin and carboplatin-based high-dose chemotherapy with autologous bone marrow rescue. *Med Pediatr Oncol*. 1996;26:95–100.

19. Miettinen S, Laurikainen E, Johansson R, et al. Radiotherapy enhanced ototoxicity of cisplatin in children. *Acta Otolaryngol Suppl*. 1997;529:90–94.

20. Schell MJ, McHaney VA, Green AA, et al. Hearing loss in children and young adults receiving cisplatin with or without prior cranial irradiation. *J Clin Oncol*. 1989;7:754–760.

21. Simon T, Hero B, Dupuis W, et al. The incidence of hearing impairment after successful treatment of neuroblastoma. *Klin Padiatr*. 2002;214:149–152.

22. Canetta R, Rozencweig M, Carter SK. Carboplatin: the clinical spectrum to date. *Cancer Treat Rev*. 1985;12 Suppl A:125–136.

23. Meyers FJ, Welborn J, Lewis JP, et al. Infusion carboplatin treatment of relapsed and refractory acute leukemia: evidence of efficacy with minimal extramedullary toxicity at intermediate doses. *J Clin Oncol*. 1989;7:173–178.

24. Ettinger LJ, Gaynon PS, Krailo MD, et al. A phase II study of carboplatin in children with recurrent or progressive solid tumors. A report from the Children's Cancer Group. *Cancer*. 1994;73:1297–1301.

25. Lambert MP, Shields C, Meadows AT. A retrospective review of hearing in children with retinoblastoma treated with carboplatin-based chemotherapy. *Pediatr Blood Cancer*. 2008;50:223–226.

26. Stern JW, Bunin N. Prospective study of carboplatin-based chemotherapy for pediatric germ cell tumors. *Med Pediatr Oncol*. 2002;39:163–167.

27. Kennedy IC, Fitzharris BM, Colls BM, et al. Carboplatin is ototoxic. *Cancer Chemother Pharmacol*. 1990;26:232–234.

28. Allen JRL. Modern-period muddy sediments in the severn estuary (Southwestern UK) – A pollutant-based model for dating and correlation. *Sedimentary Geol*. 1988;58:1.

29. Macdonald MR, Harrison RV, Wake M, et al. Ototoxicity of carboplatin: comparing animal and clinical models at the Hospital for Sick Children. *J Otolaryngol*. 1994;23:151–159.

30. Doolittle ND, Muldoon LL, Brummett RE, et al. Delayed sodium thiosulfate as an otoprotectant against carboplatin-induced hearing loss in patients with malignant brain tumors. *Clin Cancer Res*. 2001;7:493–500.

31. Williams PC, Henner WD, Roman-Goldstein S, et al. Toxicity and efficacy of carboplatin and etoposide in conjunction with disruption of the blood-brain tumor barrier in the treatment of intracranial neoplasms. *Neurosurgery*. 1995;37:17–27; discussion -8.

32. Lugassy G, Shapira A. Sensorineural hearing loss associated with vincristine treatment. *Blut*. 1990;61:320–321.

33. Aydogdu I, Ozturan O, Kuku I, et al. Bilateral transient hearing loss associated with vincristine therapy: case report. *J Chemother*. 2000;12:530–532.
34. Riga M, Psarommatis I, Korres S, et al. Neurotoxicity of vincristine on the medial olivocochlear bundle. *Int J Pediatr Otorhinolaryngol*. 2007;71:63–69.
35. Moroso MJ, Blair RL. A review of cis-platinum ototoxicity. *J Otolaryngol*. 1983;12:365–369.
36. Boheim K, Bichler E. Cisplatin-induced ototoxicity: audiometric findings and experimental cochlear pathology. *Arch Otorhinolaryngol*. 1985;242:1–6.
37. Komune S, Asakuma S, Snow JB, Jr. Pathophysiology of the ototoxicity of cis-diamminedichloroplatinum. *Otolaryngol Head Neck Surg*. 1981;89:275–282.
38. Hoistad DL, Ondrey FG, Mutlu C, et al. Histopathology of human temporal bone after cis-platinum, radiation, or both. *Otolaryngol Head Neck Surg*. 1998;118:825–832.
39. Hinojosa R, Riggs LC, Strauss M, et al. Temporal bone histopathology of cisplatin ototoxicity. *Am J Otol*. 1995;16:731–740.
40. Dehne N, Lautermann J, Petrat F, et al. Cisplatin ototoxicity: involvement of iron and enhanced formation of superoxide anion radicals. *Toxicol Appl Pharmacol*. 2001;174:27–34.
41. Takeno S, Harrison RV, Ibrahim D, et al. Cochlear function after selective inner hair cell degeneration induced by carboplatin. *Hear Res*. 1994;75:93–102.
42. Kwong DL, Wei WI, Sham JS, et al. Sensorineural hearing loss in patients treated for nasopharyngeal carcinoma: a prospective study of the effect of radiation and cisplatin treatment. *Int J Radiat Oncol Biol Phys*.1996;36:281–289.
43. Walker DA, Pillow J, Waters KD, et al. Enhanced cis-platinum ototoxicity in children with brain tumours who have received simultaneous or prior cranial irradiation. *Med Pediatr Oncol*. 1989;17:48–52.
44. Knight KR, Kraemer DF, Neuwelt EA. Ototoxicity in children receiving platinum chemotherapy: underestimating a commonly occurring toxicity that may influence academic and social development. *J Clin Oncol*. 2005;23:8588–8596.
45. Huang E, Teh BS, Strother DR, et al. Intensity-modulated radiation therapy for pediatric medulloblastoma: early report on the reduction of ototoxicity. Int J Radiat Oncol Biol Phys. 2002;52:599–605.
46. Weatherly RA, Owens JJ, Catlin FI, et al. Cis-platinum ototoxicity in children. *Laryngoscope*. 1991;101:917–924.
47. McHaney VA TG, Hayes FA. Hearing loss in children receiving cisplatin chemotherapy. *K Pediatr*. 1983;83:314–317.
48. Pasic TR, Dobie RA. Cis-platinum ototoxicity in children. *Laryngoscope*. 1991;101:985–991.
49. Rademaker-Lakhai JM, Crul M, Zuur L, et al. Relationship between cisplatin administration and the development of ototoxicity. *J Clin Oncol*. 2006;24:918–924.
50. Calvert AH, Newell DR, Gumbrell LA, et al. Carboplatin dosage: prospective evaluation of a simple formula based on renal function. *J Clin Oncol*. 1989;7:1748–1756.
51. Peng B, English MW, Boddy AV, et al. Cisplatin pharmacokinetics in children with cancer. *Eur J Cancer*. 1997;33:1823–1828.
52. Peng B BA, English MW, et al. The comparative pharmacokinetics and pharmacodynamics of cisplatin and carboplatin in paediatric patients: a review. *Anticancer Res*. 1994;14:2279–2283.
53. Posner MR, Ferrari L, Belliveau JF, et al. A phase I trial of continuous infusion cisplatin. *Cancer*. 1987;59:15–18.
54. Erdlenbruch B, Nier M, Kern W, et al. Pharmacokinetics of cisplatin and relation to nephrotoxicity in paediatric patients. *Eur J Clin Pharmacol*. 2001;57:393–402.
55. Humes HD. Insights into ototoxicity. Analogies to nephrotoxicity. *Ann N Y Acad Sci*. 1999;884:15–18.
56. Dominici C, Petrucci F, Caroli S, et al. A pharmacokinetic study of high-dose continuous infusion cisplatin in children with solid tumors. *J Clin Oncol*. 1989;7:100–107.

57. Murakami T, Inoue S, Sasaki K, et al. Studies on age-dependent plasma platinum pharmacokinetics and ototoxicity of cisplatin. *Sel Cancer Ther*. 1990;6:145–151.
58. Gupta AA, Capra M, Papaioannou V, et al. Low incidence of ototoxicity with continuous infusion of cisplatin in the treatment of pediatric germ cell tumors. *J Pediatr Hematol Oncol*. 2006;28:91–94.
59. Lanvers-Kaminsky C, Krefeld B, Dinnesen AG, et al. Continuous or repeated prolonged cisplatin infusions in children: a prospective study on ototoxicity, platinum concentrations, and standard serum parameters. *Pediatr Blood Cancer*. 2006;47:183–193.
60. Oldenburg J, Kraggerud SM, Cvancarova M, et al. Cisplatin-induced long-term hearing impairment is associated with specific glutathione s-transferase genotypes in testicular cancer survivors. *J Clin Oncol*. 2007;25:708–714.
61. Peters U, Preisler-Adams S, Hebeisen A, et al. Glutathione S-transferase genetic polymorphisms and individual sensitivity to the ototoxic effect of cisplatin. *Anticancer Drugs*. 2000;11:639–643.
62. Kohn S, Fradis M, Podoshin L, et al. Ototoxicity resulting from combined administration of cisplatin and gentamicin. *Laryngoscope*. 1997;107:407–408.
63. Coradini PP, Cigana L, Selistre SG, et al. Ototoxicity from cisplatin therapy in childhood cancer. *J Pediatr Hematol Oncol*. 2007;29:355–360.
64. Hallmark RJ, Snyder JM, Jusenius K, et al. Factors influencing ototoxicity in ovarian cancer patients treated with Cis-platinum based chemotherapy. *Eur J Gynaecol Oncol*. 1992;13:35–44.
65. Gaegcnti DL. Childhood. In: Finegold M, Beningtion J, eds. *Pathology of Neoplasia in Children and Adults*. Philadelphia: WB Saunders. 1986:282–312.
66. Buhrer C, Weinel P, Sauter S, et al. Acute onset deafness in a 4–year-old girl after a single infusion of cis-platinum. *Pediatr Hematol Oncol*. 1990;7:145–148.
67. Berg AL, Spitzer JB, Garvin JH, Jr. Ototoxic impact of cisplatin in pediatric oncology patients. *Laryngoscope*. 1999;109:1806–1814.
68. Skinner R. Best practice in assessing ototoxicity in children with cancer. *Eur J Cancer*. 2004;40:2352–2354.
69. Northern JL, Downs MP. *Hearing in Children*, ed. Baltimore, MD: Williams & Wilkins, 1991
70. American Speech-Language-Hearing Association. Guidelines for the audiologic management of individuals receiving cochleotoxic drug therapy. *ASHA*. 2004;35(Suppl 12):11–19.
71. Bess FH, Dodd-Murphy J, Parker RA. Children with minimal sensorineural hearing loss: prevalence, educational performance, and functional status. *Ear Hear*. 1998;19:339–354.
72. Schmidt CM, Bartholomäus E, Deuster D, et al. The Muenster classification of high frequency hearing loss following cisplatin chemotherapy. HNO 2007;55(4):299–306.
73. Stavroulaki P, Apostolopoulos N, Segas J, et al. Evoked otoacoustic emissions – an approach for monitoring cisplatin induced ototoxicity in children. *Int J Pediatr Otorhinolaryngol*. 2001;59:47–57.
74. Littman TA, Magruder A, Strother DR. Monitoring and predicting ototoxic damage using distortion-product otoacoustic emissions: pediatric case study. *J Am Acad Audiol*. 1998;9:257–262.
75. Smith LJ, inventor Smith, L J (SMIT-Individual), assignee. Educational kit used for teaching paleontology to child. US. 1999 August 24.
76. Sockalingam R, Freeman S, Cherny TL, et al. Effect of high-dose cisplatin on auditory brainstem responses and otoacoustic emissions in laboratory animals. *Am J Otol*. 2000;21:521–527.
77. Toral RM, Skurovitch-Bialik P, Collado-Corona MA, et al. Distortion product otoacoustic emissions test is useful in children undergoing cisplatin treatment. *Arch Med Res*. 2003;34:205–208.
78. Hotz MA, Harris FP, Probst R. Otoacoustic emissions: an approach for monitoring aminoglycoside-induced ototoxicity. *Laryngoscope*. 1994;104:1130–1134.

79. Subramaniam M, Salvi RJ, Spongr VP, et al. Changes in distortion product otoacoustic emissions and outer hair cells following interrupted noise exposures. *Hear Res.* 1994;74:204–216.
80. Dhooge I, Dhooge C, Geukens S, et al. Distortion product otoacoustic emissions: an objective technique for the screening of hearing loss in children treated with platin derivatives. *Int J Audiol.* 2006;45:337–343.
81. Campbell KC, Kelly E, Targovnik N, et al. Audiologic monitoring for potential ototoxicity in a phase I clinical trial of a new glycopeptide antibiotic. *J Am Acad Audiol.* 2003;14:157–168; quiz 70–71.
82. Ress BD, Sridhar KS, Balkany TJ, et al. Effects of cis-platinum chemotherapy on otoacoustic emissions: the development of an objective screening protocol. Third place – Resident Clinical Science Award. 1998. *Otolaryngol Head Neck Surg.* 1999;121:693–701.
83. Knight KR, Kraemer DF, Winter C, et al. Early changes in auditory function as a result of platinum chemotherapy: use of extended high-frequency audiometry and evoked distortion product otoacoustic emissions. *J Clin Oncol.* 2007;25:1190–1195.
84. A. B. Room acoustics and speech perception. http://wwwwrohansdsuedu/~aboothro/files/RoomAcoustics/Roomacousticsandspeechperceptionpdf, 2002.
85. Stelmachowicz PG, Pittman AL, Hoover BM, et al. The importance of high-frequency audibility in the speech and language development of children with hearing loss. *Arch Otolaryngol Head Neck Surg.* 2004;130:556–562.
86. Stelmachowicz PG, Pittman AL, Hoover BM, et al. Effect of stimulus bandwidth on the perception of /s/ in normal- and hearing-impaired children and adults. *J Acoust Soc Am.* 2001;110:2183–2190.
87. French NR, Steinberg J. Factors governing the intelligibility of speech sounds. *J Acoust Soc Am.* 1947;19:90–119.
88. Katz J WT. *Introduction to the Handicap of Hearing Impairment: Auditory Impairment Versus Hearing Handicap.*San Diego, CA: Singular Publishing Group; 1982.
89. Smoluk GD, Fahey RC, Calabro-Jones PM, et al. Radioprotection of cells in culture by WR-2721 and derivatives: form of the drug responsible for protection. *Cancer Res.* 1988;48:3641–3647.
90. Schiller JH. High-dose cisplatin and vinblastine plus amifostine for metastatic non-small cell lung cancer. *Semin Oncol.* 1996;23:78–82.
91. Schuchter LM. Exploration of platinum-based dose-intensive chemotherapy strategies with amifostine (Ethyol). *Eur J Cancer.* 1996;32A Suppl 4:S40–S42.
92. Hospers GA, Eisenhauer EA, de Vries EG. The sulfhydryl containing compounds WR-2721 and glutathione as radio- and chemoprotective agents. A review, indications for use and prospects. *Br J Cancer.* 1999;80:629–638.
93. Block KI GC. Commentary: the pharmacological antioxidant amifostine – implications of recent research for integrative cancer care. *Integrative Cancer Therapies.* 2005;4:325–351.
94. Hussain AE, Blakley BW, Nicolas M, et al. Assessment of the protective effects of amifostine against cisplatin-induced toxicity. *J Otolaryngol.* 2003;32:294–297.
95. Ekborn A, Hansson J, Ehrsson H, et al. High-dose Cisplatin with amifostine: ototoxicity and pharmacokinetics. *Laryngoscope.* 2004;114:1660–1667.
96. Marina N, Chang KW, Malogolowkin M, et al. Amifostine does not protect against the ototoxicity of high-dose cisplatin combined with etoposide and bleomycin in pediatric germ-cell tumors: a Children's Oncology Group study. *Cancer.* 2005;104:841–847.
97. Capizzi R. Amifostine: the preclinical basis for broad-spectrum selective cytoprotection of normal tissues from cytotoxic therapies. *Semin Oncol.* 1996;23:2–17.
98. Neuwelt EA, Brummett RE, Remsen LG, et al. In vitro and animal studies of sodium thiosulfate as a potential chemoprotectant against carboplatin-induced ototoxicity. *Cancer Res.* 1996;56:706–709.

99. Neuwelt EA, Brummett RE, Doolittle ND, et al. First evidence of otoprotection against carboplatin-induced hearing loss with a two-compartment system in patients with central nervous system malignancy using sodium thiosulfate. *J Pharmacol Exp Ther.* 1998;286: 77–84.

100. Abe R, Akiyoshi T, Tsuji H, et al. Protection of antiproliferative effect of cis-diammi-nedichloroplatinum (II) by sodium thiosulfate. *Cancer Chemother Pharmacol.* 1986;18: 98–100.

101. Elferink F, van der Vijgh WJ, Klein I, et al. Interaction of cisplatin and carboplatin with sodium thiosulfate: reaction rates and protein binding. *Clin Chem.* 1986;32:641–645.

102. Dickey DT, Wu YJ, Muldoon LL, et al. Protection against cisplatin-induced toxicities by N-acetylcysteine and sodium thiosulfate as assessed at the molecular, cellular, and in vivo levels. *J Pharmacol Exp Ther.* 2005;314:1052–1058.

103. Campbell KC, Rybak LP, Meech RP, et al. D-methionine provides excellent protection from cisplatin ototoxicity in the rat. *Hear Res.* 1996;102:90–98.

104. Reser D, Rho M, Dewan D, et al. L- and D- methionine provide equivalent long term protection against CDDP-induced ototoxicity in vivo, with partial in vitro and in vivo retention of antineoplastic activity. *Neurotoxicology.* 1999;20:731–748.

105. Korver KD, Rybak LP, Whitworth C, et al. Round window application of D-methionine provides complete cisplatin otoprotection. *Otolaryngol Head Neck Surg.* 2002;126: 683–689.

106. Campbell KC, Meech RP, Rybak LP, et al. D-Methionine protects against cisplatin damage to the stria vascularis. *Hear Res.* 1999;138:13–28.

107. Sequoia Ecosystem and Recreation Preserve Act of 1999. In. 106th Congress ed; 1999.

108. Wimmer C, Mees K, Stumpf P, et al. Round window application of D-methionine, sodium thiosulfate, brain-derived neurotrophic factor, and fibroblast growth factor-2 in cisplatin-induced ototoxicity. *Otol Neurotol.* 2004;25:33–40.

109. Church MW, Kaltenbach JA, Blakley BW, et al. The comparative effects of sodium thiosulfate, diethyldithiocarbamate, fosfomycin and WR-2721 on ameliorating cisplatin-induced ototoxicity. *Hear Res.* 1995;86:195–203.

110. Kaltenbach JA, Church MW, Blakley BW, et al. Comparison of five agents in protecting the cochlea against the ototoxic effects of cisplatin in the hamster. *Otolaryngol Head Neck Surg.* 1997;117:493–500.

111. Copeland BJ, Pillsbury HC, 3rd. Cochlear implantation for the treatment of deafness. *Annu Rev Med.* 2004;55:157–167.

112. Brock P, Pritchard J, Bellman S, Pinkerton CR. Ototoxicity of high-dose cisplatinum in children. *Med Pediatr Oncol.* 1988;16:368–369.

113. Brock P, Bellman S, Pritchard J. Ototoxicity of cisplatinum *Br J Cancer.* 1991;63: 159–161.

114. Brock PR, Bellman SC, Yeomans EC, Pinkerton CR, Pritchard J. Cisplatin ototoxicity in children; a practical grading system. *Med Pediatr Oncol.* 1991;19:295–300.

115. Brock P, Yeomans E, Bellman S, Pritchard J. Cisplatin therapy in infants: short and long-term morbidity. *Br J Cancer.* 1992;66:Suppl XVIII:S36–S40.

Chapter 14
Reproductive Health Issues in Survivors of Childhood and Adult Brain Tumors

Tress Goodwin, B. Elizabeth Delasobera, and Paul Graham Fisher

Introduction

With improving survival rates over recent decades, brain tumor patients and their doctors have now begun to focus on quality of life issues, including reproductive health. Infertility or impaired fertility is a known side effect of certain cancer therapies. Fertility issues are important to patients and their families, regardless of the patient's age, and oncology practitioners should routinely address this sensitive topic with families at tumor diagnosis in children and adults, and in long-term follow-up. Fertility preservation technologies have advanced significantly in the past decade, and these options should also be reviewed with families. However, clinicians must keep in mind that the majority of treatments remain experimental and may not be available or affordable for some patients. Knowing how and when to discuss these issues with patients and when to refer to specialists requires sensitivity on the part of the practitioner, especially in children who have been diagnosed with a brain tumor.

Infertility is defined as the inability to conceive a child after one year of regular heterosexual intercourse without the use of contraception. In the general population, infertility is estimated to affect 10% of individuals and 15% of heterosexual couples, regardless of past medical history. Perhaps one-third of infertility is due to a male factor, one-third stems from a female factor, about 20% is without known cause, and the remainder is a combination of factors.[1] A brain tumor survivor who presents to a physician with an inability to conceive should not be assumed to have infertility related to cancer therapy, but the cancer history must be considered.

P.G. Fisher (✉)
Director of Neuro-Oncology, Packard Hospital, Stanford University Medical Center, 875 Blake Wilbur Drive, Palo Alto, CA 94305-5826, USA
e-mail: pfisher@stanford.edu

S. Goldman, C.D. Turner (eds.), *Late Effects of Treatment for Brain Tumors*, Cancer Treatment and Research 150, DOI 10.1007/b109924_14,
© Springer Science+Business Media, LLC 2009

Cancer Therapy Impact on Fertility

Not all patients undergoing treatment for brain tumors are at risk for infertility. Chemotherapy can cause oligospermia or azospermia in males, and premature ovarian failure in females.[2] The relationship between cumulative dosage of specific cancer therapies and impact on fertility is not well characterized. Specific risk assessment is difficult, given the individual variability to the gonadotoxic effects of antineoplastic therapy. For instance, alkylating agent chemotherapy and pelvic or spinal radiotherapy confer a dose-related risk of gonadal injury that varies based on the patient's gender and age at treatment. While specific data about the potential for dose-related gonadal damage may not be available for each drug or treatment regimen, general risk levels for infertility or gonadal dysfunction can usually be estimated, based on previously observed outcomes.[3–5] (Table 14.1)

Spinal irradiation can affect fertility, as a total dosage greater than 4 Gy to the ovaries can cause permanent infertility in 30% of females. One group recommends that prepubertal female patients who undergo craniospinal irradiation receive an asymmetric dosimetry plan in order to reduce the dosage to one of the ovaries. That group also suggested using magnetic resonance imaging (MRI) prior to irradiation to precisely localize the ovaries, which can help guide the treatment planning for passage of radiation beams.[6] A recent report described two successful pregnancies after spinal irradiation, when pretreatment MRI was employed to locate the ovaries and eliminate one from the spine field.[7]

Table 14.1 Infertility risk based on chemotherapy treatment

High risk:
Chemotherapy conditioning for bone marrow transplantation
Cyclophosphamide (above 4,000 mg/m^2 for males; above 15,000 mg/m^2 for females)
Ifosfamide

Medium risk:
Cyclophosphamide (below 4,000 mg/m^2 for males; below 15,000 mg/m^2 for females)
Cisplatin
Carboplatin

Low Risk/No Risk:
Cytarabine
Vincristine
Methotrexate
Dactinomycin
Bleomycin
Vinblastine

Table information based on institutional experience and article by Wallace et al.[4]

Cranial irradiation can influence gonadotropic hormones secondary to damage to the hypothalamic-pituitary axis, potentially impairing the patient's reproductive capacity. The site of the damage is often hypothalamic in origin and leads to a reduction or loss of GnRH production. GnRH can be replaced exogenously in some cases. One study showed that 78% of women who presented with amenorrhea secondary to cranial irradiation responded to exogenous GnRH treatment.[8]

Fertility Preservation Prior to Therapy

A recent cross-sectional survey of both mothers and fathers and their teenage children who had been diagnosed with cancer revealed that the majority of respondents want to know more about fertility preservation options. The same respondents felt that they had not been given sufficient information about fertility-related effects prior to therapy and wished all options, even experimental ones, had been discussed before treatment.[9] Nevertheless, current recommendations advise that all men and boys able to produce sperm should be counseled about semen cryopreservation prior to starting any cancer therapy. For male patients who are unable to produce sperm, testicular tissue cryopreservation is an experimental option, though not widely available and performed only at select institutions.[10] For female patients, the only proven fertility preservation technique is oocyte and embryo cryopreservation, although this option has limited availability, too. Other experimental techniques, such as ovarian or testicular tissue cryopreservation, are beginning to be pursued at select institutions.

Evaluation of Infertility

Males

A standard infertility workup for male patients involves a semen analysis to evaluate sperm count, motility, and morphology. This service is offered at most medical centers and sperm banks for a modest fee. In addition, a full physical examination should be performed during a fertility evaluation, with particular attention to secondary sex characteristics, including body habitus, hair distribution, and breast development. Lack of appropriate traits may indicate a possible central cause of gonadal insufficiency. A genital examination of the urethral meatus, for findings such as hypospadias or condylomata, is indicated. Palpation and measurement of the testes (normal adult range 12–25 ml) should be performed to exclude the possibility of a cyst, varicocele, or mass. Small volume testes are often indicative of decreased spermatogenesis.

A standard endocrine workup includes assessment of serum FSH, LH, testosterone, prolactin, and TSH. Hypothyroidism can cause infertility, and thyroid dysfunction is common among survivors of brain tumors. The underlying etiology of infertility can be identified by the relationship of various hormone levels (Table 14.2).[11]

Table 14.2 Basal hormone levels in various clinical states

Clinical condition	FSH	LH	Testosterone	Prolactin
Normal Spermatogenesis	Normal	Normal	Normal	Normal
Hypogonadotropic hypogonadism	Low	Low	Low	Normal
Abnormal spermatogenesis	High/Normal	Normal	Normal	Normal
Complete testicular failure/ Hypergonadotropic hypogonadism	High	High	Normal/Low	Normal
Prolactin-secreting pituitary tumor	Normal/Low	Normal	Low	High

Table information from.[11]

If a male patient with prior fertility presents with recent onset of infertility, further workup for an intracranial process (e.g., prolactinoma or basilar meningioma) should be considered, due to the predilection for secondary tumors in brain tumor survivors. Erectile dysfunction (ED) can also impair fertility, and this issue should also be considered when reviewing the patient's history. ED in long-term adult survivors of primary brain tumors has been found to be more common than in the general population.[12]

Females

Female cancer patients are at increased risk for premature ovarian failure and, thus, an infertility workup should be pursued aggressively and in a timely fashion. As the general rate of infertility increases in women above age 35, patients that fall in this age group should also be advised to pursue fertility services if they plan to have children. Expedited referral to a reproductive specialist is recommended, and the standard year of unprotected intercourse without pregnancy does not need to be established in cancer survivors.

Past medical history should review menstrual history. Particular attention should be paid to any changes following cancer therapy. Resumption of menses is a reliable indicator that gonadal and pituitary function has returned after tumor treatment, but other factors could still contribute to infertility. A full physical exam should be performed, noting the woman's body mass index, signs of androgen excess, breast secretions, and any vaginal, cervical or uterine abnormality.[13] An evaluation of hormones should include serum progesterone, LH, FSH, and TSH, though these levels vary throughout the menstrual cycle. A clomiphene citrate challenge with measurement of FSH can be used to estimate ovarian reserve. An elevated FSH level on menstrual cycle day 3 is an indication of poor ovarian reserve or approaching menopause. Additional tests, such as transvaginal ultrasound and endometrial biopsies, can also be pursued to elucidate the cause of infertility.[13]

Management of Infertility

Because of the complex nature of infertility in a brain tumor survivor, referral to an infertility specialist early in management is a reasonable step. At most medical centers, an obstetrics and gynecology department or reproductive endocrinology and infertility (REI) subspecialists can evaluate and treat female infertility. Male infertility is often managed by the urology service. Infertility diagnosis and treatment is not covered by all insurance companies. Some states require that insurance companies cover costs for certain aspects of the initial workup and limited treatment. However, since infertility in cancer patients can be complicated, not all specialists will have experience managing these patients. Treatment of infertility in cancer survivors is an emerging field of medicine, since many childhood and young adult cancer patients previously did not survive to reproductive age. Referral of patients to a tertiary care or specialty center may be required if these services are not available in the institution which treated the person's cancer.

Patients who have cryopreserved tissue (e.g., sperm, eggs, embryos) in storage should be encouraged to consult with a reproductive specialist regarding implantation or fertilization when deemed appropriate by both the physician and patient. In making this decision, physicians should take into consideration medical prognosis and psychosocial issues. In men with ED, treatments and prosthetic devices are available for enhancing sexual function, and fertility can be achieved through direct fertilization. Men should be reassured that there are several options available for parenthood even if the sperm analysis reveals a low sperm count. For example, intracytoplasmic sperm injection can be achieved even from men with very low sperm counts.

Other options for parenthood certainly exist, and these should also be discussed with brain tumor patients. Adoption can be pursued nationally or internationally through a public or private agency. Men unable to produce sperm can seek donor sperm readily available in banks throughout the country. For infertile women, a surrogate can carry a child fertilized with the partner's sperm. Female patients with viable eggs who are unable to maintain a pregnancy can have an embryo implanted in the uterus of a surrogate mother (in vitro fertilization [IVF]) who will carry the fetus to term. In general, the success rate for IVF is about 18–30%, but rates vary widely within institutions. Donor eggs can be obtained through a directed donor, such as a sister or friend, or through an agency.

Understanding the costs of these choices is important, and price can certainly affect these decisions. Adoption can cost between $2,500 and $35,000. Surrogacy ranges from $10,000 to $100,000, and donor eggs cost approximately $20,000.[14]

Antiepileptic Drugs

A number of brain tumor survivors will experience seizures, requiring treatment with anticonvulsant drugs. Carbamazepine (Tegretol), felbamate (Felbatol), phenytoin (Dilantin), phenobarbital, primidone (Mysoline), oxcarbazepine (Trileptal), and topiramate (Topamax) are known to diminish the efficacy of oral contraceptives by inducting cytochrome P450 metabolism, and patients should be advised to seek other forms of contraception or to switch to a nonenzyme-inducing anticonvulsant such as gabapentin (Neurontin) or valproate (Depakote). Furthermore, many of the older anticonvulsants generate free radicals and can be teratogenic, causing birth defects such as spina bifida, complex congenital heart disease, and facial anomalies. Thus, carbamezapine, phenytoin, phenobarbitol, and valproate are all classified as Category D, signifying that there is evidence of human fetal risk, but potential benefits for an individual may still warrant use of the drug. Most other antiepileptic drugs are Category C, with only animal evidence showing risk to the fetus. Guidelines from the American Academy of Neurology suggest the use of one, newer generation anticonvulsant at the lowest dosage possible to control seizures in a woman who is pregnant or trying to conceive. Due to varying risks of neural tube defects in the fetus from any of these drugs, all postpubertal women on an antiepileptic drug are advised to be administered at least 0.4 mg of folate daily and up to 4.0 mg with certain anticonvulsants. In addition, pregnant women on antiepileptic medications should receive 10 mg per day of oral vitamin K during the last month of pregnancy to reduce the risk of neonatal hemorrhage.[15]

Other Considerations

Whether or not administered cancer treatment affects fertility, it is important to advise brain tumor survivors about the risk of sexually transmitted infections and unplanned pregnancies. Some studies have shown that cancer survivors may think they are unable to have children and then have unprotected intercourse, resulting in both unplanned pregnancies and sexually transmitted infections.[16]

Numerous studies have failed to demonstrate an excess risk of birth defects or cancer in children born to the vast majority of childhood cancer survivors, with the exception being those offspring born to parents with germ line cancer-predisposing genetic mutations.[17–19] Nervous system tumors are manifested in many cancer syndromes such as neurofibromatosis 1 and 2, tuberous sclerosis, von Hippel-Lindau disease, Gorlin syndrome, and familial retinoblastoma. Patients known to possess these genes should be appropriately counseled on their risk of transmitting the gene to their offspring. However, the vast majority of brain tumor patients have sporadic tumors that do not have a direct genetic cause and do not have a higher than average risk of having an affected child.

A study of clinicians revealed that only 53% of providers surveyed were aware of the lack of difference in pregnancy outcomes among survivors and population controls,[20] suggesting the need for education to dispel unfounded concerns. In a similar study of young male cancer survivors, 24% agreed and 33% indicated they were unsure that children born to them would have higher risks of special health problems.[21] In addition, 31% indicated they believed their offspring would have higher rates of cancer and 28% were unsure, when only 8% in fact had an attributable genetic basis to their cancer.[21] This underscores the importance of clarifying risks to alleviate unnecessary anxiety among brain tumor survivors, who may already suffer significant stressors related to their disease experience.

Summary

Many brain tumor survivors, like other cancer survivors, are at risk for infertility. This risk is related to the cumulative dosage of specific antineoplastic agents, concomitant medications (such as antiepileptic agents), location and dosage of radiation therapy exposure, and the degree of endocrine dysfunction that exists. While infertility continues to be a significant late effect for many brain tumor survivors, increasingly, advances in reproductive endocrinology and in vitro fertilization techniques are offering new options and new hope to brain tumor survivors.

References

1. American Society of Reproductive Medicine: Frequently Asked Questions. 2007. (Accessed September 27, 2008, at http://www.asrm.org/Patients/faqs.)
2. Pizzo PA, Poplack DG. *Principles and Practice of Pediatric Oncology*. 5th ed. Philadelphia, PA: Lippincott Williams & Wilkins; 2005.
3. Lee SJ, Schover LR, Partridge AH, et al. American Society of Clinical Oncology recommendations for fertility preservation in cancer patients. *J Clin Oncol*. 2006;24:2917–2931.
4. Wallace WH, Anderson RA, Irvine DS. Fertility preservation for young patients with cancer: who is at risk and what can be offered? *Lancet Oncol*. 2005;6:209–218.
5. Sklar CA, Mertens AC, Mitby P, et al. Premature menopause in survivors of childhood cancer: a report from the childhood cancer survivor study. *J Natl Cancer Inst*. 2006;98: 890–896.
6. Harden SV, Twyman N, Lomas DJ, et al. A method for reducing ovarian doses in whole neuro-axis irradiation for medulloblastoma. *Radiother Oncol*. 2003;69:183–188.

7. Shigematsu N, Shinmoto H, Ito N, et al. Successful pregnancy and normal delivery after whole craniospinal irradiation in two patients. *Anticancer Res*. 2005;25:3481–3487.
8. Hall JE, Martin KA, Whitney HA, et al. Potential for fertility with replacement of hypothalamic gonadotropin-releasing hormone in long term female survivors of cranial tumors. *J Clin Endocrinol Metab*. 1994;79:1166–72.
9. Oosterhuis BE, Goodwin T, Kiernan M, et al. Concerns about infertility risks among pediatric oncology patients and their parents. *Pediatr Blood Cancer*. 2008;50:85–89.
10. Keros V, Hultenby K, Borgstrom B, et al. Methods of cryopreservation of testicular tissue with viable spermatogonia in pre-pubertal boys undergoing gonadotoxic cancer treatment. *Hum Reprod*. 2007;22:1384–1395.
11. Male Infertility Best Practice Policy Committee of the American Urological Association and Practice Committee of the American Society for Reproductive Medicine. Report on optimal evaluation of the infertile male. *Fertil Steril*. 2006;86(5 Suppl):S202–S209.
12. Arlt W, Hove U, Muller B, et al. Frequent and frequently overlooked: treatment-induced endocrine dysfunction in adult long-term survivors of primary brain tumors. *Neurology*. 1997;49:498–506.
13. ASRM. Optimal evaluation of the infertile female. *Fertil Steril*. 2006;86:S264–S267.
14. FertileHope. http://www.fertilehope.org/. In; 2007.
15. AAN Guideline Summary for Clinicians. Management Issues for Women with Epilepsy. http://www.aan.com/professionals/practice/pdfs/women_epilepsy.pdf. Accessed September 27, 2008
16. Zebrack BJ, Casillas J, Nohr L, et al. Fertility issues for young adult survivors of childhood cancer. *Psychooncology*. 2004;13:689–699.
17. Byrne J, Rasmussen SA, Steinhorn SC, et al. Genetic disease in offspring of long-term survivors of childhood and adolescent cancer. *Am J Hum Genet*. 1998;62:45–52.
18. Sankila R, Olsen JH, Anderson H, et al. Risk of cancer among offspring of childhood-cancer survivors. Association of the Nordic Cancer Registries and the Nordic Society of Paediatric Haematology and Oncology. *N Engl J Med*. 1998;338:1339–1344.
19. Nicholson HS, Byrne J. Fertility and pregnancy after treatment for cancer during childhood or adolescence. *Cancer*. 1993;71:3392–3399.
20. Goodwin T, Oosterhuis B, Kiernan M, et al. Attitudes and practices of pediatric oncology providers regarding fertility issues. *Pediatr Blood Cancer*. 2007;48:80–85.
21. Schover LR, Brey K, Lichtin A, et al. Knowledge and experience regarding cancer, infertility, and sperm banking in younger male survivors. *J Clin Oncol*. 2002;20:1880–1889.

Chapter 15
Cancer Predisposition Syndromes

Joanna L. Weinstein, Kanyalakshmi Ayyanar, and Melody A. Watral

Introduction

Several decades ago, genetic predisposition was first identified as a risk factor for the development of secondary malignant neoplasms (SMN) with the observation of second tumors, namely sarcomas, in survivors of hereditary retinoblastoma.[1–4] The two-hit hypothesis, originally proposed in 1971 by Knudson, may explain why some individuals may be more prone to the development of primary tumors, or of subsequent tumors after tumorigenic therapies, as a result of inheriting a cancer-associated gene mutation.[2,5] Such a germline mutation is the first of the two "hits" required for tumorigenesis. This model has since been applied to other cancer susceptibility syndromes, such as Li-Fraumeni, associated with early-onset cancers.[6–8] Some recent publications suggest that the two-hit model may be overly simplistic and that other chromosomal and epigenetic phenomena drive cancer tumorigenesis.[9]

Though only a small proportion of primary brain tumors appear to be due to a genetic predisposition syndrome in adults, genetic predisposition syndromes may account for a larger portion of primary brain cancers in children.[10–13] In some series of cancer survivors who have developed SMN, nearly one-third had confirmed genetic abnormalities or suspected cancer predisposition syndromes.[10,11,13–16]

Prospective search for a genetic predisposition can involve complex and conflicting ethical, legal, social, and medical issues for patients and may have wide-ranging repercussions for patients and family members.[17–23] Although these syndromes are uncommon, genetic testing for cancer susceptibility syndromes in particular individuals may assist patient management, influence family screening, and guide clinicians about surveillance protocols in affected individuals and 'at risk' family members; this information may strongly impact outcomes in some cases.[17]

J.L. Weinstein (✉)
Division of Hematology, Oncology and Stem Cell Transplantation,
Children's Memorial Hospital, Chicago, IL, USA
e-mail: jweinstein@childrensmemorial.org

S. Goldman, C.D. Turner (eds.), *Late Effects of Treatment for Brain Tumors*, 223
Cancer Treatment and Research 150, DOI 10.1007/b109924_15,
© Springer Science+Business Media, LLC 2009

In this section, the most common cancer predisposition syndromes having increased risk of brain tumors will be discussed.

Neurofibromatoses

The neurofibromatoses, including Neurofibromatosis Type 1 (von Recklinghausen disease; NF1) and Neurofibromatosis Type 2 (NF2) are autosomal-dominant neurocutaneous disorders that carry a high risk of tumor formation.[24–26] Half of cases lack a family history.[27] These two syndromes differ in genetics, penetrance, phenotypic features, and cells most commonly affected.[25,28–31]

NF1, estimated to affect 1:3,500, is caused by mutations in the *NF1* gene (at 17q11), coding for a protein called neurofibromin.[25] The clinical diagnosis of NF1 is confirmed by identifying characteristic combinations of cutaneous, ocular and skeletal features.[25,27,32] Though genetic testing is available and is used in select situations, the detection rate with current techniques is not high enough to justify routine use for screening.[17,33–35]

The most common neoplasms associated with NF-1 are low-grade glial tumors of the optic pathway, occurring in approximately 15–20% of patients with NF1.[36–38] Typically arising during the preschool years,[37,39–41] the majority of patients with optic pathway tumors (OPTs) are asymptomatic at the time of detection.[38,42,43] These lesions are usually slow growing and indolent;[44] in fact, some tumors may spontaneously regress.[45–47] The low-grade histopathology of these OPTs is typically stable over many years, with only rare examples of these lesions undergoing malignant transformation; most of these unfortunate cases have been associated with prior RT treatment.[48] Because of this typical clinically benign behavior, treatment is recommended only in specific clinical situations, for instance, when there is presence of symptoms such as abnormal vision or proptosis.[44,49]

In addition to OPTs, common malignancies in NF-1 include other CNS tumors,[50–53] leukemias and myelodysplasia,[54,55] pheochromocytomas,[56] as well as malignant peripheral nerve sheath tumors (MPNST).[25,57] Various series confirm high risk of second BTs in patients with NF1 and OPTs, estimating risk of approximately 11–50%.[52,53] It is not clear if the phenotype of patients with OPT will be more likely to develop CNS tumors based on a genotypic difference or if secondary tumors arise due to treatment of the OPT. In a series of NF1 patients with OPTs, Sharif et al. confirmed this high incidence of second CNS tumors; this risk was highest if radiotherapy was administered for the OPT.[50,51] Of the 18 patients with OPTs who received RT for treatment of their OPT, half of these patients developed 12 second tumors; all received their RT during childhood. The remaining eight patients who developed nine second tumors had not been treated with RT. Additionally, the irradiated patients seemed to have a higher risk of dying from their later tumor.[15] Other studies have suggested a higher incidence of subsequent CNS tumors developing within the RT field of NF1 patients with OPTs.[50]

Patients with NF1 have a lifetime risk of approximately 10% of developing a malignant peripheral nerve sheath tumor (MPNST), an aggressive and often fatal malignancy.[57] In adults with NF1, MPNSTs tend to arise due to malignant transformation within a neurofibroma;[54] this diagnosis must be considered if neurofibroma undergoes rapid change in size or symptoms. MPNSTs frequently arise in previously irradiated fields.[51] In the series by Sharif, all five MPNSTs that developed in NF1 patients with OPTs treated with RT arose within the radiation field, while the single MPNST in the nonirradiated group arose distant from original the OPT.[51]

Neurofibromatosis-2, a condition less common than NF1, is caused by mutations in the *NF2* gene which codes for a tumor suppressor protein called merlin.[58,59] Some have reported genotypic-phenotypic correlations between the type of constitutional NF2 mutation and the number of NF2-associated tumors.[60] NF2 is clinically characterized by vestibular schwannomas (also known as acoustic neuromas) and other CNS tumors, including meningiomas. The presence of bilateral acoustic neuromas is pathognomonic of NF2; a single early-onset acoustic neuroma, combined with a family history or with other NF2 features such as schwannomas, meningiomas or juvenile cataracts, may be diagnostic.[61] Although the tumors of NF2 can cause significant morbidity and can be life-threatening, they rarely display malignant histology.[24,25] Patients with NF-2 require regular, thorough audiologic, neurologic, ophthalmologic and dermatologic examinations that include periodic screening MRI of the brain and spine. Brain stem auditory evoked responses may detect tumors of the vestibular nerves prior to their visualization on MRI.[41,61]

Clinical presentations of NF2 in children are typically related to meningiomas or schwannomas. Pediatric meningiomas can be histologically and clinically aggressive.[62] Ninety-eight percent of adults with NF2 develop an acoustic neuroma.[63] which usually manifests clinically with deafness, tinnitus and balance disturbance, though some are asymptomatic.

Tuberous Sclerosis

Tuberous sclerosis complex (TS) is characterized by multiple tumors (hamartomas) affecting the skin, central nervous system, kidneys, heart, eyes, blood vessels, lungs, bones, and gastrointestinal tract.[64-66] This autosomal dominant systemic disorder, whose genetic defect has been localized to mutations in two gene loci, *TSC1* (9q34) and *TSC2* (16p13.3),[64,66] demonstrates almost complete penetrance, but variable expressivity.[65] Approximately 60% of patients present with new sporadic mutations.[67]

Central nervous system involvement in TS consists of benign epileptogenic cortical tubers, subependymal nodules, and subependymal giant cell astrocytomas (SEGAs).[65] The latter are considered to be low-grade glial tumors, occurring in about 5–15% of individuals with TS. A multidisciplinary management approach is necessary for TS patients.[68,69] Surgery is the routine mode of treatment for the typically chemoresistant SEGAs;[69] radiation therapy is reserved for cases when there is no surgical alternative in order to avoid long-term complications.[68,70]

Screening recommendations for patients with TS include a cranial MRI screening at the time of diagnosis, and then every 1–3 years through adolescence.[68] Additional screening includes ophthalmologic, dermatologic, cardiac, and renal evaluations as clinically indicated. TS patients and their families should also be referred for genetic counseling, although molecular testing is not commercially available.

Von Hippel Lindau Disease

Von Hippel–Lindau disease (VHL), a rare autosomal dominant cancer syndrome, is characterized by multiple benign and malignant tumors.[71] It is characterized by hemangioblastomas of the retina, cerebellum or spinal cord; retinal angiomas; renal cell carcinoma (RCC), and pheochromocytomas.[72] Less common associated lesions include renal and pancreatic cysts, pancreatic carcinoma, cysts of the epididymus and broad ligament, and endolymphatic sac tumors.[72–74] CNS hemangioblastomas account for 80% of the lesions in VHL[74–78] and most frequently occur in the cerebellum, spinal cord, and brain stem.[75,77] Since these tumors rarely present sporadically, any patient diagnosed with a hemangioblastoma should be evaluated for VHL disease and associated lesions. Retinal angiomas, if untreated, may cause retinal detachment and hemorrhage, leading to blindness. Multiple renal cysts may develop in the third or fourth decade and may be associated with renal impairment, and these cysts bear a lifelong risk of transformation into renal cell carcinoma.[79] Pheochromocytomas may occur in young patients; often are bilateral and multiple; may cause hypertension, sweating, palpitations, and headaches, or may be asymptomatic. Pancreatic cysts are often multiple and rarely cause endocrine or exocrine insufficiency. Endolymphatic sac tumors are slow growing, low-grade papillary adenocarcinomas that can cause hearing loss.[73] Cerebellar hemangioblastoma and RCC are the leading causes of mortality in patients with VHL disease.[72]

Von Hippel–Lindau disease arises from germline mutations in the *VHL* gene (3p25.15).[71,80,81] Approximately 80% of patients have an affected parent, while approximately 20% of patients with VHL have new mutations.[71] The functions of the *VHL* gene are under investigation;[82] loss of this tumor suppressor appears to affect angiogenesis and hypoxia-induced genes.[83] Mutations in the *VHL* gene are detectable in the vast majority of patients,[84] allowing for gene testing and distinction of family members requiring tumor surveillance.[72] Surveillance guidelines focus on screening of at-risk individuals to permit early detection of tumors.[17,85,86]

Nevoid Basal Cell Carcinoma Syndrome (Gorlin Syndrome)

Nevoid basal cell carcinoma syndrome (NBCCS), also known as Gorlin syndrome, is an autosomal dominant syndrome characterized by the development of multiple neoplasms, including basal cell carcinoma in children and adolescents, medulloblastoma (MB), ovarian fibromas and carcinomas, fetal rhabdomyosarcoma and others.[87–91] Developmental defects such as odontogenic keratocyst of the jaws, plantar or palmar pits, congenital anomalies such as cleft lip and palate and other facial dysmorphisms, calcification of the falx cerebri, and skeletal deformities also characterize these patients.[91–93] Affected patients are extremely sensitive to ionizing radiation, including sunlight.

The genetic locus for NBCCS has been shown to be linked to germline mutations in the Patched gene (*PTCH*) (9q22.3–q31).[94–98] The prevalence of NBCCS is estimated to be one in 60,000, with about 40% of NBCCS cases representing new mutations.[93] Murine models of PTCH mutations develop MB,[99] while the majority of sporadic MB do not demonstrate such mutations.[100–102]

In patients with NBCCS, medulloblastoma (MB) presents at a median age of two years, younger than the median presenting age in sporadic cases.[72,93] Screening for NBCCS should be considered in the youngest children diagnosed with MB and in any patient presenting with basal cell carcinomas at an early age (i.e., younger than 30 years) or in atypical locations (i.e., non-sun-exposed).[103] Suspicion for NBCCS should be high if basal cell carcinomas are detected in a child. For patients with suspected or confirmed NBCCS, screening neurological exams and MRIs of the brain are recommended for children to detect MB early.[93]

Because of their excessive sensitivity to sunlight, patients with NBCCS should be counseled to avoid sun exposure, since virtually every patient develops basal cell carcinomas. Additionally, since the use of therapeutic irradiation may lead to potentially thousands of basal cell carcinomas in patients with this syndrome,[91,104,105] nonstandard management should be considered for children with NBCCS and MB, including limited-field radiation or treatments that exclude radiation therapy.

Li-Fraumeni Syndrome, Germline p53 Mutations, and Variants

Li-Fraumeni syndrome (LFS) is a cancer predisposition syndrome, characterized by autosomal dominant inheritance and a wide variety of cancer types.[6,106–112] The most prevalent tumors include breast cancer (especially premenopausal), brain tumors, acute leukemias, bone and soft tissue sarcomas, and adrenocortical carcinoma.[6,106,108] Though breast cancer is the most common cancer seen in LFS, a history of childhood adrenocortical carcinoma, rhabdomyosarcoma, and some other childhood tumors is most strongly associated with the presence of the germline p53 mutation.[17] The characterization of additional families affected by LFS and Li-Fraumeni-like syndrome (LFLS) has expanded the associated cancers to include gastric cancer, lymphoma, choroid plexus carcinoma, and colorectal cancer, and early-onset lung cancer and others.[6,106,113]

LFS has been linked to germline mutations of the tumor suppressor gene *TP53*, which codes for a transcription factor that regulates cell proliferation and homeostasis, DNA repair processes, and apoptosis. Mutations of *p53* have been described in approximately 50–80% of LFS cases, while the majority of kindreds with LFLS do not harbor mutations in the coding regions of this gene.[7,72,109,114–116] Non-germline *TP53* mutations are common in sporadic human cancers, suggesting that *TP53* alterations play an important role in the development of cancer.[117,118] Investigations have been extensive examining the role of other tumor suppressor genes and targets in the p53 and related growth regulatory pathways in these patients with LFS or LFLS.

Because of the significantly increased risk of cancer associated with LFS, obtaining a thorough family cancer history is critical; this history should screen for all tumor types, particularly soft tissue sarcomas, osteosarcoma, and adrenocortical carcinoma. Periodic reevaluation of family health status may expose additional cancers which may increase suspicion of cancer suscept-ibility and guide management in affected families. Cancers in LFS/LFLS typically present at a younger age compared with those occurring due to sporadic mutations. The mean age at presentation varies for different tumor types: five years for adrenocortical carcinomas, 16 years for sarcomas, 25 years for brain tumors, 37 years for breast cancer, and 50 years for lung cancer.[109] Children in families with LFS who survive an initial cancer have a substantially high relative risk of developing a second cancer – more than 80 times greater than that of the general population – and a cumulative probability of second cancer development of 57% at 30 years.[113]

This inherent cancer predisposition must be taken into consideration when cancer therapy is indicated for these patients; radiation therapy should be avoided if at all possible because of the high likelihood of inducing secondary cancers.[6,17,119,120] Patients and families with histories consistent with LFS, or with presentations of cancer suggestive of a possible germline *TP53* mutation, should be counseled regarding genetic testing.[17] At first, testing for a *TP53* mutation should be limited to the proband, followed by testing of the at-risk family for the specific mutation documented. Nevertheless, the range of malig-nancies, their early onset and the lack of highly effective cancer screening raises questions and issues regarding the usefulness of genetic testing in this predis-position syndrome.[17]

Brain Tumor-Polyposis Syndrome (Turcot Syndrome)

Turcot syndrome is a rare inherited disorder characterized by benign adeno-matous polyps in the gastrointestinal tract, an increased risk of colon cancer, and tumors of the central nervous system.[72,121] Since early reports, there is considerable controversy regarding the mode of genetic transmission and the distinction from other syndromes like familial adenomatous polyposis (FAP).[122,123]

From a molecular standpoint, Turcot syndrome has been reported in association with two genotypic-phenotypic variants, those affecting the adenomatous polyposis coli (*APC*) gene and those involving Hereditary Non-polyposis Colon Cancer (*HNPCC*)-associated genes.[124–126] The more common type having *APC* abnormalities and autosomal dominant inheritance is associated with medulloblastoma, whereas Turcot families, whose susceptibility is linked with *HNPCC*-associated, mismatch repair genes and microsatellite instability, tend to develop glioblastoma multiforme.[125]

The clinical diagnosis of Turcot syndrome is made in a patient with multiple colonic polyps and a primary brain tumor, with or without a family history. Treatment of affected patients includes: screening for and management of colonic polyps by an experienced gastroenterologist, appropriate management of the primary brain tumor by a neuro-oncology team, and genetic counseling. Family members of affected patients should be screened accordingly.[8,121]

Multiple Endocrine Neoplasia Type 1 (Wermer Syndrome)

Multiple endocrine neoplasia type 1 (MEN1, Wermer syndrome) is a disorder characterized by tumors of the pituitary gland, parathyroid adenomas with associated hyperparathyroidism, and enteropancreatic tumors.[17,127] Most of the pituitary tumors are prolactinomas, but other secreting and non-functioning tumors are also seen.[127] Treatment for pituitary adenomas is similar to those with sporadic disease. Mutation testing, available for patients suspected to have this condition, is important to confirm the diagnosis and appropriateness of screening, and to test at-risk family members.[17]

Hereditary (Germline) Retinoblastoma

Germline *RB1* mutations are identified in the majority of retinoblastoma (RB) cases with bilateral or multifocal disease or/and with positive family history, whereas 10–15% patients with unilateral disease lacking family history will have detectable germline mutations.[128,129] There are also rare cases of 13q deletion syndrome, characterized by malformations and varying degrees of developmental and growth delays, in addition to RB tumors.[130] Hereditary patients are at risk for developing intracranial (pineal) neuroectodermal tumors known as trilateral disease[131,132] and of second primary tumor[1,3–5,133–156] based on the absence of this tumor suppressor gene, which regulates cell proliferation and other critical cellular processes.[157–160]

Retinoblastoma is frequently the first cancer in various series of survivors affected by secondary malignancies,[4,14] though some late effects registries (CCSS) explicitly exclude RB patients because of their genetic predisposition and very high risk of SMN.[161] The incidence of SMN in all survivors of RB ranges from 2 to 20% at 10 years from initial diagnosis and, with longer follow-up, the incidence increases dramatically.[143,147,156] Kleinerman et al. showed that the cumulative incidence for developing a new cancer at 50 years after diagnosis of RB was 36% for hereditary patients versus 5.7% for nonhereditary patients.[144]

The most common secondary tumors in hereditary RB are bone and soft tissue sarcomas, brain tumors, and melanomas.[1,133,135,139,141,143,144,146–154,162,163] Radiation therapy dramatically increases the risk of SMN in RB patients.[1,5,135,142–144,149,150,154–156,164] Studies clearly demonstrate a high incidence of cancers in nonirradiated RB patients and at nonirradiated sites, suggesting that these survivors have a high lifetime risk of cancer in adulthood, irrespective of their primary treatment for their initial RB. In a study of secondary sarcomas developing after RB, uterine leiomyosarcoma was found as a common second cancer in these RB patients.[139] Of those patients who did receive RT, there was a statistically significant increased risk of soft tissue sarcomas in the RT field as well as an increased risk of sarcomas, namely leiomyosarcomas, outside the field. Reports also suggest an increased susceptibility to carcinogenic effects of smoking in RB patients as the risk of tobacco-related cancers, namely of the lung and bladder, appears to be increased in hereditary RB patients.[141,144,153,154,163]

Trilateral retinoblastoma (TRb) is the association of hereditary retinoblastoma with a primary intracranial neuroectodermal neoplasm in the pineal or parasellar regions.[131] Occurring in about 5% of patients with germline disease, TRb usually presents within a few years of the original RB's diagnosis.[132] Prognosis is poor,[132] so many centers recommend brain imaging to screen at the time of retinoblastoma diagnosis, and at least yearly until at least five years of age,[132] but it is not known whether earlier detection improves outcome. Interestingly, there may be a decreasing incidence of trilateral disease in RB survivors; this decline may be related to recent avoidance of RT, which has been hypothesized to trigger these tumors, while others propose that the use of chemoreduction to treat RB in the past decade (coincident with decline in use of RT) may alter potentially malignant cells of the pineal gland in these susceptible individuals.[144,151,165]

While RB is one of the most curable childhood cancers in developed cancers, mortality rates in RB survivors are significantly affected by SMN. In the case of hereditary RB in developed countries, more patients die of secondary cancers than from their initial eye tumor.[155] Eng et al. found a statistically significant excess mortality for second cancers of bone and connective tissue, malignant melanoma, and benign and malignant CNS neoplasms.[150] In this study, the cumulative probability of death from SMN was 26% at 40 years after bilateral RB diagnosis, and RT as initial treatment further increased the risk.

It is unclear whether distinct genotypes in RB patients correlate with phenotypic variations of RB and the risk of SMN.[128,145,166] In general, genetic testing is recommended for patients with suspected germline disease, in those presenting with RB at a very young age and in any patients with tumor tissue available.[17] For patients with hereditary or suspected germline disease, awareness of the lifelong cancer susceptibility is crucial, and the need for long-term follow-up must be emphasized with education and counseling.[4,153,154]

Conclusion

It is important for clinicians to be aware of genetic predisposition syndromes at the time of initial primary diagnosis in order to implement risk-adapted therapies. Avoiding radiation therapy or leukomogenic therapy in patients with a cancer susceptibility may be an appropriate approach in some cases.[167] Likewise, those who treat cancer survivors must understand the added risks of secondary malignancies in these patients and increase surveillance appropriately. Appropriateness of genetic screening should be discussed with patients suspected to have cancer susceptibility and considered for at-risk family members, if indicated.

References

1. Wong FL, Boice JD, Jr., Abramson DH, et al. Cancer incidence after retinoblastoma. Radiation dose and sarcoma risk. *JAMA*. 1997;278:1262–1267.
2. Knudson AG, Jr. Mutation and cancer: statistical study of retinoblastoma. *Proc Natl Acad Sci USA*. 1971;68:820–823.
3. Moll AC, Imhof SM, Bouter LM, et al. Second primary tumors in patients with hereditary retinoblastoma: a register-based follow-up study, 1945–1994. *Int J Cancer*. 1996;67:515–519.
4. Meadows AT. Retinoblastoma survivors: sarcomas and surveillance. *J Natl Cancer Inst*. 2007;99:3–5.
5. Sagerman RH, Cassady JR, Tretter P, et al. Radiation induced neoplasia following external beam therapy for children with retinoblastoma. *Am J Roentgenol Radium Ther Nucl Med*. 1969;105:529–535.
6. Varley JM, Evans DG, Birch JM. Li-Fraumeni syndrome – a molecular and clinical review. *Br J Cancer*. 1997;76:1–14.
7. Varley JM, McGown G, Thorncroft M, et al. Germ-line mutations of TP53 in Li-Fraumeni families: an extended study of 39 families. *Cancer Res*. 1997;57:3245–3252.
8. Hottinger AF, Khakoo Y. Update on the management of familial central nervous system tumor syndromes. *Curr Neurol Neurosci Rep*. 2007;7:200–207.
9. Mastrangelo D, De Francesco S, Di Leonardo A, et al. Does the evidence matter in medicine? The retinoblastoma paradigm. *Int J Cancer*. 2007;121:2501–2505.
10. Broniscer A, Ke W, Fuller CE, et al. Second neoplasms in pediatric patients with primary central nervous system tumors: the St. Jude Children's Research Hospital experience. *Cancer*. 2004;100:2246–2252.
11. Stavrou T, Bromley CM, Nicholson HS, et al. Prognostic factors and secondary malignancies in childhood medulloblastoma. *J Pediatr Hematol Oncol*. 2001;23:431–436.
12. Narod SA, Stiller C, Lenoir GM. An estimate of the heritable fraction of childhood cancer. *Br J Cancer*. 1991;63:993–999.

13. Kingston JE, Hawkins MM, Draper GJ, et al. Patterns of multiple primary tumours in patients treated for cancer during childhood. *Br J Cancer*. 1987;56:331–338.
14. Meadows AT, Baum E, Fossati-Bellani F, et al. Second malignant neoplasms in children: an update from the Late Effects Study Group. *J Clin Oncol*. 1985;3:532–538.
15. Little MP, de Vathaire F, Shamsaldin A, et al. Risks of brain tumour following treatment for cancer in childhood: modification by genetic factors, radiotherapy and chemotherapy. *Int J Cancer*. 1998;78:269–275.
16. Garwicz S, Anderson H, Olsen JH, et al. Second malignant neoplasms after cancer in childhood and adolescence: a population-based case-control study in the 5 Nordic countries. The Nordic Society for Pediatric Hematology and Oncology. The Association of the Nordic Cancer Registries. *Int J Cancer*. 2000;88:672–678.
17. Field M, Shanley S, Kirk J. Inherited cancer susceptibility syndromes in paediatric practice. *J Paediatr Child Health*. 2007;43:219–229.
18. Clayton EW. Ethical, legal, and social implications of genomic medicine. *N Engl J Med*. 2003;349:562–569.
19. Eng CM, Schechter C, Robinowitz J, et al. Prenatal genetic carrier testing using triple disease screening. *JAMA*. 1997;278:1268–1272.
20. Wilfond BS, Fost N. The cystic fibrosis gene: medical and social implications for heterozygote detection. *JAMA*. 1990;263:2777–2783.
21. Pyeritz RE. Family history and genetic risk factors: forward to the future. *JAMA*. 1997;278:1284–1285.
22. Statement of the American Society of Clinical Oncology: genetic testing for cancer susceptibility, Adopted on February 20, 1996. *J Clin Oncol*. 1996;14:1730–1736; discussion 7–40.
23. American Society of Clinical Oncology policy statement update: genetic testing for cancer susceptibility. *J Clin Oncol*. 2003;21:2397–2406.
24. Ferner RE. Neurofibromatosis 1 and neurofibromatosis 2: a twenty first century perspective. *Lancet Neurol*. 2007;6:340–351.
25. Korf BR. Malignancy in neurofibromatosis type 1. *Oncologist*. 2000;5:477–485.
26. Rasmussen SA, Friedman JM. NF1 gene and neurofibromatosis 1. *Am J Epidemiol*. 2000;151:33–40.
27. Neurofibromatosis. Conference statement. National Institutes of Health Consensus Development Conference. *Arc Neurol*. 1988;45:575–578.
28. Wu BL, Austin MA, Schneider GH, et al. Deletion of the entire NF1 gene detected by the FISH: four deletion patients associated with severe manifestations. *Am J Med Genet*. 1995;59:528–535.
29. Leppig KA, Kaplan P, Viskochil D, et al. Familial neurofibromatosis 1 microdeletions: cosegregation with distinct facial phenotype and early onset of cutaneous neurofibromata. *Am J Med Genet*. 1997;73:197–204.7
30. Carey JC, Laub JM, Hall BD. Penetrance and variability in neurofibromatosis: a genetic study of 60 families. *Birth Defects Original Article Series*. 1979;15:271–281.
31. Friedman JM, Birch PH. Type 1 neurofibromatosis: a descriptive analysis of the disorder in 1,728 patients. *Am J Med Genet*. 1997;70:138–143.
32. National Institutes of Health Consensus Development Conference Statement: neurofibromatosis. Bethesda, Md., USA, July 13–15, 1987. *Neurofibromatosis*. 1988;1:172–178.
33. Griffiths S, Thompson P, Frayling I, et al. Molecular diagnosis of neurofibromatosis type 1: 2 years experience. *Familial Cancer*. 2007;6:21–34.
34. Upadhyaya M, Osborn MJ, Maynard J, et al. Mutational and functional analysis of the neurofibromatosis type 1 (NF1) gene. *Human Genet*. 1997;99:88–92.
35. Fahsold R, Hoffmeyer S, Mischung C, et al. Minor lesion mutational spectrum of the entire NF1 gene does not explain its high mutability but points to a functional domain upstream of the GAP-related domain. *Am J Human Genet*. 2000;66:790–818.

36. Listernick R, Louis DN, Packer RJ, et al. Optic pathway gliomas in children with neurofibromatosis 1: consensus statement from the NF1 optic pathway glioma task force. *Ann Neurol.* 1997;41:143–149.
37. Listernick R, Charrow J, Greenwald M, et al. Natural history of optic pathway tumors in children with neurofibromatosis type 1: a longitudinal study. *J Pediatr.* 1994;125:63–66.
38. Listernick R, Darling C, Greenwald M, et al. Optic pathway tumors in children: the effect of neurofibromatosis type 1 on clinical manifestations and natural history. *J Pediatr.* 1995;127:718–722.
39. Gutmann DH, Aylsworth A, Carey JC, et al. The diagnostic evaluation and multidisciplinary management of neurofibromatosis 1 and neurofibromatosis 2. *JAMA.* 1997;278:51–57.
40. Pollack IF, Shultz B, Mulvihill JJ. The management of brainstem gliomas in patients with neurofibromatosis 1. *Neurology.* 1996;46:1652–1660.
41. Baser ME, DG RE, Gutmann DH. Neurofibromatosis 2. *Curr Opin Neurol.* 2003;16:27–33.
42. Singhal S, Birch JM, Kerr B, et al. Neurofibromatosis type 1 and sporadic optic gliomas. *Arch Dis Child.* 2002;87:65–70.
43. Guillamo JS, Creange A, Kalifa C, et al. Prognostic factors of CNS tumours in Neurofi-bromatosis 1 (NF1): a retrospective study of 104 patients. *Brain.* 2003;126:152–160.
44. Hoyt WF, Baghdassarian SA. Optic glioma of childhood. Natural history and rationale for conservative management. *Br J Ophthalmol.* 1969;53:793–798.
45. Allen JC. Initial management of children with hypothalamic and thalamic tumors and the modifying role of neurofibromatosis-1. *Pediatric Neurosurg.* 2000;32:154–162.
46. Brzowski AE, Bazan C, 3rd, Mumma JV, et al. Spontaneous regression of optic glioma in a patient with neurofibromatosis. *Neurology.* 1992;42:679–681.
47. Perilongo G, Moras P, Carollo C, et al. Spontaneous partial regression of low-grade glioma in children with neurofibromatosis-1: a real possibility. *J Child Neurol.* 1999;14:352–356.
48. Jamjoom AB, Malabarey T, Jamjoom ZA, et al. Cerebro-vasculopathy and malignancy: catastrophic complications of radiotherapy for optic nerve glioma in a von Recklinghausen neurofibromatosis patient. *Neurosurg Rev.* 1996;19:47–51.
49. Listernick R, Ferner RE, Liu GT, et al. Optic pathway gliomas in neurofibromatosis-1: controversies and recommendations. *Ann Neurol.* 2007;61:189–198.
50. Korones DN, Padowski J, Factor BA, et al. Do children with optic pathway tumors have an increased frequency of other central nervous system tumors? *Neuro-oncology.* 2003;5:116–120.
51. Sharif S, Ferner R, Birch JM, et al. Second primary tumors in neurofibromatosis 1 patients treated for optic glioma: substantial risks after radiotherapy. *J Clin Oncol.* 2006;24:2570–2575.
52. Shearer P, Parham D, Kovnar E, et al. Neurofibromatosis type I and malignancy: review of 32 pediatric cases treated at a single institution. *Medical Pediatric Oncol.* 1994;22:78–83.
53. Kuenzle C, Weissert M, Roulet E, et al. Follow-up of optic pathway gliomas in children with neurofibromatosis type 1. *Neuropediatrics.* 1994;25:295–300.
54. McGaughran JM, Harris DI, Donnai D, et al. A clinical study of type 1 neurofibroma-tosis in northwest England. *J Med Genet.* 1999;36:197–203.
55. Brodeur GM. The NF1 gene in myelopoiesis and childhood myelodysplastic syndromes. *N Engl J Med.* 1994;330:637–639.
56. Walther MM, Herring J, Enquist E, et al. von Recklinghausen's disease and pheochro-mocytomas. *J Urol.* 1999;162:1582–1586.
57. Evans DG, Baser ME, McGaughran J, et al. Malignant peripheral nerve sheath tumours in neurofibromatosis 1. *J Med Genet.* 2002;39:311–314.
58. Ruttledge MH, Rouleau GA. Role of the neurofibromatosis type 2 gene in the development of tumors of the nervous system. *Neurosurg Focus.* 2005;19:E6.
59. Trofatter JA, MacCollin MM, Rutter JL, et al. A novel moesin-, ezrin-, radixin-like gene is a candidate for the neurofibromatosis 2 tumor suppressor. *Cell.* 1993;72:791–800.

60. Baser ME, Kuramoto L, Joe H, et al. Genotype-phenotype correlations for nervous system tumors in neurofibromatosis 2: a population-based study. *Am J Human Genet.* 2004;75:231–239.

61. Mautner VF, Tatagiba M, Guthoff R, et al. Neurofibromatosis 2 in the pediatric age group. *Neurosurgery.* 1993;33:92–96.

62. Perry A, Giannini C, Raghavan R, et al. Aggressive phenotypic and genotypic features in pediatric and NF2-associated meningiomas: a clinicopathologic study of 53 cases. *J Neuropathol Exp Neurol.* 2001;60:994–1003.

63. Parry DM, Eldridge R, Kaiser-Kupfer MI, et al. Neurofibromatosis 2 (NF2): clinical characteristics of 63 affected individuals and clinical evidence for heterogeneity. *Am J Med Genet.* 1994;52:450–461.

64. van Slegtenhorst M, de Hoogt R, Hermans C, et al. Identification of the tuberous sclerosis gene TSC1 on chromosome 9q34. *Scienc* (New York, NY). 1997;277:805–808.

65. Narayanan V. Tuberous sclerosis complex: genetics to pathogenesis. *Pediatric Neurol.* 2003;29:404–409.

66. Identification and characterization of the tuberous sclerosis gene on chromosome 16. *Cell.* 1993;75:1305–1315.

67. Au KS, Rodriguez JA, Finch JL, et al. Germ-line mutational analysis of the TSC2 gene in 90 tuberous-sclerosis patients. *Am J Human Genet.* 1998;62:286–294.

68. Roach ES, DiMario FJ, Kandt RS, et al. Tuberous Sclerosis Consensus Conference: recommendations for diagnostic evaluation. National Tuberous Sclerosis Association. *J Child Neurol.* 1999;14:401–407.8

69. de Ribaupierre S, Dorfmuller G, Bulteau C, et al. Subependymal giant-cell astrocytomas in pediatric tuberous sclerosis disease: when should we operate? *Neurosurgery.* 2007;60:83–89; discussion 9–90.

70. Hyman MH, Whittemore VH. National Institutes of Health consensus conference: tuberous sclerosis complex. *Arc Neurol.* 2000;57:662–665.

71. Maher ER, Iselius L, Yates JR, et al. Von Hippel-Lindau disease: a genetic study. *J Med Genet.* 1991;28:443–447.

72. Pizzo PAP, D.G., ed. *Principles & Practice of Pediatric Oncology.* 5th ed. Philadelphia, PA: Lippincott Williams & Wilkins; 2005.

73. Lonser RR, Kim HJ, Butman JA, et al. Tumors of the endolymphatic sac in von Hippel-Lindau disease. *N Engl J Med.* 2004;350:2481–2486.

74. Maher ER, Yates JR, Harries R, et al. Clinical features and natural history of von Hippel-Lindau disease. *Quart J Med.* 1990;77:1151–1163.

75. Hanse MC, Vincent A, van den Bent MJ. Hemangioblastomatosis in a patient with von Hippel-Lindau disease. *J Neuro-Oncol.* 2007;82:163–164.

76. Maddock IR, Moran A, Maher ER, et al. A genetic register for von Hippel-Lindau disease. *J Med Genet.* 1996;33:120–127.

77. Filling-Katz MR, Choyke PL, Oldfield E, et al. Central nervous system involvement in Von Hippel-Lindau disease. *Neurology.* 1991;41:41–46.

78. Richard S, David P, Marsot-Dupuch K, et al. Central nervous system hemangioblastomas, endolymphatic sac tumors, and von Hippel-Lindau disease. *Neurosurg Rev.* 2000;23:1–22; discussion 3–4.

79. Steinbach F, Novick AC, Zincke H, et al. Treatment of renal cell carcinoma in von Hippel-Lindau disease: a multicenter study. *J Urol.* 1995;153:1812–1816.

80. Maher ER, Bentley E, Yates JR, et al. Mapping of von Hippel-Lindau disease to chromosome 3p confirmed by genetic linkage analysis. *J Neurological Sci.* 1990;100:27–30.

81. Latif F, Tory K, Gnarra J, et al. Identification of the von Hippel-Lindau disease tumor suppressor gene. *Scienc* (New York, NY). 1993;260:1317–1320.

82. Ohh M, Kaelin WG, Jr. The von Hippel-Lindau tumour suppressor protein: new perspectives. *Mol Med Today.* 1999;5:257–263.

83. Sufan RI, Jewett MA, Ohh M. The role of von Hippel-Lindau tumor suppressor protein and hypoxia in renal clear cell carcinoma. *Am J Physiol.* 2004;287:F1–F6.

84. Stolle C, Glenn G, Zbar B, et al. Improved detection of germline mutations in the von Hippel-Lindau disease tumor suppressor gene. *Human Mutation.* 1998;12:417–423.

85. Choyke PL, Glenn GM, Walther MM, et al. von Hippel-Lindau disease: genetic, clinical, and imaging features. *Radiology.* 1995;194:629–642.

86. Eisenhofer G, Lenders JW, Linehan WM, et al. Plasma normetanephrine and metanephrine for detecting pheochromocytoma in von Hippel-Lindau disease and multiple endocrine neoplasia type 2. *N Engl J Med.* 1999;340:1872–1879.

87. Gorlin RJ, Goltz RW. Multiple nevoid basal-cell epithelioma, jaw cysts and bifid rib. A syndrome. *N Engl J Med.* 1960;262:908–912.

88. Cawson RA, Kerr GA. The Syndrome of Jaw Cysts, Basal Cell Tumours and Skeletal Abnormalities. *Proc Roy Soc Med.* 1964;57:799–801.

89. Berlin NI, Van Scott EJ, Clendenning WE, et al. Basal cell nevus syndrome. Combined clinical staff conference at the National Institutes of Health. *Ann Int Med.* 1966;64:403–421.

90. Gorlin RJ. Nevoid basal cell carcinoma (Gorlin) syndrome. *Genet Med.* 2004;6:530–539.

91. Evans DG, Ladusans EJ, Rimmer S, et al. Complications of the naevoid basal cell carcinoma syndrome: results of a population based study. *J Med Genet.* 1993;30:460–464.

92. Gorlin RJ. Nevoid basal cell carcinoma (Gorlin) syndrome: unanswered issues. *J Lab Clin Med.* 1999;134:551–552.

93. Kimonis VE, Goldstein AM, Pastakia B, et al. Clinical manifestations in 105 persons with nevoid basal cell carcinoma syndrome. *Am J Med Genet.* 1997;69:299–308.

94. Johnson RL, Rothman AL, Xie J, et al. Human homolog of patched, a candidate gene for the basal cell nevus syndrome. *Scienc* (New York, NY). 1996;272:1668–1671.

95. Gailani MR, Stahle-Backdahl M, Leffell DJ, et al. The role of the human homologue of Drosophila patched in sporadic basal cell carcinomas. *Nature Genet.* 1996;14:78–81.

96. Gailani MR, Bale AE. Acquired and inherited basal cell carcinomas and the patched gene. *Adv Dermatol.* 1999;14:261–283; discussion 84.

97. Farndon PA, Del Mastro RG, Evans DG, et al. Location of gene for Gorlin syndrome. *Lancet.* 1992;339:581–582.

98. Hahn H, Wicking C, Zaphiropoulous PG, et al. Mutations of the human homolog of Drosophila patched in the nevoid basal cell carcinoma syndrome. *Cell.* 1996;85:841–851.

99. Goodrich LV, Milenkovic L, Higgins KM, et al. Altered neural cell fates and medulloblastoma in mouse patched mutants. *Scienc* (New York, NY). 1997;277:1109–1113.

100. Raffel C, Jenkins RB, Frederick L, et al. Sporadic medulloblastomas contain PTCH mutations. *Cancer Res.* 1997;57:842–845.

101. Zurawel RH, Allen C, Chiappa S, et al. Analysis of PTCH/SMO/SHH pathway genes in medulloblastoma. *Genes, Chromosomes Cancer.* 2000;27:44–51.

102. Booth DR. The hedgehog signaling pathway and its role in basal cell carcinoma. *Cancer Metastasis Rev.* 1999;18:261–284.

103. Cowan R, Hoban P, Kelsey A, et al. The gene for the naevoid basal cell carcinoma syndrome acts as a tumour-suppressor gene in medulloblastoma. *Br J Cancer.* 1997;76:141–145.

104. Korczak JF, Brahim JS, DiGiovanna JJ, et al. Nevoid basal cell carcinoma syndrome with medulloblastoma in an African-American boy: a rare case illustrating gene-environment interaction. *Am J Med Genet.* 1997;69:309–314.

105. Walter AW, Pivnick EK, Bale AE, et al. Complications of the nevoid basal cell carcinoma syndrome: a case report. *J Pediatr Hematol Oncol.* 1997;19:258–262.

106. Nichols KE, Malkin D, Garber JE, et al. Germ-line p53 mutations predispose to a wide spectrum of early-onset cancers. *Cancer Epidemiol Biomarkers Prev.* 2001;10:83–87.

107. Bottomley RH, Trainer AL, Condit PT. Chromosome studies in a "cancer family". *Cancer.* 1971;28:519–528.

108. Lynch HT, McComb RD, Osborn NK, et al. Predominance of brain tumors in an extended Li-Fraumeni (SBLA) kindred, including a case of Sturge-Weber syndrome. *Cancer*. 2000;88:433–439.
109. Kleihues P, Schauble B, zur Hausen A, et al. Tumors associated with p53 germline mutations: a synopsis of 91 families. *Am J Pathol*. 1997;150:1–13.
110. Chompret A. The Li-Fraumeni syndrome. *Biochimie*. 2002;84:75–82.
111. Malkin D. p53 and the Li-Fraumeni syndrome. *Cancer Genet Cytogenet*. 1993;66:83–92.
112. Malkin D, Li FP, Strong LC, et al. Germ line p53 mutations in a familial syndrome of breast cancer, sarcomas, and other neoplasms. *Scienc* (New York, NY). 1990;250:1233–1238.
113. Hisada M, Garber JE, Fung CY, et al. Multiple primary cancers in families with Li-Fraumeni syndrome. *J Natl Cancer Inst*. 1998;90:606–611.
114. Srivastava S, Zou ZQ, Pirollo K, et al. Germ-line transmission of a mutated p53 gene in a cancer-prone family with Li-Fraumeni syndrome. *Nature*. 1990;348:747–749.
115. Frebourg T, Barbier N, Yan YX, et al. Germ-line p53 mutations in 15 families with Li-Fraumeni syndrome. *Am J Human Genet*. 1995;56:608–615.
116. Birch JM, Hartley AL, Tricker KJ, et al. Prevalence and diversity of constitutional mutations in the p53 gene among 21 Li-Fraumeni families. *Cancer Res*. 1994;54:1298–1304.
117. Rasheed BK, McLendon RE, Herndon JE, et al. Alterations of the TP53 gene in human gliomas. *Cancer Res*. 1994;54:1324–1330.
118. Poeta ML, Manola J, Goldwasser MA, et al. TP53 mutations and survival in squamous-cell carcinoma of the head and neck. *N Engl J Med*. 2007;357:2552–2561.
119. Nutting C, Camplejohn RS, Gilchrist R, et al. A patient with 17 primary tumours and a germ line mutation in TP53: tumour induction by adjuvant therapy? *Clin Onco* (Royal College of Radiologists (Great Britain)). 2000;12:300–304.
120. Limacher JM, Frebourg T, Natarajan-Ame S, et al. Two metachronous tumors in the radiotherapy fields of a patient with Li-Fraumeni syndrome. *Int J Cancer*. 2001;96:238–242.
121. Mullins KJ, Rubio A, Myers SP, et al. Malignant ependymomas in a patient with Turcot's syndrome: case report and management guidelines. *Surg Neurol*. 1998;49:290–294.
122. Costa OL, Silva DM, Colnago FA, et al. Turcot syndrome. Autosomal dominant or recessive transmission? *Dis Colon Rectum*. 1987;30:391–394.
123. Foulkes WD. A tale of four syndromes: familial adenomatous polyposis, Gardner syndrome, attenuated APC and Turcot syndrome. *Qjm*. 1995;88:853–863.
124. Mori T, Nagase H, Horii A, et al. Germ-line and somatic mutations of the APC gene in patients with Turcot syndrome and analysis of APC mutations in brain tumors. *Genes Chromosomes Cancer*. 1994;9:168–172.
125. Hamilton SR, Liu B, Parsons RE, et al. The molecular basis of Turcot's syndrome. *N Engl J Med*. 1995;332:839–847.
126. De Rosa M, Fasano C, Panariello L, et al. Evidence for a recessive inheritance of Turcot's syndrome caused by compound heterozygous mutations within the PMS2 gene. *Oncogene*. 2000;19:1719–1723.
127. Thakker RV. Multiple endocrine neoplasia – syndromes of the twentieth century. *J Clin Endocrinol Metabolism*. 1998;83:2617–2620.
128. Lohmann DR, Brandt B, Hopping W, et al. The spectrum of RB1 germ-line mutations in hereditary retinoblastoma. *Am J Human Genet*. 1996;58:940–949.
129. Richter S, Vandezande K, Chen N, et al. Sensitive and efficient detection of RB1 gene mutations enhances care for families with retinoblastoma. *Am J Human Genet*. 2003;72:253–269.
130. Lance EI, DuPont BR, Holden KR. Expansion of the deletion 13q syndrome phenotype: a case report. *J Child Neurol*. 2007;22:1124–1127.
131. Meadows A. Trilateral retinoblastoma. *Med Pediatric Oncol*. 1986;14:323–326.

132. Kivela T. Trilateral retinoblastoma: a meta-analysis of hereditary retinoblastoma associated with primary ectopic intracranial retinoblastoma. *J Clin Oncol.* 1999;17:1829–1837.

133. Abramson DH, Melson MR, Dunkel IJ, et al. Third (fourth and fifth) nonocular tumors in survivors of retinoblastoma. *Ophthalmology.* 2001;108:1868–1876.

134. Albert LS, Sober AJ, Rhodes AR. Cutaneous melanoma and bilateral retinoblastoma. *J Am Acad Dermatol.* 1990;23:1001–1004.

135. Abramson DH, Frank CM. Second nonocular tumors in survivors of bilateral retinoblastoma: a possible age effect on radiation-related risk. *Ophthalmology.* 1998;105:573–579; discussion 9–80.

136. Dorfmuller G, Wurtz FG, Kleinert R, et al. Cerebral primitive neuro-ectodermal tumour following treatment of a unilateral retinoblastoma. *Acta Neurochirurgica.* 1997;139:749–755.

137. Traboulsi EI, Zimmerman LE, Manz HJ. Cutaneous malignant melanoma in survivors of heritable retinoblastoma. *Arc Ophthalmol.* 1988;106:1059–1061.

138. Belt PJ, Smithers M, Elston T. The triad of bilateral retinoblastoma, dysplastic naevus syndrome and multiple cutaneous malignant melanomas: a case report and review of the literature. *Melanoma Res.* 2002;12:179–182.

139. Kleinerman RA, Tucker MA, Abramson DH, et al. Risk of soft tissue sarcomas by individual subtype in survivors of hereditary retinoblastoma. *J Natl Cancer Inst.* 2007;99:24–31.

140. Wenzel CT, Halperin EC, Fisher SR. Second malignant neoplasms of the head and neck in survivors of retinoblastoma. *Ear Nose Throat J.* 2001;80:106, 9–12.

141. Kleinerman RA, Tarone RE, Abramson DH, et al. Hereditary retinoblastoma and risk of lung cancer. *J Natl Cancer Inst.* 2000;92:2037–2039.

142. Soloway HB. Radiation-induced neoplasms following curative therapy for retinoblastoma. *Cancer.* 1966;19:1984–1988.

143. Abramson DH, Ellsworth RM, Kitchin FD, et al. Second nonocular tumors in retinoblastoma survivors. Are they radiation-induced? *Ophthalmology.* 1984;91:1351–1355.

144. Kleinerman RA, Tucker MA, Tarone RE, et al. Risk of new cancers after radiotherapy in long-term survivors of retinoblastoma: an extended follow-up. *J Clin Oncol.* 2005;23:2272–2279.

145. Acquaviva A, Ciccolallo L, Rondelli R, et al. Mortality from second tumour among long-term survivors of retinoblastoma: a retrospective analysis of the Italian retinoblastoma registry. *Oncogene.* 2006;25:5350–5357.

146. Abramson DH, Ronner HJ, Ellsworth RM. Second tumors in nonirradiated bilateral retinoblastoma. *Am J Ophthalmol.* 1979;87:624–627.

147. Lueder GT, Judisch F, O'Gorman TW. Second nonocular tumors in survivors of heritable retinoblastoma. *Arc Ophthalmol.* 1986;104:372–373.

148. Derkinderen DJ, Koten JW, Wolterbeek R, et al. Non-ocular cancer in hereditary retinoblastoma survivors and relatives. *Ophthalmic Paediatrics Genet.* 1987;8:23–25.

149. Roarty JD, McLean IW, Zimmerman LE. Incidence of second neoplasms in patients with bilateral retinoblastoma. *Ophthalmology.* 1988;95:1583–1587.

150. Eng C, Li FP, Abramson DH, et al. Mortality from second tumors among long-term survivors of retinoblastoma. *J Natl Cancer Inst.* 1993;85:1121–1128.

151. Moll AC, Imhof SM, Bouter LM, et al. Second primary tumors in patients with retinoblastoma. A review of the literature. *Ophthalmic Genet.* 1997;18:27–34.

152. Imhof SM, Moll AC, Hofman P, et al. Second primary tumours in hereditary- and nonhereditary retinoblastoma patients treated with megavoltage external beam irradiation. *Documenta Ophthalmologica.* 1997;93:337–344.

153. Kaye FJ, Harbour JW. For whom the bell tolls: susceptibility to common adult cancers in retinoblastoma survivors. *J Natl Cancer Inst.* 2004;96:342–343.

154. Fletcher O, Easton D, Anderson K, et al. Lifetime risks of common cancers among retinoblastoma survivors. *J Natl Cancer Inst.* 2004;96:357–363.

155. Mohney BG, Robertson DM, Schomberg PJ, et al. Second nonocular tumors in survivors of heritable retinoblastoma and prior radiation therapy. *Am J Ophthalmol.* 1998;126:269–277.
156. Draper GJ, Sanders BM, Kingston JE. Second primary neoplasms in patients with retinoblastoma. *Br J Cancer.* 1986;53:661–671.
157. Markey MP, Bergseid J, Bosco EE, et al. Loss of the retinoblastoma tumor suppressor: differential action on transcriptional programs related to cell cycle control and immune function. *Oncogene.* 2007;26:6307–6318.
158. Sharma A, Comstock CE, Knudsen ES, et al. Retinoblastoma tumor suppressor status is a critical determinant of therapeutic response in prostate cancer cells. *Cancer Res.* 2007;67:6192–6203.
159. Agoston AT, Argani P, De Marzo AM, et al. Retinoblastoma pathway dysregulation causes DNA methyltransferase 1 overexpression in cancer via MAD2-mediated inhibition of the anaphase-promoting complex. *Am J Pathol.* 2007;170:1585–1593.
160. Friend SH, Bernards R, Rogelj S, et al. A human DNA segment with properties of the gene that predisposes to retinoblastoma and osteosarcoma. *Nature.* 1986;323:643–646.
161. Neglia JP, Friedman DL, Yasui Y, et al. Second malignant neoplasms in five-year survivors of childhood cancer: childhood cancer survivor study. *J Natl Cancer Inst.* 2001;93:618–629.
162. Strong LC, Herson J, Haas C, et al. Cancer mortality in relatives of retinoblastoma patients. *J Natl Cancer Inst.* 1984;73:303–311.
163. Sanders BM, Jay M, Draper GJ, et al. Non-ocular cancer in relatives of retinoblastoma patients. *Br J Cancer.* 1989;60:358–365.
164. Forrest AW. Tumors following radiation about the eye. *Trans – Am Acad Ophthalmol Otolaryngol.* 1961;65:694–717.
165. Meadows AT, Shields CL. Regarding chemoreduction for retinoblastoma and intracranial neoplasms. *Arch Ophthalmol.* 2004;122:1570–1571; author reply 1.
166. Blanquet V, Turleau C, Gross-Morand MS, et al. Spectrum of germline mutations in the RB1 gene: a study of 232 patients with hereditary and non hereditary retinoblastoma. *Human Molecular Genet.* 1995;4:383–388.
167. Bassal M, Mertens AC, Taylor L, et al. Risk of selected subsequent carcinomas in survivors of childhood cancer: a report from the Childhood Cancer Survivor Study. *J Clin Oncol.* 2006;24:476–483.

Chapter 16
Secondary Neoplasms Following Treatment for Brain Tumors

Joanna L. Weinstein, Kanyalakshmi Ayyanar, and Melody A. Watral

Introduction

Secondary malignant neoplasms (SMNs) are considered one of the most devastating late effects of cancer therapies, as they are associated with significant morbidity and mortality. Defined as histologically distinct neoplasms that develop after a first cancer, SMNs are estimated to account for 6–10% of all cancer diagnoses in the United States.[1,2] In particular, survivors with a history of cancers during childhood and adolescence have a significantly increased risk of developing a SMN. The therapeutic advances that have improved survival in these pediatric patients have resulted in a 5–10-fold increased risk of developing additional tumors.[3–16] Additionally, as survival rates continue to improve, it is predicted that the occurrence of SMN will increase accordingly.[9,15,17–24]

Overview and Epidemiology

Incidence data regarding SMNs varies depending on the inclusion and exclusion criteria of various studies.[9,14,15] For instance, many of the largest registries that track "late effects" by definition exclude early-onset SMN that occur within the first five years after primary diagnosis; thereby a significant proportion of the secondary hematologic conditions and other events that tend to occur early are not accounted for.[9,23,25,26] Additionally, some series exclude cancer predisposition syndromes that are associated with multiple cancers, such as germline RB and NF1,[9] while others exclude certain "benign" tumors or conditions, such as nonmelanoma skin cancer and meningiomas.[9,27]

J.L. Weinstein (✉)
Division of Hematology, Oncology and Stem Cell Transplantation, Children's
Memorial Hospital, Chicago, IL, USA
e-mail: jweinstein@childrensmemorial.org

S. Goldman, C.D. Turner (eds.), *Late Effects of Treatment for Brain Tumors*,
Cancer Treatment and Research 150, DOI 10.1007/b109924_16,
© Springer Science+Business Media, LLC 2009

When considering all age groups, SMN account for the fourth or fifth most common cancer in the United States.[1,28] If the risk of developing a SMN is examined for all age groups, some studies have suggested that the overall increased risk is not substantial, compared to the general population as has been seen for survivors in younger age groups.[29–31] One large series from Finland of cancer patients registered between 1953 and 1991 demonstrated a 1.7-fold increased risk of developing a second cancer for patients less than 50 years of age at their primary cancer diagnosis; however, when all age groups were examined, there was no demonstrable overall increased risk of developing a second cancer, when compared to the age- and gender-matched healthy population.[29] Similarly, at least two other studies of cancer patients revealed a less than 2-fold increased risk of development of subsequent cancers developing a second cancer when compared to the general population.[30,31]

These data examining cancer patients of all ages are in distinct contrast to the results for patients treated for cancer at younger ages. For those treated for cancer when younger than 21 years, the risk of developing SMN is dramatically higher, with multiple studies confirming a 3–6-fold increased risk compared to the general population.[1,9,10,14,15] For children diagnosed with any primary malignancy, the overall incidence of SMN ranges from 8 to 12% up to 20 years following the occurrence of their primary cancer.[32] Additionally, this risk of developing SMN continues to increase as these cohorts of survivors age.[9,15,17,20,21]

The analysis from the Childhood Cancer Survivor Study (CCSS), which reported on SMN in 13,581 patients, originally diagnosed and treated for childhood cancer between 1970 and 1986 and surviving five or more years from original diagnosis, found an estimated cumulative incidence of SMN of 3.2% at 20 years after the initial diagnosis.[9] Specifically, 314 SMNs occurred in 298 participants, with 16 patients developing multiple SMNs. In an update of this data, Neglia et al. reported that 116 of the survivors developed subsequent tumors in the brain and central nervous system.[33] Notably, the CCSS excluded individuals who developed and died of an SMN after less than five years of follow-up, and excluded secondary malignant diagnoses of meningiomas and nonmalignant CNS tumors, nonmelanoma skin cancer, as well as premalignant or dysplastic conditions.

For patients with an original diagnosis of pediatric brain tumors, the SEER database from 1973 to 1998 showed that 39 of 2,056 long-term survivors developed a SMN.[32] More recent treatment eras, which have included more frequent use of chemotherapies and often higher cumulative doses of chemotherapies, seem to show an increased risk of developing SMN than earlier eras; researchers surmise that greater exposure to chemotherapies implemented in the more modern treatment era may be, in part, to blame.[1,32,34]

Whereas primary tumor recurrence generally occurs within five years, SMNs can develop from months to decades after initial tumor diagnosis and treatment.[3,9,16,20,21,23,35–37] After primary brain tumor treatment, secondary solid tumors can develop in the CNS or other sites. With increasing use of chemotherapies in CNS and other primary cancers, hematologic malignances are occurring as well.[34,35,38,39] In general, the risk of chemotherapy-induced secondary leukemia is associated with a relatively short latency period (i.e., within 10 years) in contrast to radiation-induced solid malignancies which tend to occur later and are detectable in series with longer follow-up.[14,25,34,40–43] A Nordic series of 25,120 cancer survivors demonstrated a mean interval between first and second diagnosis of 12.0 years, with a short latency of approximately five years to development of leukemia as the secondary tumor, versus eight or more years for development of other secondary solid tumors, not limited to tumors of the brain and breast.[25] Similarly, the CCSS cohort demonstrated a median time from primary diagnosis to SMN was 11.7 years, with the shortest time to develop secondary AML (6.1 years) and a longer time to the development of breast cancer (15.7 years).[9]

The specific cohort population under study may affect the latency period to the development of SMN. For example, patients with tumor predisposition syndromes, such as germline p53 mutations (Li-Fraumeni), hereditary retinoblastoma or Gorlin syndrome, often present with second cancer with a shorter latency than in those patients without such susceptibility.[36,44–48] For instance, in Gorlin syndrome, the young patient with medulloblastoma may develop multiple basal cell carcinomas relatively soon after therapeutic radiation;[49,50] similarly, certain secondary sarcomas tend to develop at a younger age in hereditary RB patients than those with sporadic disease.[46,51–54]

With extended follow-up and longer survivorship, these patterns of SMN may change, and the occurrence of SMN will undoubtedly increase.[14,16,18,19,21,23,55] For instance, cumulative risk of developing SMN in a study of childhood cancer survivors in the Netherlands showed 1.6%, 4.4%, and 11.1% risk at follow-up of 10, 20, and 30 years, respectively.[23] A recent report from St. Jude Children's Research Hospital suggests that the cumulative incidence of SMN in patients in remission does not plateau at 20 years of follow-up, but continues to increase.[21] This latter study suggests that although many of the late-onset SMN are low-grade lesions, such as basal cell carcinoma (BCC) and meningioma, a substantial portion of these "later-onset" neoplasms are histologically aggressive tumors, including carcinomas and soft tissue sarcomas.[21]

Effect on Mortality and Morbidity

Though less common than other late effects seen in survivors of cancer, secondary malignancies have a most profound impact on cancer survivor mortality and morbidity.[22,26,56–63] In most studies, secondary malignancies account for the most common cause of death in long-term survivors after recurrence of the primary tumor.[59,61,62,64–69] The CCSS data reported by Mertens et al. demonstrated a 19-fold increased risk of death due to a secondary or subsequent neoplasm;[59,68] 15% of the deaths in these long-term survivors were attributed to second neoplasms, which is at least twice that was attributable to other treatment–related sequelae (i.e., cardiac or pulmonary).[59,68] Nordic, British, and other series confirm this degree of excess second cancer-related mortality as well.[62,66,70]

Developing SMN was associated with an increased risk of mortality in the CCSS cohort of individuals surviving more than five years from original cancer diagnosis; 91.9% of the cohort members who had not developed a SMN were alive, whereas only 59.4% who had developed a SMN were alive.[9] Likewise, data from a series from the Netherlands documented a 20-year actuarial risk of death in survivors who developed SMN to be 31.7, versus 9% in those who did not.[23]

Diagnosis-, treatment- and host-related factors variably impact the risk of mortality due to these second cancers. Most studies show that standardized mortality ratios (SMRs) varied according to the original cancer diagnosis,[59,60,64,66,68] with the highest SMRs due to all causes most commonly seen in survivors of Hodgkin lymphoma,[95,66,68] CNS tumors,[59,68] and retinoblastoma.[66]

The excess mortality rates attributable to SMN are seen for all age groups and in both genders.[59,66,68] Female survivors have a higher SMR due to SMN than males in most studies.[68,70] A report from the Roswell Park Cancer Institute demonstrated deaths due to SMN accounted for half of female survivor deaths, versus one-third of male survivor deaths.[62] This increased risk of mortality for female cancer survivors is due, in part, to excess breast cancers; hormonal factors may contribute as well.

In multiple studies, the risk of death due to SMN is increased for patients treated with radiotherapy,[26,59,61,68,71] with higher doses of alkylators[72] and epipodophyllotoxins,[59,68,73] and, particularly, chemoradiotherapy regimens.[57]

Though much of this mortality risk is due to these therapeutic exposures, genetic factors clearly contribute to the risk of mortality from the second cancer.[62,74,76] The increased likelihood of death due to SMN affects both those patients with an overt genetic cancer predisposition syndrome, such as germline retinoblastoma patients, and those without clearly identifiable genetic predisposition.[74] In an Italian series, RB patients had a 10-fold increased risk of mortality compared to the general population, and those with confirmed or suspected germline disease had overall cumulative mortality at least twice that of the sporadic RB patients.[75] Eng et al. found that the cumulative probability of death specifically due to SMN in survivors of bilateral RB was 26% at 40 years.[74] For RB patients, much of this excess mortality is attributable to fatal sarcomas in these high risk patients.[51–53,74,75,77]

It is well accepted that with longer duration of follow-up, these observed patterns of mortality in these survivor cohorts may change, along with changes in the observed pattern and incidence of SMNs.[68] These mortality trends may vary depending on characteristics of the survivor cohort and on the era of treatment.[55,66,78] Whereas deaths due to recurrence of primary cancer rose between five and 15 years post-diagnosis, deaths due to SMN and other treatment-related sequelae increased more rapidly in the period 15–30 years after diagnosis.[68] Though deaths due to secondary brain tumors were not different between these two follow-up periods, there were notable increases in deaths due to lung cancer, breast cancer, and melanoma in this North American cohort.[68] Some, but not all, of this may be due to an underlying increase in these particular cancers within the general population.

Specifically, in patients with brain tumors as their primary diagnosis, Jenkin et al. showed that the actuarial cumulative incidence of death due to SMN was 1, 5, and 13%, respectively, at 10, 20, and 30 years.[67] The Pediatric Oncology Group found that five of their 198 infant patients treated with prolonged chemotherapy with or without radiotherapy for CNS tumors developed SMN, and only one of these five was alive at follow-up.[34] Investigations are ongoing to examine these patterns of mortality due to SMN and other secondary complications, and to determine whether external factors, either modifiable or not, are at play.

In addition to a significant effect on the mortality, secondary malignancies also impact survivor morbidity.[79] For the adult survivor cohort of the CCSS, the survivors affected by a SMN were more likely than their siblings to report modest to extreme adverse outcomes in general health, mental health, functional impairment, activity limitations, pain as a result of cancer, and anxiety as a result of the cancer compared to survivors without a second cancer.[79] Additional therapy required for treatment of SMN further increased the likelihood of morbidity and mortality due to other late effects.[80,81] Another study demonstrated that adult survivors of multiple primary cancers experience modest, but lasting deficits in quality of life, including reduced functioning in psychosocial domains, including global QOL, vitality, cancer-specific stress reactions, and existential well-being, when compared to the functioning in controls who had a single cancer;[82] the experience of cancer can have long-term effects, and the experience of multiple cancers may amplify this risk.

Risk Factors for Secondary Malignant Neoplasms

Risk factors for the development of SMN are multifactorial and include host- and cancer-related factors (See Table 16.1).[1,17,83,84] The degree of increased risk, as well as the types of subsequent neoplasms, differ according to the following and other less well-defined factors: original cancer diagnosis; patient age at primary cancer diagnosis and treatment; treatment modality directed against the primary tumor; family history, and presence of known genetic conditions and other less well-defined genetic features (e.g., polymorphisms); environmental and behavioral factors, and other unknown contributing factors.[1,4,9,17,25,83–86] Host-related factors include age at diagnosis, gender, genetics (e.g., inherited predisposition and less well-defined genetics related to drug metabolism) as well as behavioral and environmental exposures (e.g., smoking, sun exposure), whereas cancer-related factors include original cancer diagnosis, tumor location, tumor biology, tumor response, and treatment modality.[1,17,86]

Table 16.1 Risk factors for developing secondary malignant neoplasms after childhood cancer

Host-related
Age
Gender
Predisposition syndromes
Gene-environment interactions; other genetics
Lifestyle, Environmental (sun, tobacco use, alcohol consumption)
Therapy-related
Chemotherapy (dose, schedule)
Radiotherapy (location, dose, modality)
Stem Cell Transplantation (conditioning, RT, complications)
Other therapies, endocrine or other complications
Primary cancer diagnosis
Brain tumors
Retinoblastoma
Hodgkin's lymphoma
Soft tissue sarcomas
Acute lymphoblastic leukemia (ALL)
NHL, other hematologic malignancies

Host-Related Factors

Most studies of long-term survivors report that young age at primary cancer diagnosis is associated with an increased risk of secondary cancers.[9,10,27,87,88] This finding excludes secondary myelodysplasia and acute myeloid leukemia in which risk of their development has consistently been shown to correlate with an older age at the diagnosis and treatment of the primary cancer.[89–91] In many studies, pediatric patients with a primary diagnosis of ALL, brain tumors, and Hodgkin's lymphoma treated at a younger age had a higher risk of developing secondary brain tumors than those treated at an older age.[9,38,87,92,93] In the CCSS, younger age was independently and significantly associated with the occurrence of malignant CNS tumors, sarcoma, and thyroid cancers in particular.[9] Rare studies do not support this association.[35,94]

Children under age five years appear to be especially vulnerable to the development of secondary brain tumors, implying that the developing brain of a young child is very susceptible to the effects of radiation.[33,38,95–97] Underlying genetics may also be at play since youngest children may have an underlying predisposition to develop their cancer in the first place.[38,98,99] Broniscer et al., in an analysis of SMN in CNS tumor survivors, demonstrated that patients two years or younger had a significantly greater risk of developing a SMN, compared with those older than two years;[38] when patients with identifiable genetic syndromes such as Gorlin syndrome, NF-2, and Gardner syndrome, and germline TP53 mutation were excluded, though, this specific age cutoff lost its significance. In most studies, the basis for this relation with younger age has not been well-characterized; some have reasoned that these age-associated effects may be related to (1) increased vulnerability of younger tissue to mutagenicity of cancer-directed therapies, (2) the higher proliferative rate of tissues during younger stages of development, (3) inherent genetic susceptibility, or (4) longer follow-up of the surviving cohort, allowing second cancers of longer latency to become apparent.[1]

In contrast to other SMNs, development of treatment-related leukemia and myelodysplasia (MDS/sAML) is associated with older age at primary treatment;[89–91] this relationship may be due to a greater susceptibility of the older hematopoietic stem cells to cumulative mutagenic effects of chemoradiotherapies, as well as environmental exposures and mutagens.[1,90,91,100]

Most studies demonstrate that female gender is associated with an increased risk of developing SMN.[9,16,20,23,88,92,101] This is largely due to the excess occurrence of secondary breast cancer and the increased risk of thyroid cancer in female survivors.[9,87,92,101–103] Even when women with breast cancer as the SMN were excluded, multivariate analysis revealed that female sex was associated with an increased risk of developing SMN in general, but not of specific neoplasms.[92] At least one study demonstrated an increased risk of basal cell carcinoma in female compared to male survivors.[23] In one study of brain tumor survivors, after adjusting for radiation exposure, females were 3.6 times more likely to develop a SMN.[35] Some data suggests that women may be more susceptible to carcinogenic effects of radiotherapy than men, possibly related to gender differences of cytochrome-450 enzymatic activity and of *TP53* mutations and the effects of hormones on tumor promotion.[101,104]

Genetic Factors

Convincing evidence has established that cancer is the result of multiple mutations in DNA, and underlying genetic predisposition clearly contributes to the development of cancer in many cases.[17,105–107] Although the proportion of pediatric cancers that have a clear hereditary factor is small,[12] children can have a cancer susceptibility with a noncontributory family history because of a constitutional chromosome disorder or a de novo mutation in a cancer predisposition gene. For instance, a significant portion of RB patients are affected by a new germline mutation without a family history of RB.[17,108,109] In many series, patients whose cancer was treated with surgery alone (i.e., not exposed to chemoradiotherapies) have a higher than general population risk to develop SMN,[23] suggesting an inherent predisposition of multiple cancers in those affected by a first. Other genetic factors may be at play with development of the primary and subsequent neoplasms; several studies have suggested that siblings of patients with childhood malignancy are at an increased risk of cancer development, even in the absence of a recognizable cancer predisposition syndrome or family history.[99,110]

These genetic factors, which contribute to the development of a patient's first malignancy, also appear to increase the risk of second primary tumors as well as the risk of therapy-induced secondary malignancies.[17] In addition to the overtly recognized genetic susceptibilities (to be discussed in detail later), there is emerging evidence suggesting that various genetic polymorphisms predispose patients to the develop treatment-related secondary neoplasia. Polymorphisms in genes linked to metabolic activation, detoxification, and DNA repair enzymes have been associated with susceptibility to various treatment-related malignancies.[111–117] For instance, patients with secondary AML are more likely than patients with de novo AML to have an inactivating gene polymorphism in NAD(P)H:quinone oxidoreductase, an enzyme capable of metabolizing anticancer drugs, suggesting that hematopoietic stem cells of patients with this polymorphism are more sensitive to the carcinogenic effects of treatment.[111] Similarly, investigations of the metabolizing enzyme CYP3A4 suggest that individuals possessing a particular variant polymorphism of this enzyme may be at higher risk of developing treatment-related leukemia, hypothetically related to the higher accumulation of potentially DNA-damaging reactive intermediates.[113] Polymorphisms in genes that encode glutathione S-transferases (GSTs), a detoxification enzyme, may alter susceptibility to chemotherapy-induced carcinogenesis, specifically to therapy-related AML.[114,116]

Relling et al. examined patients who developed brain tumors after radiotherapy and concomitant thiopurine therapy for acute lymphoblastic leukemia.[118] Three of the six patients who developed secondary brain tumors after RT and chemotherapy were heterozygous- or homozygous-deficient for thiopurine methyltransferase, an enzyme crucial for the inactivation of 6-mercaptopurine; patients with this polymorphism thus had greater accumulations of thioguanine nucleotide metabolites of 6MP. This data suggests that a higher cumulative exposure to antimetabolite therapy, namely during the RT portion of treatment, may predispose to SMN, namely BTs and AML.[118,119] This phenomenon has not been well-characterized by larger registries.[33,120,121]

If an inherited syndrome is suspected, this susceptibility to develop second tumors must be acknowledged when considering treatment decisions regarding the patient's primary cancer. In risk-adapted therapy, goals may include avoiding RT and leukemogenic therapy for patients with malignant predisposition. For instance, in patients with germline RB or p53, treatment options that avoid radiotherapy may be most appropriate, because the risk of RT-induced tumors is exceptionally high in these predisposed patients.[97,122] For patients with NF-1 who have CNS lesions and optic pathway tumors, therapies using non-alkylator chemotherapies and avoiding radiation therapy are preferred in order to decrease risk of developing secondary malignancies.[122,123]

Behavioral or modifiable host risk factors likely contribute to the development of second neoplasms. These include tobacco use,[124–130] sun exposure,[131,132] alcohol consumption,[86,133,134] activity and exercise levels, dietary practices, and hormonal factors. To date, the contribution of these lifestyle factors has not been well studied in pediatric survivor cohorts. Ideally, these modifiable factors should be a focus of long-term follow-up clinics.[131,132,135–138]

Cancer- and Treatment-Related Factors

Specific types of primary cancers of childhood are clearly associated with a higher risk of secondary cancers: Hodgkin lymphoma (HL), retinoblastoma (RB), sarcomas and, in some series, brain tumors are consistently overrepresented as primary diagnoses among patients with SMNs.[1,4,5,8,9,14,20,41,76,139–146] In some disorders, this trend is related to the genetics of the underlying cancer and its therapy (i.e., hereditary RB and secondary sarcomas induced by RT), whereas in other cancers, such as HL or various soft tissue sarcomas, it is unclear whether the primary disease process is an independent risk factor for the development of secondary cancer, or whether the specific therapy required to treat the primary cancer is the main contributor.

Cancer-related factors include the tumor site, tumor biology, treatment modality with their associated systemic effects, treatment response and relapse status. For instance, in pediatric brain tumors, histology per se does not appear to be a major determinant in the occurrence of late effects; however, because treatments vary considerably according to specific tumor types, histology plays a strong *indirect* role since it dictates therapeutic approach.[35] Also, different organs vary in their vulnerability to the mutagenic effects of chemoradiotherapies. Relapse of primary disease is associated with a higher risk of SMN; most likely this increased risk is due to the fact that recurrence must be treated with additional and more aggressive therapies, though it is possible that biologic features inherent to a tumor destined to recur are part of any cancer predisposition.[23,147,148]

Therapeutic exposures during cancer therapy, including chemotherapy, radiation therapy, and other supportive care modalities, directly affect the treatment and the therapeutic sequelae. Prior therapeutic exposure to radiation and chemotherapy clearly predispose patients to develop secondary malignancies.[9,14,20,23,33,34,47,48,92,147,149,150] In many examples, the cumulative dose of chemoradiotherapies affects risk of development of SMN.

Radiation treatment for childhood cancer is unmistakably linked to a higher risk for developing secondary tumors, both benign and malignant.[33,62,147] Factors related to the use of radiation that clearly affect the risk for SMN induction consist of radiation dose,[25,33,54,104,146–148,151–153] age at time of RT,[9,23,87,92,97,154] underlying genetic risk factors,[54,122,155,156] and other concurrent therapies (e.g., chemotherapy).[7,53,71,118,150,151,153,157,158]

Most data suggests a greater risk of a secondary tumor with an increasing cumulative dose of therapeutic radiation.[25,33,54,71,94,104,146,148,150–153,159,160] Most, but certainly not all, radiation-induced malignancies occur within or near the radiation field;[53,161–163] and in some cases, genetic factors may contribute to tumors occurring in nonirradiated locations.[51,52]

The threshold dose required to produce tissue damage and be tumorigenic is not known.[35,164] Based on the follow-up data for children treated with low-dose radiotherapy for tinea capitis who later developed brain neoplasms (e.g., meningiomas, gliomas, nerve sheath tumors), the estimated mean radiation dose to the neural tissue was 1.5 Gy; even this low dose of radiation was not "safe" against tumor induction.[161] Some have suggested that low-dose cranial RT (i.e., 500 cGy) causes predominantly extra-axial tumors, while higher doses of cranial RT (>1,000) are more likely to cause malignant brain tumors.[161] Additionally, different modalities of radiation may offer different tumorigenic risk; after orthovoltage radiation, the predominant modality used prior to 1960, the cumulative incidence at 40 years for germline RB patients was 32.9%, compared to 26.3% for patients treated in later eras with other types of RT modalities that have fewer scatter rays.[53] New advances in radiotherapy technology, including intensity-modulated RT and proton beam radiotherapy, may mitigate some of the known side effects of therapy.[165] Lessening doses and changing modalities may decrease the risk of SMN, although a risk of tumor induction will remain.[161]

Interestingly, the histologic subtypes of radiation-induced malignancies appear to differ with different durations of follow-up; that is, gliomas, namely high-grade gliomas, usually occur with a shorter latency (within a decade) following radiation, while meningiomas tend to occur after a longer latency (usually after a decade).[33,95]

In many studies, chemotherapy appears to be a significant risk factor for the development of SMNs, even in those patients not treated with radiotherapy.[9,34,71,72,90,143,151,166–174] This risk may be even higher in genetically susceptible populations.[175–177] Certain chemotherapeutic agents, in particular alkylators[9,170,172] and topoisomerase inhibitors,[178] including anthracyclines,[172,174] epipodophyllotoxins, and platinum agents,[166,170] predisposed patients to secondary cancers. In some, but not all, studies an increasing cumulative dose of specific agents increases risk.[9,153,170] Controlled studies suggest that there is not a clear dose-response relationship for epipodophyllotoxins.[168,170] In other studies, agents in combination, for example alkylating agents along with doxorubicin[179–181] or 6MP with dexamethasone,[170] increased the risk of SMN in nonirradiated patients.

Treatment-induced metabolic and endocrinologic effects are commonly seen after treatment of childhood cancer (discussed in Chapter 11). The resultant hormonal defects following childhood cancer therapy, such as obesity, early menarche, premature menopause, and hypopituitarism, may be associated with the development of subsequent cancers, though it is unclear whether these conditions and the associated endocrinopathies directly contribute, or if hormone replacement and other therapies required to treat them lead to this increased risk.[1,182,183] For instance, estrogen, endogenous or as part of hormone replacement therapy, are tied to an increased risk of breast cancer.[184,185] Hormonal factors are also suspected to be involved in the pathogenesis of prostate, thyroid and other cancers.[186,187] Additionally, obesity, a disorder that commonly affects survivors of childhood brain tumors and other cancers,[102] is a known risk factor for the development of cancers in general.[188–190]

Reports from the CCSS suggested an increased risk of secondary malignancies in childhood cancer survivors treated with growth hormone (GH),[182] compared to survivors not so treated, though an updated report suggests this elevation of risk related to the use of GH may diminish with longer follow-up.[183] However, a large study of medulloblastoma survivors treated with GH failed to show any increased risk of relapse or secondary malignancy.[191] The overall risk, if any, appears to be low and may be overestimated; the authors suggest that other factors, including closer imaging surveillance, may have contributed to the increased detection of tumors, most commonly meningiomas, in the GH-treated group.

When considering the original diagnosis of brain tumors, secondary tumors can originate in the CNS or elsewhere. Though early publications suggested that the incidence of SMN in survivors of BT was low (approximately 1–2%, 2–8 years after therapy),[192] more recent series with longer follow-up suggest a significant risk of SMNs.[32,34,39,67] Much of this observation may be related to the fact that patients are surviving longer, to a point where these late SMNs are observed.

In a series of young children treated with chemotherapy to avoid or postpone RT, Duffner et al. reported five SMNs in 198 treated patients:[34,193] three hematologic malignancies, one meningioma and one sarcoma. The estimated risk of developing a SMN eight years after diagnosis was 11.3%. Though all the children who developed hematologic malignancies were less than 24 months of age at initial treatment, small numbers of patients and events preclude conclusions to determine if the youngest age predisposes to these SMNs, or whether the youngest patients were those destined to receive the longer duration and thus higher cumulative dose of chemotherapy.

Jenkin et al. reported on the follow-up of children irradiated for brain tumors,[67] and SMN was the cause of death in 11 of these 912 patients. Nearly half of the SMNs arose in radiation portals, while two were in irradiated patients outside RT field; the remainder were hematologic malignancies. The actuarial cumulative incidence of death due to SMN was 1, 5, and 13%, at 10, 20, and 30 years, respectively.[67]

A retrospective analysis of SMN in primary BT patients from St. Jude Children's Research Hospital showed 24 of 1,283 BT patients developed SMN. This series, which excluded patients with NF1, found suspected or confirmed genetic predisposition in nearly one-third of those who developed SMN.[38] This study showed a higher risk of SMN in youngest patients, but once genetic predisposition was addressed, age lost independent significance. Follow-up in this study is relatively short (median 3.5 years), so occurrence of SMN may increase with time. At least two other studies suggest that a generous proportion of pediatric BT patients with SMN have an underlying genetic susceptibility.[142,194]

In a study of adult patients with pituitary adenomas, 11 of 426 patients developed a second intracranial tumor after surgery and radiotherapy.

Histology of the subsequent tumor was meningioma in five patients, high-grade astrocytoma in four, and other high-grade lesions in two. These secondary tumors were diagnosed 6–34 years after radiotherapy, all within RT fields.[195]

Types of Secondary Tumors

Secondary malignant neoplasms may develop in cancer survivors include solid and hematologic malignancies. The location and the histologic subtypes range widely, and the predisposing factors vary accordingly (See Table 16.2).

Table 16.2 Risk factors for secondary cancers

Second cancer	Risk factors and associations
Breast cancer	Primary cancer (i.e., HL, CNS, STS, ALL, WT, NHL) Female gender RT (i.e., chest) Age (i.e., stage of breast development)* Genetics*
Thyroid cancer	Primary diagnosis RT Younger age Female gender
Skin cancer	RT CT UV exposure Underlying skin features Genetics (e.g., RB, Gorlin)
Soft tissue Sarcoma	Primary diagnosis (i.e., germ line RB, STS, HL, WT, bone tumors, ALL) Radiation Younger age CT (i.e., anthracyclines)
Bone tumors	Primary diagnosis (i.e., germ line RB, STS, HD, WT, bone tumors, ALL) RT Genetics (i.e., p53, RB) CT (i.e., alkylators)
Brain (CNS) Tumors	Primary diagnosis (CNS tumors, ALL, HL, RB) Age Genetics (i.e., RB, Gorlin, p53, NF; polymorphisms*) Growth hormone therapy*
MDS/t-AML	Primary diagnosis (ALL, HL, NHL, bone tumors, STS) Older Age CT (Topoisomerase II inhibitors, alkylators) Genetics (polymorphisms)

Abbreviations: HL = Hodgkin Lymphoma , ALL = acute lymphoblastic lymphoma, STS thinsp;= soft tissue sarcoma, RB = retinoblastoma, CNS = central nervous system tumors; WT = Wilms' tumor, RT = radiation therapy, CT = chemotherapy, NHL = Non-Hodgkin lymphoma, NF = neurofibromatosis, * = controversial.

In the SEER report of 2,056 long-term survivors of primary malignant brain tumors diagnosed during childhood, the most frequent histologically defined second neoplasms among all primary brain tumors combined were CNS tumors, sarcomas, and melanomas;[32] this data is consistent with other published reports.[55,196,197] In particular, secondary bone cancers and soft tissue sarcomas have been found to be in excess after treating any childhood cancer with radiation therapy.[1,9,92,151,172] Other commonly documented secondary tumors after primary brain tumor treatment are basal cell carcinoma, desmoid tumors, salivary gland tumors, and thyroid carcinoma.[7,8]

Secondary Brain Tumors

Secondary neoplasms of the central nervous system (CNS) have frequently been described as late events following treatment for primary brain tumors and other malignancies.[9,19,21,33,34,38,39,67,93,98,161,195,198–203] These CNS tumors are considered especially devastating, as a large proportion display malignant histology and behavior, are associated with significant morbidity, and may be fatal.

Numerous reports suggest that a large proportion of brain tumors developing after treatment of childhood cancers are high-grade glial lesions.[33,38,96,204–210] Broniscer et al. reported the single-institution experience from St. Jude Children's Research Hospital with second neoplasms after the diagnosis of a primary CNS tumor in children and adolescents.[38] Of 1,283 patients younger than 22 years treated for primary CNS tumors, excluding patients with NF1, 24 developed SMN. Ten (42%) were gliomas, the majority of which were high-grade lesions such as anaplastic astrocytoma and glioblastoma multiforme. The median interval from original diagnosis to the development of these secondary glial tumors was 6.6 years (range, 3.3–17.9 years). All 10 of these survivors had received RT as part of their primary cancer treatment, with three patients also receiving multi-agent chemotherapy.

Patients with secondary malignant CNS tumors, and secondary high-grade gliomas, in particular, may fare worse than those patients treated for primary high-grade gliomas.[209] It is unclear whether this inferior outcome is due to distinct biologic differences between secondary and radiation-induced gliomas compared to de novo/primary tumors, due to differences in resistance to therapy in secondary tumors or due to therapeutic limitations of a previously irradiated location.[209,211,212] Additionally, it is not clear whether earlier detection of these secondary glial tumors will improve survival.

In various studies, especially those with longer follow-up, meningiomas have been recognized as one of the most common RT-induced neoplasms of the CNS.[21,23,38,95,213] In the series from St. Jude, of those survivors with follow-up greater than 10 years, meningiomas were found to account for two-thirds of all second BTs.[38] Unlike the acute presenting symptoms of high-grade lesions, meningiomas tend to be asymptomatic for a prolonged period of time, so the possibility of detection bias needs to be considered when estimating incidence of this secondary tumor.[183] Meningiomas are clearly linked with prior exposure to ionizing radiation[214–217] at any dose level. Secondary meningiomas have been seen after the relatively low-dose cranial radiation (<10 Gy) used in the treatment for tinea capitis used in the mid-20th century,[218] and after doses employed (>10 Gy) for treatment of intracranial tumors and as prophylactic radiation for acute lymphoblastic leukemia. Compared to sporadic meningiomas in the general population, radiation-induced meningiomas are more likely to behave more aggressively,[219] to be multiple,[220] to recur after surgery, and to demonstrate malignant or atypical histology.[216,220] The average latency between radiation exposure and development of radiation-induced meningiomas is 15–20 years, ranging from two to 63 years.[33,214] Primitive neuroectodermal tumors have been reported occurring 5–18 years after therapeutic chemoradiotherapy,[39,93,95,160,161,198,199,203,221,222] and other histologic subtypes of secondary CNS tumors have been described, though less commonly.[34,198,199,203]

Secondary Skin Cancer

Skin cancers, including basal cell carcinoma (BCC), squamous cell carcinoma (SCC), and melanoma, are well-known SMN occurring after treatment for cancer.[223–226] In the general population, risk factors associated with the development of skin cancers include artificial and environmental exposure to ultraviolet (UV) radiation – especially at an early age, exposure to ionizing radiation for malignant or nonmalignant disorders,[32,223–225,227–231] medical conditions or therapies that suppress the immune system,[232] the presence of dysplastic nevi and/or greater than 50 moles on the body,[233] and various familial or genetic factors.[50,234] As previously mentioned, genetic syndromes, such as Gorlin Syndrome, are associated with medulloblastoma in young children and numerous nevi in radiation fields within a few years of radiotherapy.[49,50,235] In several series, survivors of germline retinoblastoma had a high risk of developing dysplastic nevi and malignant melanoma, with or without exposure to therapeutic RT.[230,236,239]

Chemoradiotherapies used in the treatment of CNS tumors appear to greatly contribute to the development of skin cancer as a SMN.[21,23,24,32,158,231,236,240] Guerin et al. reported that treating children with ionizing radiation significantly increased the risk of developing malignant melanoma as a secondary malignant neoplasm, especially at local doses greater than 15 Gy.[158,241] As reported by the CCSS, approximately 90% of the reported nonmelanoma skin cancers previously occurred in irradiated portals, with BCC being the most commonly reported histologic subtype.[9] In a Swiss series of 766 patients younger than 20 years of age treated for primary CNS and non-CNS tumors, only cases of BCC were observed, all occurring within the RT field,[226] suggesting the key etiology is RT. Other series support this strong link with RT.[225,242,243]

In a series examining malignant melanoma as a SMN after childhood cancer, 11 secondary melanomas were identified from a cohort of over 7,000 survivors of childhood cancers.[24] Of these, four developed an average of 13.1 years (2.3–39.5 years) after RT in or adjacent to the radiation field for previous diagnosis of Hodgkin's lymphoma or brain tumors. The authors note that predisposition genetic syndromes (i.e., xeroderma pigmentosum) may have contributed to the development of melanoma in some cases.[24] Several series have confirmed a high risk of melanoma in survivors of RB, with melanoma affecting 3–25% of various cohorts; these lesions were not limited to the field of RT.[53,54,175,236,244]

In some series, concomitant chemoradiotherapy with cytotoxic agents, alkylating or microtubule-inhibiting agents, such as vinca alkaloids, significantly increased the risk of skin malignancies, including melanoma, after treatment for childhood cancers.[150,158,241] Several studies have shown that patients develop an increased number of melanocytic nevi after receiving chemotherapy for hematological malignancies,[245,246] and that total body nevi counts were higher in such patients treated with chemoradiotherapies compared to their untreated siblings.[247] Since high numbers of benign nevi are associated with an increased risk for subsequent development of malignant melanoma,[233] one can conclude that survivors at risk should be monitored regularly for development of such secondary skin lesions in order to detect them early, and that preventive measures should be emphasized in follow-up clinics.

Most studies support that the relative risk of developing skin cancers was higher after receiving RT as a child or adolescent, compared to RT as an adult, suggesting a higher predisposition in younger patients.[248,249]

Early diagnosis plays an important role in the morbidity and mortality associated with all types of skin cancer, and survivors of childhood cancers should undergo lifelong surveillance of their skin by a knowledgeable practitioner. Those further from diagnosis and those previously treated with radiation therapy are at highest risk of developing skin cancers, particularly in, but not exclusive to, previously irradiated areas.[225] Patients and especially those treated as young children should be counseled about measures to minimize undue sun exposure, including avoiding tanning booths, wearing protective gear when outside including hats and UV-absorbent sunglasses, and applying of sunblock with an adequate SPF.[243] The Children's Oncology Group has developed guidelines for the long-term surveillance of survivors of childhood, adolescent and young adult cancers.[131]

Secondary Breast Cancer

Breast cancer has been clearly identified as a SMN after treatment of many childhood malignancies;[9,47,92,152,250] much of the relevant data stems from the recognition of the significantly increased risk of breast cancer in female survivors of Hodgkin lymphoma treated with RT.[47,92,250] Female survivors in the

Late Effects Study Group (LESG) cohort had a risk of breast cancer 75 times greater than that in the general population, and the estimated cumulative probability of breast cancer among the women in this cohort approached 35% at 40 years of age.[92] Not surprisingly, the majority of breast cancers in the survivors arose within the radiation field, and the risk of breast cancer development increased with the dose of radiation therapy, with most occurring in patients receiving at least 2,000 cGy in the mantle region. Kleinerman et al. point out that the risk of breast cancer was elevated in the young patients who received RT for retinoblastoma,[53] even though scatter radiation dose to the breast was estimated at approximately 0.4 Gy. The risk of RT-related breast cancer is heightened when the exposure occurs at very young ages, as observed in cases where RT was used for nonmalignant disorders (0.5–0.7 Gy), and with atomic bomb exposure (0.3 Gy).[251]

In the CCSS study of 6,068 eligible female survivors, 95 had 111 confirmed cases of secondary breast cancer after childhood cancer diagnosis.[47] Most of these women had initial diagnosis of HD, and nearly all had received chest RT. Other primary diagnoses included bone and soft tissue sarcomas, NHL, Wilms' tumor, leukemia and brain tumors; surprisingly, the majority of these patients had not received RT to the chest for their primary cancer. Whereas survivors of childhood bone sarcoma and STS who were not treated with previous chest RT had increased risk, in this particular study this increased risk was not seen in survivors of leukemia or brain tumors. Genetic and hereditary factors may be at play, since breast cancer risk in this study was elevated in those patients with a family history of breast cancer or sarcoma, especially in those survivors who did not previously receive chest RT.

Interestingly, cancer-predisposing genes such as TP53, BRCA1, BRCA2, or ATM genes, which have been commonly identified in patients with primary breast cancer, have not been identified in survivors with secondary breast cancers;[17,252,254] studies of these genes and other genes involved in cellular DNA damage response pathways may identify host genetic factors that contribute to secondary tumorigenesis.

Cases of secondary and, namely, RT-induced breast cancer tend to present in much younger women relative to the general population;[47,255,256] Kenney et al. and others found a median age of 35 years at breast cancer diagnosis (range 20–49), compared to older than 50 years for sporadic breast cancer,[47] and others have found remarkably similar results.[9,47,92,250,252,255–258]

There are inconsistent results when assessing the relationship between age at primary cancer diagnosis and treatment exposure and risk of subsequent breast cancer development.[47,92,250,255,257,258] Conclusions made by the LESG noted that the increased risk of breast cancer after treatment for HD was related to younger age at the time of radiation exposure,[92] whereas data from the CCSS did not demonstrate that age modifies this risk.[47] These discrepant results may be explained by differences in follow-up or in methodology.[140,259] Even though sensitivity to radiation of tissues in general may be higher in infancy and childhood, puberty may be the most radiosensitive period for the breast, when the tissue is proliferating.[250] Moreover, precise estimation of the delivered radiation dose to different parts of the breast is technically challenging.[258] Also, the effects of other antineoplastic treatments, genetic factors, hormonal alterations including future pregnancy and hormone replacement are highly difficult to assess as contributing factors in secondary breast cancer development.

Based on this elevated risk of breast cancer, most profoundly in those treated with chest RT, female survivors should be carefully monitored in the long-term by clinical examination, mammography and ultrasonography; mammography should start at a younger age, compared to the general population. Patient education and awareness of this increased risk is a critical component of follow-up.[250,260]

Secondary Thyroid Cancer

In addition to metabolic and endocrine abnormalities commonly resulting from treatment of brain tumors and other cancers during childhood, long-term survivors have an increased risk of developing cancers of the thyroid gland,[9,87,93,102,160,261,262] with some studies estimating a greater than 50-fold increased risk of thyroid cancer in childhood cancer survivors compared to the general population.[87] Radiation therapy and young age at the time of treatment have been identified as risk factors for the development of second thyroid cancers,[9,87,93,102,103,149,262–265] but chemotherapy has not.[103,140] Patients younger than 10 years had substantially higher thyroid cancer risk at all radiation doses than did patients age 10 and older.[103] Tumorigenic radiation fields may involve anywhere in the head and neck region, including the craniospinal axis.[1,9,87,93,102,103,140,261] Additionally, not all patients with secondary thyroid tumors received RT, so other factors may be involved in its pathogenesis.[266] For instance, radiation-induced thyroid tumors demonstrate distinct chromosomal abnormalities compared with sporadic cases, suggesting that the genetics and mechanisms of carcinogenesis may be unique.[267–270]

The CCSS was one of several studies to definitively confirm the increased risk of thyroid cancer at moderate RT doses (up to 20–29 Gy), versus a reduced risk at higher doses.[103,140] Some have surmised that this dose-response relationship is consistent with a "cell-killing effect" at the higher doses, rather than a mutagenic effect seen at the low-moderate doses.[140,271]

Other Secondary Solid Tumors

In addition to carcinomas of the breast, thyroid and skin, other carcinomas are not uncommon following treatment of childhood cancer.[48] Of the 677 SMNS in 14,372 CCSS cohort survivors, 71 other carcinomas were identified:[48] these patients tended to be older at the time of primary tumor diagnosis;

had a primary diagnosis of Hodgkin lymphoma, soft tissue sarcomas, or neuroblastoma; had a family history of a first degree relative with cancer, and were more likely to report alcohol use. The overall standardized incidence ratio of a subsequent carcinoma was found to increase for all primary childhood cancer diagnoses, including brain tumors. Most notably, patients with CNS tumors had an elevated risk of developing carcinomas of the head and neck and kidney. In most cases, patients initially diagnosed at an age younger than 10 years had the greatest risk.[48] These secondary carcinomas developed at a younger age than sporadic cases arising in the general population. Radiation therapy was associated with an increased risk of all carcinomas except those arising in the genitourinary tract, and was most marked for carcinomas of the head and neck. While not all patients with secondary carcinomas had a history of prior chemoradiotherapy, most but not all of the tumors developed within the prior radiation portal.

Salivary tumors were one of the common carcinomas occurring after therapeutic radiation.[272] In one study, more than half of head and neck carcinomas developed in the parotid gland, the majority of which were of mucoepidermoid histology; of the parotid tumors, most occurred within a prior RT field.[273] Of the carcinomas that developed outside of a radiation field, half were in patients without any RT exposure. The majority of those patients who developed carcinoma outside of an RT field had received alkylating agents or other chemotherapies[48,273] as part of their initial cancer treatment. In light of these findings, the CCSS group is investigating genetic factors that may predispose to subsequent malignant neoplasms, including carcinomas, in this CCSS cohort.[48,140]

Lung cancer is increasingly recognized after the cure of cancer, notably after Hodgkin disease.[9,20,41,124–126,130,274] The risk of developing lung cancer appeared to increase with the increasing cumulative dose of radiation,[125,126] tobacco use,[125,126] and, in some studies, exposure to alkylating agents.[125,274] Smoking had a multiplicative effect, most notably for patients who received radiotherapy.[124,125,274] This increased risk is not limited to patients with known genetic predisposition,[275] though inactivation of the RB1 gene is frequently identified in common cancers of adulthood, including cancers of the lung and bladder.[276,277]

Secondary soft tissue sarcomas are estimated to make up 10% of SMN.[9] Recent publications have reported a 9–54-fold increased risk of developing secondary sarcomas in survivors of pediatric cancers compared to the general population.[153,172] These secondary sarcomas, namely osteosarcomas and soft tissue sarcomas, tended to occur an average of 11 years after the patient's original diagnosis.[172] Much of this increased risk has been attributed to radiation therapy as the vast majority of second sarcomas occurred within or at the border of the RT field[4,54,153,172] with most studies supporting a dose-dependent relationship. The study from the CCSS also demonstrated an increased risk of subsequent sarcoma development with higher cumulative doses of either anthracyclines or alkylating agents; a primary diagnosis of soft tissue sarcoma, bone sarcoma, and Hodgkin lymphoma; a family history of cancer, and a history of other secondary cancers. Recognized and less well-understood genetic factors may be at play in the risk of developing secondary sarcomas.[53,54,106,156,278] Much of the data on secondary sarcomas stems from observations regarding patients with germline RB who have demonstrated an increased (up to 400-fold) risk of bone cancer,[52–54] whether treated with RT or not. These sarcomas, which are not limited to irradiated patients or the RT field,[53] have significant effects on mortality in affected patients.[74,75]

Secondary Hematopoietic Disorders, Secondary Leukemia and Myelodysplastic Syndrome

Secondary hematologic malignancies, most commonly myelodysplasia and acute myeloid leukemia (MDS/AML), are recognized SMN in survivors following treatment of cancers, including CNS tumors.[9,14,21,124,166,171,181,279–283] Secondary AML (sAML) may account for up to 10% of all AML cases.[280,284] Since most late effects registries examining SMN include survivors of greater than five years since diagnosis, and since a sizable proportion of secondary hematologic malignancies have a relatively short latency period,[34,41,42,285] relative and absolute risks for these hematopoietic disorders cannot be completely extrapolated from many of the biggest and often-cited late effects registries and long-term survivors follow-up series.[23] For instance, in the CCSS cohort, the risk of secondary leukemias was highest 5–9 years after diagnosis with incidence decreasing thereafter, and this cohort does not include any treatment-related effect with onset at less than five years after diagnosis.[9]

Risk of therapy-induced secondary leukemia is most frequently, but not exclusively,[286] associated with exposure to certain chemotherapeutic agents,[71,145,176,282,287] including alkylating agents such as temozolomide,[288] busulfan, chlorambucil, CCNU, cyclophosphamide,[171,280,281] platinum agents,[166] and epipodophyllotoxins, such as etoposide and teniposide.[113,167,178,285,289] For instance, estimates of cumulative risk for sAML after treatment with the chemotherapeutic agent etoposide range from 5 to 10% (2–12% for epipodophyllotoxins) in patients with hematologic malignancy.[167]

Most studies suggest that radiation therapy, along with exposure to alkylators, does not appear to further increase the risk of developing secondary leukemia,[21,71,72,100,166] though in one study the relative risk of secondary leukemia increased significantly with exposure to epipodophyllotoxins and the dose of RT averaged over patients' active bone marrow.[169] Exposure to other chemotherapeutic agents, such as anthracyclines and others, may be a possible risk factor as well. While young age at the time of primary cancer diagnosis has been shown to be associated with an increased risk of developing other types of SMN,[9] older age at treatment of the primary cancer has been consistently shown to be associated with an increased risk of secondary MDS and AML.[90,91,100]

Several groups of investigators have identified genetic polymorphisms of enzymes responsible for metabolic activation or detoxification of antineoplastic agents that appear to be associated with an increased risk of therapy-related leukemia/MDS. It is hypothesized that these intrinsic polymorphisms may lead to increased production of reactive intermediates that damage DNA, thereby disturbing hematopoietic stem cells.[17,112,115,290,291]

Therapy-related MDS/AML is often associated with characteristic chromosomal alterations.[287] One frequently described group of tMDS/AML is characterized by abnormalities of chromosome 5 or 7, that may include whole chromosome loss, as well as long arm deletions and unbalanced trans-locations of the long arm.[292] Most, but not all, patients who develop these cytogenetic disorders have been exposed to alkylators with or without radiotherapy, often have a myelodysplasia preceding the emergence of overt leukemia, and have trilineage BM dysplasia.[100] In one series of pediatric patients with tMDS/sAML, for instance, 12/20 patients had cytogenetic abnormalities of chromosome 5 or 7, and 10 of these 12 had been previously treated with alkylating agents.[287] Alkylator-induced secondary MDS/AML tends to occur 5–10 years (range 3 months to 21 years) after exposure to alkylating agents;[113] again, these may be missed by some late effects registries.

Another group of therapy-related AML demonstrates rearrangement of chromosome 11 at band q23 and/or MLL gene involvement,[280,289,293] typically with translocations and deletions involving the 11q23 locus, but other chromo-somal variants have been seen.[178,294] Most patients with this sAML have been previously exposed to epipodophyllotoxins, such as etoposide or teniposide, but there are clearly cases with such 11q23 abnormalities that may be attributed to prior exposure to non-epipodophyllotoxin topoisomerase inhibitors;[283] in these cases low cumulative doses of doxorubicin, cyclophosphamide, plus RT were cited as causative agents. In contrast to therapy-related leukemias following alkylator exposure, these 11q23 cases usually present with a more acute presentation, without a preceding myelodysplastic phase, with a shorter latency period, and commonly have M4 or M5 FAB subtype.

A dose-dependent relationship between alkylating agents and sAML/MDS leukemia has been clearly established,[71,100,282] whereas epipodophyllotoxin expo-sure has not consistently shown this dose-response relationship.[73,143,167,168,295] Some have suggested that the risk of epipodophyllotoxin-related leukemia may be dependent on the schedule of drug administration,[295,296] on concomitant administration of other agents,[113,143,168,169,296] and with exposure of bone mar-row to radiotherapy.[169]

The incidence of sAML/MDS in patients with brain tumors has been increasing due to improved survival after treatment for their brain tumors and more common exposure to leukemogenic chemotherapies in recent treat-ment eras.[297] In a report by Duffner et al., five of 198 children less than three years of age treated for CNS tumors developed second SMNs, of which three were MDS/AML that were considered to be the result of prolonged postoperative alkylating agents and topoisomerase II inhibitors.[34] In an effort to postpone or avoid RT, these youngest patients were treated with long periods of chemotherapy containing etoposide, cyclophosphamide, and cisplatinum; these secondary hematologic malignancies developed approximately 2–7 years following initial therapy. Similar results were demonstrated in a study from St. Jude Children's Research Hospital in which two of 1,283 children and adolescents treated for primary CNS tumors developed MDS;[38] both patients had primary diagnoses of choroid plexus tumors, were treated with prolonged chemotherapy, including high cumulative doses of alkylating agents (one received craniospinal RT, too), and both patients, interestingly, had *p53* germline mutations.

The prognosis for patients with secondary leukemia and myelodysplasia tends to be poor;[298] patients may have an initial response to salvage chemo,[296] but standard chemotherapy is not effective in achieving long-term remission or survival.[100,299,300] Even with stem cell transplantation, outcomes are not ideal.[301,302] It is not clear whether this poor prognosis for patients with therapy-related leukemia represents a true biologic phenomenon or is related to antecedent disease and treatment, and therapeutic restrictions therein.

Other secondary hematopoietic malignancies have rarely been reported; treatment-related AML can involve t(15;17) translocation with the formation of acute promyelocytic leukemia.[294] Reports of secondary lymphoblastic leukemia are uncommon, and the correlation with antecedent therapies is not definitive.[285,303] There have been case reports of secondary non-Hodgkin lymphoma in patients with primary brain tumors.[304]

Conclusion

Long-term surveillance is critical for following survivors of brain tumors and other cancers. Awareness of this increased risk of SMN in cancer survivors is one of the most critical pieces for long-term follow-up care.[48] Programs should educate clinicians, including primary care physicians, and survivors about the risk of SMN. Patients and health care providers must be cognizant of the risk factors of SMN, so that healthy lifestyle behaviors (e.g., reducing sun exposure, avoiding tobacco) are emphasized and early prevention strategies and appropriate surveillance plans (e.g., earlier mammography in female survivors treated with RT) are implemented if indicated.

References

1. Bhatia S, Sklar C. Second cancers in survivors of childhood cancer. *Nature Rev.* 2002; 2:124–132.
2. Neugut AI, Meadows, AT, Robinson E, ed. *Multiple Primary Cancers.* 1st ed. Philadelphia: Lippincott Williams & Wilkins; 1999.

3. Li FP, Cassady JR, Jaffe N. Risk of second tumors in survivors of childhood cancer. *Cancer*. 1975;35:1230–1235.
4. Meadows AT, Baum E, Fossati-Bellani F, et al. Second malignant neoplasms in children: an update from the Late Effects Study Group. *J Clin Oncol*. 1985;3:532–538.
5. Hawkins MM, Draper GJ, Kingston JE. Incidence of second primary tumours among childhood cancer survivors. *Br J Cancer*. 1987;56:339–347.
6. Blatt J, Olshan A, Gula MJ, et al. Second malignancies in very-long-term survivors of childhood cancer. *Am J Med*. 1992;93:57–60.
7. de Vathaire F, Hawkins M, Campbell S, et al. Second malignant neoplasms after a first cancer in childhood: temporal pattern of risk according to type of treatment. *Br J Cancer*. 1999;79:1884–1893.
8. de Vathaire F, Schweisguth O, Rodary C, et al. Long-term risk of second malignant neoplasm after a cancer in childhood. *Br J Cancer*. 1989;59:448–452.
9. Neglia JP, Friedman DL, Yasui Y, et al. Second malignant neoplasms in five-year survivors of childhood cancer: childhood cancer survivor study. *J Natl Cancer Inst*. 2001;93:618–629.
10. Jenkinson HC, Hawkins MM, Stiller CA, et al. Long-term population-based risks of second malignant neoplasms after childhood cancer in Britain. *Br J Cancer*. 2004;91:1905–1910.
11. Knudson AG, Jr. Mutation and cancer: statistical study of retinoblastoma. *Proc Natl Acad Sci USA*. 1971;68:820–823.
12. Narod SA, Stiller C, Lenoir GM. An estimate of the heritable fraction of childhood cancer. *Br J Cancer*. 1991;63:993–999.
13. Ferner RE. Neurofibromatosis 1 and neurofibromatosis 2: a twenty first century perspective. *Lancet Neurol*. 2007;6:340–351.
14. Inskip PD, Curtis RE. New malignancies following childhood cancer in the United States, 1973–2002. *Int J Cancer*. 2007;121:2233–2240.
15. Olsen JH, Garwicz S, Hertz H, et al. Second malignant neoplasms after cancer in childhood or adolescence. Nordic Society of Paediatric Haematology and Oncology Association of the Nordic Cancer Registries. *BMJ* (Clin Res) ed. 1993;307:1030–1036.
16. MacArthur AC, Spinelli JJ, Rogers PC, et al. Risk of a second malignant neoplasm among 5-year survivors of cancer in childhood and adolescence in British Columbia, Canada. *Pediatr Blood Cancer*. 2007;48:453–459.
17. Pizzo PA, Poplack, DG, ed. *Principles & Practice of Pediatric Oncology*. 5th ed: Philadelphia: Lippincott Williams & Wilkins; 2005.
18. Jenkin D. Long-term survival of children with brain tumors. *Oncology* (Williston Park, NY). 1996;10:715–719; discussion 20, 22, 28.
19. Devarahally SR, Severson RK, Chuba P, et al. Second malignant neoplasms after primary central nervous system malignancies of childhood and adolescence. *Pediatr Hematol Oncol*. 2003;20:617–625.
20. Bhatia S, Yasui Y, Robison LL, et al. High risk of subsequent neoplasms continues with extended follow-up of childhood Hodgkin's disease: report from the Late Effects Study Group. *J Clin Oncol*. 2003;21:4386–4394.
21. Hijiya N, Hudson MM, Lensing S, et al. Cumulative incidence of secondary neoplasms as a first event after childhood acute lymphoblastic leukemia. *JAMA*. 2007;297:1207–1215.
22. Smith MB, Xue H, Strong L, et al. Forty-year experience with second malignancies after treatment of childhood cancer: analysis of outcome following the development of the second malignancy. *J Pediatr Surg*. 1993;28:1342–1348; discussion 8–9.
23. Cardous-Ubbink MC, Heinen RC, Bakker PJ, et al. Risk of second malignancies in long-term survivors of childhood cancer. *Eur J Cancer*. 2007;43:351–362.
24. Corpron CA, Black CT, Ross MI, et al. Melanoma as a second malignant neoplasm after childhood cancer. *Am J Surg*. 1996;172:459–461; discussion 61–62.
25. Garwicz S, Anderson H, Olsen JH, et al. Second malignant neoplasms after cancer in childhood and adolescence: a population-based case-control study in the 5 Nordic

countries. The Nordic Society for Pediatric Hematology and Oncology. The Association of the Nordic Cancer Registries. *Int J Cancer*. 2000;88:672–678.

26. Li FP, Myers MH, Heise HW, et al. The course of five-year survivors of cancer in childhood. *J Pediatr*. 1978;93:185–187.

27. Baker KS, DeFor TE, Burns LJ, et al. New malignancies after blood or marrow stem-cell transplantation in children and adults: incidence and risk factors. *J Clin Oncol*. 2003;21: 1352–1358.

28. Neuget AI, Meadows AT, Robinson E, ed. *Multiple Primary Cancers*. Philadelphia: Lippincott Williams & Wilkins; 1999.

29. Sankila R, Pukkala E, Teppo L. Risk of subsequent malignant neoplasms among 470,000 cancer patients in Finland, 1953–1991. *Int J Cancer*. 1995;60:464–470.

30. Dong C, Hemminki K. Second primary neoplasms in 633,964 cancer patients in Sweden, 1958–1996. *Int J Cancer*. 2001;93:155–161.

31. Curtis RE, Boice JD, Jr., Kleinerman RA, et al. Summary: multiple primary cancers in Connecticut, 1935–82. *Natl Cancer Inst Monograph*. 1985;68:219–242.

32. Peterson KM, Shao C, McCarter R, et al. An analysis of SEER data of increasing risk of secondary malignant neoplasms among long-term survivors of childhood brain tumors. *Pediatr Blood Cancer*. 2006;47:83–88.

33. Neglia JP, Robison LL, Stovall M, et al. New primary neoplasms of the central nervous system in survivors of childhood cancer: a report from the Childhood Cancer Survivor Study. *J Natl Cancer Inst*. 2006;98:1528–1537.

34. Duffner PK, Krischer JP, Horowitz ME, et al. Second malignancies in young children with primary brain tumors following treatment with prolonged postoperative chemotherapy and delayed irradiation: a Pediatric Oncology Group study. *Ann Neurol*. 1998;44:313–316.

35. Anderson DM, Rennie KM, Ziegler RS, et al. Medical and neurocognitive late effects among survivors of childhood central nervous system tumors. *Cancer*. 2001;92:2709–2719.

36. Bhatia S. Late effects among survivors of leukemia during childhood and adolescence. *Blood Cells Mol Dis*. 2003;31:84–92.

37. Albright AL. Pediatric brain tumors. *CA: A Cancer J Clin*. 1993;43:272–288.

38. Broniscer A, Ke W, Fuller CE, et al. Second neoplasms in pediatric patients with primary central nervous system tumors: the St. Jude Children's Research Hospital experience. *Cancer*. 2004;100:2246–2252.

39. Buyukpamukcu M, Varan A, Yazici N, et al. Second malignant neoplasms following the treatment of brain tumors in children. *J Child Neurol*. 2006;21:433–436.

40. Fisher PG, Jenab J, Gopldthwaite PT, et al. Outcomes and failure patterns in childhood craniopharyngiomas. *Childs Nerv Syst*. 1998;14:558–563.

41. Donaldson SS, Hancock SL. Second cancers after Hodgkin's disease in childhood. *N Engl J Med*. 1996;334:792–794.

42. Inskip HM, Kinlen LJ, Taylor AM, et al. Risk of breast cancer and other cancers in heterozygotes for ataxia-telangiectasia. *Br J Cancer*. 1999;79:1304–1307.

43. Caglar K, Varan A, Akyuz C, et al. Second neoplasms in pediatric patients treated for cancer: a center's 30-year experience. *J Pediatr Hematol Oncol*. 2006;28:374–378.

44. Nichols KE, Malkin D, Garber JE, et al. Germ-line p53 mutations predispose to a wide spectrum of early-onset cancers. *Cancer Epidemiol Biomarkers Prev*. 2001;10:83–87.

45. Evans SC, Lozano G. The Li-Fraumeni syndrome: an inherited susceptibility to cancer. *Mol Med Today*. 1997;3:390–395.

46. Strong LC, Knudson AG, Jr. Letter: Second cancers in retinoblastoma. *Lancet*. 1973; 2:1086.

47. Kenney LB, Yasui Y, Inskip PD, et al. Breast cancer after childhood cancer: a report from the Childhood Cancer Survivor Study. *Ann Int Med*. 2004;141:590–597.

48. Bassal M, Mertens AC, Taylor L, et al. Risk of selected subsequent carcinomas in survivors of childhood cancer: a report from the Childhood Cancer Survivor Study. *J Clin Oncol*. 2006;24:476–483.

49. Kimonis VE, Goldstein AM, Pastakia B, et al. Clinical manifestations in 105 persons with nevoid basal cell carcinoma syndrome. *Am J Med Genet.* 1997;69:299–308.
50. Walter AW, Pivnick EK, Bale AE, et al. Complications of the nevoid basal cell carcinoma syndrome: a case report. *J Pediatr Hematol Oncol.* 1997;19:258–262.
51. Meadows AT. Retinoblastoma survivors: sarcomas and surveillance. *J Natl Cancer Inst.* 2007;99:3–5.
52. Kleinerman RA, Tucker MA, Abramson DH, et al. Risk of soft tissue sarcomas by individual subtype in survivors of hereditary retinoblastoma. *J Natl Cancer Inst.* 2007;99:24–31.
53. Kleinerman RA, Tucker MA, Tarone RE, et al. Risk of new cancers after radiotherapy in long-term survivors of retinoblastoma: an extended follow-up. *J Clin Oncol.* 2005;23: 2272–2279.
54. Wong FL, Boice JD, Jr., Abramson DH, et al. Cancer incidence after retinoblastoma. Radiation dose and sarcoma risk. *JAMA.* 1997;278:1262–1267.
55. Inskip PD. Multiple primary tumors involving cancer of the brain and central nervous system as the first or subsequent cancer. *Cancer.* 2003;98:562–570.
56. Sklar CA. Overview of the effects of cancer therapies: the nature, scale and breadth of the problem. *Acta Paediatr Suppl.* 1999;88:1–4.
57. Nicholson HS, Fears TR, Byrne J. Death during adulthood in survivors of childhood and adolescent cancer. *Cancer.* 1994;73:3094–3102.
58. Green DM, Zevon MA, Reese PA, et al. Factors that influence the further survival of patients who survive for five years after the diagnosis of cancer in childhood or adolescence. *Med Pediatr Oncol.* 1994;22:91–96.
59. Mertens AC, Yasui Y, Neglia JP, et al. Late mortality experience in five-year survivors of childhood and adolescent cancer: the Childhood Cancer Survivor Study. *J Clin Oncol.* 2001;19:3163–3172.
60. Robertson CM, Hawkins MM, Kingston JE. Late deaths and survival after childhood cancer: implications for cure. *BMJ* (Clin Res) ed. 1994;309:162–166.
61. Hudson MM, Jones D, Boyett J, et al. Late mortality of long-term survivors of childhood cancer. *J Clin Oncol.* 1997;15:2205–2213.
62. Lawless SC, Verma P, Green DM, et al. Mortality experiences among 15 + year survivors of childhood and adolescent cancers. *Pediatr Blood Cancer.* 2007;48:333–338.
63. Hoppe RT. Hodgkin's disease: complications of therapy and excess mortality. *Ann Oncol.* 1997;8 Suppl 1:115–118.
64. Hawkins MM, Kingston JE, Kinnier Wilson LM. Late deaths after treatment for childhood cancer. *Arch Dis Child.* 1990;65:1356–1363.
65. Green DM, Hyland A, Chung CS, et al. Cancer and cardiac mortality among 15-year survivors of cancer diagnosed during childhood or adolescence. *J Clin Oncol.* 1999;17: 3207–3215.
66. Moller TR, Garwicz S, Barlow L, et al. Decreasing late mortality among five-year survivors of cancer in childhood and adolescence: a population-based study in the Nordic countries. *J Clin Oncol.* 2001;19:3173–3181.
67. Jenkin D, Greenberg M, Hoffman H, et al. Brain tumors in children: long-term survival after radiation treatment. *Int J Radiat Oncol Biol Phys.* 1995;31:445–451.
68. Mertens AC. Cause of mortality in 5-year survivors of childhood cancer. *Pediatr Blood Cancer.* 2007;48:723–726.
69. Cardous-Ubbink MC, Heinen RC, Langeveld NE, et al. Long-term cause-specific mortality among five-year survivors of childhood cancer. *Pediatr Blood Cancer.* 2004; 42:563–573.
70. MacArthur AC, Spinelli JJ, Rogers PC, et al. Mortality among 5-year survivors of cancer diagnosed during childhood or adolescence in British Columbia, Canada. *Pediatr Blood Cancer.* 2007;48:460–467.
71. Tucker MA, D'Angio GJ, Boice JD, Jr., et al. Bone sarcomas linked to radiotherapy and chemotherapy in children. *N Engl J Med.* 1987;317:588–593.

72. Tucker MA, Meadows AT, Boice JD, Jr., et al. Leukemia after therapy with alkylating agents for childhood cancer. *J Natl Cancer Inst.* 1987;78:459–464.
73. Pui CH. Epipodophyllotoxin-related acute myeloid leukaemia. *Lancet.* 1991;338:1468.
74. Eng C, Li FP, Abramson DH, et al. Mortality from second tumors among long-term survivors of retinoblastoma. *J Natl Cancer Inst.* 1993;85:1121–1128.
75. Acquaviva A, Ciccolallo L, Rondelli R, et al. Mortality from second tumour among long-term survivors of retinoblastoma: a retrospective analysis of the Italian retinoblastoma registry. *Oncogene.* 2006;25:5350–5357.
76. Fletcher O, Easton D, Anderson K, et al. Lifetime risks of common cancers among retinoblastoma survivors. *J Natl Cancer Inst.* 2004;96:357–363.
77. Abramson DH, Ellsworth RM, Kitchin FD, et al. Second nonocular tumors in retinoblastoma survivors. Are they radiation-induced? *Ophthalmology.* 1984;91:1351–1355.
78. Simone JV. Late mortality in childhood cancer: two excellent studies bring good news tempered by room for improvement. *J Clin Oncol.* 2001;19:3161–3162.
79. Hudson MM, Mertens AC, Yasui Y, et al. Health status of adult long-term survivors of childhood cancer: a report from the Childhood Cancer Survivor Study. *JAMA.* 2003;290:1583–1592.
80. Zebrack BJ, Gurney JG, Oeffinger K, et al. Psychological outcomes in long-term survivors of childhood brain cancer: a report from the childhood cancer survivor study. *J Clin Oncol.* 2004;22:999–1006.
81. Zebrack BJ, Zevon MA, Turk N, et al. Psychological distress in long-term survivors of solid tumors diagnosed in childhood: a report from the childhood cancer survivor study. *Pediatr Blood Cancer.* 2007;49:47–51.
82. Gotay CC, Ransom S, Pagano IS. Quality of life in survivors of multiple primary cancers compared with cancer survivor controls. *Cancer.* 2007;110:2101–2109.
83. Green DM. Late effects of treatment for cancer during childhood and adolescence. *Curr Probl Cancer.* 2003;27:127–142.
84. Schwartz CL. Long-term survivors of childhood cancer: the late effects of therapy. *Oncologist.* 1999;4:45–54.
85. Mike V, Meadows AT, D'Angio GJ. Incidence of second malignant neoplasms in children: results of an international study. *Lancet.* 1982;2:1326–1331.
86. Rothman K, Keller A. The effect of joint exposure to alcohol and tobacco on risk of cancer of the mouth and pharynx. *J Chronic Dis.* 1972;25:711–716.
87. Tucker MA, Jones PH, Boice JD, Jr., et al. Therapeutic radiation at a young age is linked to secondary thyroid cancer. The Late Effects Study Group. *Cancer Res.* 1991;51:2885–2888.
88. Hammal DM, Bell CL, Craft AW, et al. Second primary tumors in children and young adults in the North of England (1968–99). *Pediatr Blood Cancer.* 2005;45:155–161.
89. Beaty O, 3rd, Hudson MM, Greenwald C, et al. Subsequent malignancies in children and adolescents after treatment for Hodgkin's disease. *J Clin Oncol.* 1995;13:603–609.
90. Bhatia S, Ramsay NK, Steinbuch M, et al. Malignant neoplasms following bone marrow transplantation. *Blood.* 1996;87:3633–3639.
91. Darrington DL, Vose JM, Anderson JR, et al. Incidence and characterization of secondary myelodysplastic syndrome and acute myelogenous leukemia following high-dose chemoradiotherapy and autologous stem-cell transplantation for lymphoid malignancies. *J Clin Oncol.* 1994;12:2527–2534.
92. Bhatia S, Robison LL, Oberlin O, et al. Breast cancer and other second neoplasms after childhood Hodgkin's disease. *N Engl J Med.* 1996;334:745–751.
93. Neglia JP, Meadows AT, Robison LL, et al. Second neoplasms after acute lymphoblastic leukemia in childhood. *N Engl J Med.* 1991;325:1330–1336.
94. Nygaard R, Garwicz S, Haldorsen T, et al. Second malignant neoplasms in patients treated for childhood leukemia. A population-based cohort study from the Nordic countries. The Nordic Society of Pediatric Oncology and Hematology (NOPHO). *Acta Paediatrica Scandinavica.* 1991;80:1220–1228.

95. Walter AW, Hancock ML, Pui CH, et al. Secondary brain tumors in children treated for acute lymphoblastic leukemia at St. Jude Children's Research Hospital. *J Clin Oncol.* 1998;16:3761–3767.
96. Shapiro S, Mealey J, Jr., Sartorius C. Radiation-induced intracranial malignant gliomas. *J Neurosurg.* 1989;71:77–82.
97. Abramson DH, Frank CM. Second nonocular tumors in survivors of bilateral retinoblastoma: a possible age effect on radiation-related risk. *Ophthalmology.* 1998;105: 573–579; discussion 9–80.
98. Jenkin D, Angyalfi S, Becker L, et al. Optic glioma in children: surveillance, resection, or irradiation? *Int J Radiat Oncol Biol Phys.* 1993;25:215–225.
99. Sussman A, Leviton A, Allred EN, et al. Childhood brain tumor: presentation at younger age is associated with a family tumor history. *Cancer Causes Control.* 1990;1:75–79.
100. Levine EG, Bloomfield CD. Leukemias and myelodysplastic syndromes secondary to drug, radiation, and environmental exposure. *Semin Oncol.* 1992;19:47–84.
101. Armstrong GT, Sklar CA, Hudson MM, et al. Long-term health status among survivors of childhood cancer: does sex matter? *J Clin Oncol.* 2007;25:4477–4489.
102. Sklar C, Whitton J, Mertens A, et al. Abnormalities of the thyroid in survivors of Hodgkin's disease: data from the Childhood Cancer Survivor Study. *J Clin Endocrinol Metab.* 2000;85:3227–3232.
103. Sigurdson AJ, Ronckers CM, Mertens AC, et al. Primary thyroid cancer after a first tumour in childhood (the Childhood Cancer Survivor Study): a nested case-control study. *Lancet.* 2005;365:2014–2023.
104. Zang EA, Wynder EL. Differences in lung cancer risk between men and women: examination of the evidence. *J Natl Cancer Inst.* 1996;88:183–192.
105. Ganjavi H, Malkin D. Genetics of childhood cancer. *Clin Orthop Relat Res* 2002:75–87.
106. Stratton MR, Williams S, Fisher C, et al. Structural alterations of the RB1 gene in human soft tissue tumours. *Br J Cancer.* 1989;60:202–205.
107. Eng C, Ponder BA. The role of gene mutations in the genesis of familial cancers. *FASEB J.* 1993;7:910–919.
108. Lohmann DR, Gerick M, Brandt B, et al. Constitutional RB1-gene mutations in patients with isolated unilateral retinoblastoma. *Am J Human Genet.* 1997;61:282–294.
109. Klutz M, Horsthemke B, Lohmann DR. RB1 gene mutations in peripheral blood DNA of patients with isolated unilateral retinoblastoma. *Am J Human Genet.* 1999;64: 667–668.
110. Farwell J, Flannery JT. Cancer in relatives of children with central-nervous-system neoplasms. *N Engl J Med.* 1984;311:749–753.
111. Larson RA, Wang Y, Banerjee M, et al. Prevalence of the inactivating 609C→T polymorphism in the NAD(P)H:quinone oxidoreductase (NQO1) gene in patients with primary and therapy-related myeloid leukemia. *Blood.* 1999;94:803–807.
112. Naoe T, Takeyama K, Yokozawa T, et al. Analysis of genetic polymorphism in NQO1, GST-M1, GST-T1, and CYP3A4 in 469 Japanese patients with therapy-related leukemia/ myelodysplastic syndrome and de novo acute myeloid leukemia. *Clin Cancer Res.* 2000;6:4091–4095.
113. Felix CA. Secondary leukemias induced by topoisomerase-targeted drugs. *Biochimica et Biophysica Acta.* 1998;1400:233–255.
114. Allan JM, Wild CP, Rollinson S, et al. Polymorphism in glutathione S-transferase P1 is associated with susceptibility to chemotherapy-induced leukemia. *Proc Natl Acad Sci USA.* 2001;98:11592–11597.
115. Felix CA, Walker AH, Lange BJ, et al. Association of CYP3A4 genotype with treatment-related leukemia. *Proc Natl Acad Sci USA.* 1998;95:13176–13181.
116. Woo MH, Shuster JJ, Chen C, et al. Glutathione S-transferase genotypes in children who develop treatment-related acute myeloid malignancies. *Leukemia.* 2000;14: 232–237.

117. Perentesis JP. Genetic predisposition and treatment-related leukemia. *Med Pediatr Oncol.* 2001;36:541–548.
118. Relling MV, Rubnitz JE, Rivera GK, et al. High incidence of secondary brain tumours after radiotherapy and antimetabolites. *Lancet.* 1999;354:34–39.
119. Relling MV, Yanishevski Y, Nemec J, et al. Etoposide and antimetabolite pharmacology in patients who develop secondary acute myeloid leukemia. *Leukemia.* 1998;12: 346–352.
120. Jenkinson H, Hawkins M. Secondary brain tumours in children with ALL. *Lancet.* 1999;354:1126.
121. Stanulla M, Loning L, Welte K, et al. Secondary brain tumours in children with ALL. *Lancet.* 1999;354:1126–1127.
122. Sharif S, Ferner R, Birch JM, et al. Second primary tumors in neurofibromatosis 1 patients treated for optic glioma: substantial risks after radiotherapy. *J Clin Oncol.* 2006;24:2570–2575.
123. Hottinger AF, Khakoo Y. Update on the management of familial central nervous system tumor syndromes. *Curr Neurol Neurosci Rep.* 2007;7:200–207.
124. van Leeuwen FE, Somers R, Taal BG, et al. Increased risk of lung cancer, non-Hodgkin's lymphoma, and leukemia following Hodgkin's disease. *J Clin Oncol.* 1989;7: 1046–1058.
125. Travis LB, Gospodarowicz M, Curtis RE, et al. Lung cancer following chemotherapy and radiotherapy for Hodgkin's disease. *J Natl Cancer Inst.* 2002;94:182–192.
126. van Leeuwen FE, Klokman WJ, Stovall M, et al. Roles of radiotherapy and smoking in lung cancer following Hodgkin's disease. *J Natl Cancer Inst.* 1995;87:1530–1537.
127. Tucker MA, Murray N, Shaw EG, et al. Second primary cancers related to smoking and treatment of small-cell lung cancer. Lung Cancer Working Cadre. *J Natl Cancer Inst.* 1997;89:1782–1788.
128. Inskip PD, Boice JD, Jr. Radiotherapy-induced lung cancer among women who smoke. *Cancer.* 1994;73:1541–1543.
129. Neugut AI, Murray T, Santos J, et al. Increased risk of lung cancer after breast cancer radiation therapy in cigarette smokers. *Cancer.* 1994;73:1615–1620.
130. Boivin JF. Smoking, treatment for Hodgkin's disease, and subsequent lung cancer risk. *J Natl Cancer Inst.* 1995;87:1502–1503.
131. Landier W, Bhatia S, Eshelman DA, et al. Development of risk-based guidelines for pediatric cancer survivors: the Children's Oncology Group Long-Term Follow-Up Guidelines from the Children's Oncology Group Late Effects Committee and Nursing Discipline. *J Clin Oncol.* 2004;22:4979–4990.
132. Laughlin-Richard N. Sun exposure and skin cancer prevention in children and adolescents. *J Sch Nurs.* 2000;16:20–26.
133. Flanders WD, Rothman KJ. Interaction of alcohol and tobacco in laryngeal cancer. *Am J Epidemiol.* 1982;115:371–379.
134. La Vecchia C, Negri E. The role of alcohol in oesophageal cancer in non-smokers, and of tobacco in non-drinkers. *Int J Cancer.* 1989;43:784–785.
135. Emmons KM, Puleo E, Park E, et al. Peer-delivered smoking counseling for childhood cancer survivors increases rate of cessation: the partnership for health study. *J Clin Oncol.* 2005;23:6516–6523.
136. Tyc VL, Hudson MM, Hinds P, et al. Tobacco use among pediatric cancer patients: recommendations for developing clinical smoking interventions. *J Clin Oncol.* 1997;15: 2194–2204.
137. Tyc VL, Lensing S, Klosky J, et al. A comparison of tobacco-related risk factors between adolescents with and without cancer. *J Pediatr Psychol.* 2005;30:359–370.
138. Tyc VL, Throckmorton-Belzer L. Smoking rates and the state of smoking interventions for children and adolescents with chronic illness. *Pediatrics.* 2006;118:e471–e487.
139. Green DM, Hyland A, Barcos MP, et al. Second malignant neoplasms after treatment for Hodgkin's disease in childhood or adolescence. *J Clin Oncol.* 2000;18:1492–1499.

140. Davies SM. Subsequent malignant neoplasms in survivors of childhood cancer: Childhood Cancer Survivor Study (CCSS) studies. *Pediatr Blood Cancer.* 2007;48:727–730.

141. Kaye FJ, Harbour JW. For whom the bell tolls: susceptibility to common adult cancers in retinoblastoma survivors. *J Natl Cancer Inst.* 2004;96:342–343.

142. Kingston JE, Hawkins MM, Draper GJ, et al. Patterns of multiple primary tumours in patients treated for cancer during childhood. *Br J Cancer.* 1987;56:331–338.

143. Le Deley MC, Leblanc T, Shamsaldin A, et al. Risk of secondary leukemia after a solid tumor in childhood according to the dose of epipodophyllotoxins and anthracyclines: a case-control study by the Societe Francaise d'Oncologie Pediatrique. *J Clin Oncol.* 2003;21:1074–1081.

144. Wenzel CT, Halperin EC, Fisher SR. Second malignant neoplasms of the head and neck in survivors of retinoblastoma. *Ear Nose Throat J.* 2001;80:106, 9–12.

145. Dunst J, Ahrens S, Paulussen M, et al. Second malignancies after treatment for Ewing's sarcoma: a report of the CESS-studies. *Int J Radiat Oncol Biol Phys.* 1998;42:379–384.

146. Kuttesch JF, Jr., Wexler LH, Marcus RB, et al. Second malignancies after Ewing's sarcoma: radiation dose-dependency of secondary sarcomas. *J Clin Oncol.* 1996;14: 2818–2825.

147. Svahn-Tapper G, Garwicz S, Anderson H, et al. Radiation dose and relapse are predictors for development of second malignant solid tumors after cancer in childhood and adolescence: a population-based case-control study in the five Nordic countries. *Acta Oncologica* (Stockholm, Sweden). 2006;45:438–448.

148. Bhatia S, Sather HN, Pabustan OB, et al. Low incidence of second neoplasms among children diagnosed with acute lymphoblastic leukemia after 1983. *Blood.* 2002;99: 4257–4264.

149. Ronckers CM, Sigurdson AJ, Stovall M, et al. Thyroid cancer in childhood cancer survivors: a detailed evaluation of radiation dose response and its modifiers. *Radiat Res.* 2006;166:618–628.

150. de Vathaire F, Francois P, Hill C, et al. Role of radiotherapy and chemotherapy in the risk of second malignant neoplasms after cancer in childhood. *Br J Cancer.* 1989;59:792–796.

151. Hawkins MM, Wilson LM, Burton HS, et al. Radiotherapy, alkylating agents, and risk of bone cancer after childhood cancer. *J Natl Cancer Inst.* 1996;88:270–278.

152. Breslow NE, Takashima JR, Whitton JA, et al. Second malignant neoplasms following treatment for Wilm's tumor: a report from the National Wilms' Tumor Study Group. *J Clin Oncol.* 1995;13:1851–1859.

153. Menu-Branthomme A, Rubino C, Shamsaldin A, et al. Radiation dose, chemotherapy and risk of soft tissue sarcoma after solid tumours during childhood. *Int J Cancer.* 2004;110:87–93.

154. Karlsson P, Holmberg E, Lundell M, et al. Intracranial tumors after exposure to ionizing radiation during infancy: a pooled analysis of two Swedish cohorts of 28,008 infants with skin hemangioma. *Radiat Res.* 1998;150:357–364.

155. Little MP, de Vathaire F, Shamsaldin A, et al. Risks of brain tumour following treatment for cancer in childhood: modification by genetic factors, radiotherapy and chemotherapy. *Int J Cancer.* 1998;78:269–275.

156. Kony SJ, de Vathaire F, Chompret A, et al. Radiation and genetic factors in the risk of second malignant neoplasms after a first cancer in childhood. *Lancet.* 1997;350:91–95.

157. Kleinerman RA, Stovall M, Tarone RE, et al. Gene environment interactions in a cohort of irradiated retinoblastoma patients. *Radiat Res.* 2005;163:701–702.

158. Guerin S, Guibout C, Shamsaldin A, et al. Concomitant chemo-radiotherapy and local dose of radiation as risk factors for second malignant neoplasms after solid cancer in childhood: a case-control study. *Int J Cancer.* 2007;120:96–102.

159. Sagerman RH, Cassady JR, Tretter P, et al. Radiation induced neoplasia following external beam therapy for children with retinoblastoma. *Am J Roentgenol Radium Ther Nucl Med.* 1969;105:529–535.

160. Loning L, Zimmermann M, Reiter A, et al. Secondary neoplasms subsequent to Berlin-Frankfurt-Munster therapy of acute lymphoblastic leukemia in childhood: significantly lower risk without cranial radiotherapy. *Blood.* 2000;95:2770 2775.

161. Ron E, Modan B, Boice JD, Jr., et al. Tumors of the brain and nervous system after radiotherapy in childhood. *N Engl J Med.* 1988;319:1033–1039.

162. Sadetzki S, Flint-Richter P, Ben-Tal T, et al. Radiation-induced meningioma: a descriptive study of 253 cases. *J Neurosurg.* 2002;97:1078–1082.

163. Brada M, Ford D, Ashley S, et al. Risk of second brain tumour after conservative surgery and radiotherapy for pituitary adenoma. *BMJ* (Clin Res) ed. 1992;304: 1343–1346.

164. Shalet SM, Beardwell CG, MacFarlane IA, et al. Endocrine morbidity in adults treated with cerebral irradiation for brain tumours during childhood. Acta endocrinologica. 1977;84:673–680.

165. Hall EJ. Intensity-modulated radiation therapy, protons, and the risk of second cancers. *Int J Radiat Oncol Biol Phys.* 2006;65:1–7.

166. Travis LB, Holowaty EJ, Bergfeldt K, et al. Risk of leukemia after platinum-based chemotherapy for ovarian cancer. *N Engl J Med.* 1999;340:351–357.

167. Smith MA, Rubinstein L, Anderson JR, et al. Secondary leukemia or myelodysplastic syndrome after treatment with epipodophyllotoxins. *J Clin Oncol.* 1999;17:569–577.

168. Smith MA, Rubinstein L, Ungerleider RS. Therapy-related acute myeloid leukemia following treatment with epipodophyllotoxins: estimating the risks. *Med Pediatr Oncol.* 1994;23:86–98.

169. Hawkins MM, Wilson LM, Stovall MA, et al. Epipodophyllotoxins, alkylating agents, and radiation and risk of secondary leukaemia after childhood cancer. *BMJ* (Clin Res) ed. 1992;304:951–958.

170. Klein G, Michaelis J, Spix C, et al. Second malignant neoplasms after treatment of childhood cancer. *Eur J Cancer.* 2003;39:808–817.

171. Haas JF, Kittelmann B, Mehnert WH, et al. Risk of leukaemia in ovarian tumour and breast cancer patients following treatment by cyclophosphamide. *Br J Cancer.* 1987;55:213–218.

172. Henderson TO, Whitton J, Stovall M, et al. Secondary sarcomas in childhood cancer survivors: a report from the Childhood Cancer Survivor Study. *J Natl Cancer Inst.* 2007;99:300–308.

173. Hawkins MM. Risks of myeloid leukaemia in children treated for solid tumours. *Lancet.* 1990;336:887.

174. Green DM, Zevon MA, Reese PA, et al. Second malignant tumors following treatment during childhood and adolescence for cancer. *Med Pediatr Oncol.* 1994;22:1–10.

175. Draper GJ, Sanders BM, Kingston JE. Second primary neoplasms in patients with retinoblastoma. *Br J Cancer.* 1986;53:661–671.

176. Gombos DS, Hungerford J, Abramson DH, et al. Secondary acute myelogenous leukemia in patients with retinoblastoma: is chemotherapy a factor? Ophthalmology. 2007;114: 1378–1383.

177. Shannon KM, O'Connell P, Martin GA, et al. Loss of the normal NF1 allele from the bone marrow of children with type 1 neurofibromatosis and malignant myeloid disorders. *N Engl J Med.* 1994;330:597–601.

178. Hoffmann L, Moller P, Pedersen-Bjergaard J, et al. Therapy-related acute promyelocytic leukemia with t(15;17) (q22;q12) following chemotherapy with drugs targeting DNA topoisomerase II. A report of two cases and a review of the literature. *Ann Oncol.* 1995;6: 781–788.

179. Bisogno G, Sotti G, Nowicki Y, et al. Soft tissue sarcoma as a second malignant neoplasm in the pediatric age group. *Cancer.* 2004;100:1758–1765.

180. Pedersen-Bjergaard J, Sigsgaard TC, Nielsen D, et al. Acute monocytic or myelomonocytic leukemia with balanced chromosome translocations to band 11q23 after therapy with 4-epi-doxorubicin and cisplatin or cyclophosphamide for breast cancer. *J Clin Oncol.* 1992;10:1444–1451.

181. Diamandidou E, Buzdar AU, Smith TL, et al. Treatment-related leukemia in breast cancer patients treated with fluorouracil-doxorubicin-cyclophosphamide combination adjuvant chemotherapy: the University of Texas M.D. Anderson Cancer Center experience. *J Clin Oncol.* 1996;14:2722–2730.

182. Sklar CA, Mertens AC, Mitby P, et al. Risk of disease recurrence and second neoplasms in survivors of childhood cancer treated with growth hormone: a report from the Childhood Cancer Survivor Study. *J Clin Endocrinol Metab.* 2002;87:3136–3141.

183. Ergun-Longmire B, Mertens AC, Mitby P, et al. Growth hormone treatment and risk of second neoplasms in the childhood cancer survivor. *J Clin Endocrinol Metab.* 2006;91: 3494–3498.

184. Toniolo PG, Levitz M, Zeleniuch-Jacquotte A, et al. A prospective study of endogenous estrogens and breast cancer in postmenopausal women. *J Natl Cancer Inst.* 1995;87: 190–197.

185. Pike MC, Spicer DV, Dahmoush L, et al. Estrogens, progestogens, normal breast cell proliferation, and breast cancer risk. *Epidemiol Rev.* 1993;15:17–35.

186. Bosland MC. Sex steroids and prostate carcinogenesis: integrated, multifactorial working hypothesis. *Ann N Y Acad Sci.* 2006;1089:168–176.

187. Schottenfeld DF, Joseph F, ed. *Cancer Epidemiology and Prevention.* 2nd ed: Oxford, USA: Oxford University Press; 1996.

188. Park SM, Lim MK, Jung KW, et al. Prediagnosis smoking, obesity, insulin resistance, and second primary cancer risk in male cancer survivors: National Health Insurance Corporation Study. *J Clin Oncol.* 2007;25:4835–4843.

189. Irigaray P, Newby JA, Lacomme S, et al. Overweight/obesity and cancer genesis: More than a biological link. *Biomed Pharmacotherapy.* 2007;61:665–678.

190. McTiernan A. Obesity and cancer: the risks, science, and potential management strategies. *Oncology* (Williston Park, NY). 2005;19:871–881; discussion 81–82, 85–86.

191. Packer RJ, Boyett JM, Janss AJ, et al. Growth hormone replacement therapy in children with medulloblastoma: use and effect on tumor control. *J Clin Oncol.* 2001;19:480–487.

192. Danoff BF, Cowchock FS, Marquette C, et al. Assessment of the long-term effects of primary radiation therapy for brain tumors in children. *Cancer.* 1982;49:1580–1586.

193. Duffner PK, Horowitz ME, Krischer JP, et al. Postoperative chemotherapy and delayed radiation in children less than three years of age with malignant brain tumors. *N Engl J Med.* 1993;328:1725–1731.

194. Stavrou T, Bromley CM, Nicholson HS, et al. Prognostic factors and secondary malignancies in childhood medulloblastoma. *J Pediatr Hematol Oncol.* 2001;23:431–436.

195. Minniti G, Traish D, Ashley S, et al. Risk of second brain tumor after conservative surgery and radiotherapy for pituitary adenoma: update after an additional 10 years. *J Clin Endocrinol Metab.* 2005;90:800–804.

196. Salminen E, Pukkala E, Teppo L. Second cancers in patients with brain tumours – impact of treatment. *Eur J Cancer.* 1999;35:102–105.

197. Goldstein AM, Yuen J, Tucker MA. Second cancers after medulloblastoma: population-based results from the United States and Sweden. *Cancer Causes Contr.* 1997;8:865–871.

198. Hader WJ, Drovini-Zis K, Maguire JA. Primitive neuroectodermal tumors in the central nervous system following cranial irradiation: a report of four cases. *Cancer.* 2003;97: 1072–1076.

199. Barasch ES, Altieri D, Decker RE, et al. Primitive neuroectodermal tumor presenting as a delayed sequela to cranial irradiation and intrathecal methotrexate. *Pediatr Neurol.* 1988;4:375–378.

200. Rittinger O, Kranzinger M, Jones R, et al. Malignant astrocytoma arising 10 years after combined treatment of craniopharyngioma. *J Pediatr Endocrinol Metab.* 2003;16:97–101.

201. Kranzinger M, Jones N, Rittinger O, et al. Malignant glioma as a secondary malignant neoplasm after radiation therapy for craniopharyngioma: report of a case and review of reported cases. *Onkologie.* 2001;24:66–72.

202. Liwnicz BH, Berger TS, Liwnicz RG, et al. Radiation-associated gliomas: a report of four cases and analysis of postradiation tumors of the central nervous system. *Neurosurgery*. 1985;17:436–445.
203. Kantar M, Cetingul N, Kansoy S, et al. Radiotherapy-induced secondary cranial neoplasms in children. *Childs Nerv Syst*. 2004;20:46–49.
204. Iyer RS, Soman CS, Nair CN, et al. Brain tumors following cure of acute lymphoblastic leukemia. *Leukemia Lymphoma*. 1994;13:183–186.
205. Kitanaka C, Shitara N, Nakagomi T, et al. Postradiation astrocytoma. Report of two cases. *J Neurosurg*. 1989;70:469–474.
206. Salvati M, Puzzilli F, Bristot R, et al. Post-radiation gliomas. *Tumori*. 1994;80:220–223.
207. Salvati M, Artico M, Caruso R, et al. A report on radiation-induced gliomas. *Cancer*. 1991;67:392–397.
208. Fontana M, Stanton C, Pompili A, et al. Late multifocal gliomas in adolescents previously treated for acute lymphoblastic leukemia. *Cancer*. 1987;60:1510–1518.
209. Stragliotto G, Packer RJ, Rausen AR, et al. "Outcome of post-radiation secondary glioblastoma in children". *Med Pediatr Oncol*. 1998;30:194–195.
210. Postovsky S, Vlodavsky E, Eran A, et al. Secondary glioblastoma multiforme after treatment for primary choroid plexus carcinoma in childhood. *J Pediatr Hematol Oncol*. 2007;29:248–252.
211. Tsang RW, Laperriere NJ, Simpson WJ, et al. Glioma arising after radiation therapy for pituitary adenoma. A report of four patients and estimation of risk. *Cancer*. 1993;72: 2227–2233.
212. Donson AM, Erwin NS, Kleinschmidt-DeMasters BK, et al. Unique molecular characteristics of radiation-induced glioblastoma. *J Neuropathol Exp Neurol*. 2007;66:740–749.
213. Pui CH, Cheng C, Leung W, et al. Extended follow-up of long-term survivors of childhood acute lymphoblastic leukemia. *N Engl J Med*. 2003;349:640–649.
214. Boljesikova E, Chorvath M. Radiation-induced meningiomas. *Neoplasma*. 2001;48: 442–444.
215. Harrison MJ, Wolfe DE, Lau TS, et al. Radiation-induced meningiomas: experience at the Mount Sinai Hospital and review of the literature. *J Neurosurg*. 1991;75:564–574.
216. Soffer D, Pittaluga S, Feiner M, et al. Intracranial meningiomas following low-dose irradiation to the head. *J Neurosurg*. 1983;59:1048–1053.
217. Korenkov AI, Imhof HG, Brandner S, et al. Growth retardation and bilateral cataracts followed by anaplastic meningioma 23 years after high-dose cranial and whole-body irradiation for acute lymphoblastic leukemia: case report and review of the literature. *J Neuro-oncol*. 2005;74:195–199.
218. Longstreth WT, Jr., Dennis LK, McGuire VM, et al. Epidemiology of intracranial meningioma. *Cancer*. 1993;72:639–648.
219. Strojan P, Popovic M, Jereb B. Secondary intracranial meningiomas after high-dose cranial irradiation: report of five cases and review of the literature. *Int J Radiat Oncol Biol Phys*. 2000;48:65–73.
220. Musa BS, Pople IK, Cummins BH. Intracranial meningiomas following irradiation – a growing problem? *Br J Neurosurg*. 1995;9:629–637.
221. Dorfmuller G, Wurtz FG, Kleinert R, et al. Cerebral primitive neuro-ectodermal tumour following treatment of a unilateral retinoblastoma. *Acta Neurochirurgica*. 1997;139:749–755.
222. Brustle O, Ohgaki H, Schmitt HP, et al. Primitive neuroectodermal tumors after prophylactic central nervous system irradiation in children. Association with an activated K-ras gene. *Cancer*. 1992;69:2385–2392.
223. Shore RE, Albert RE, Reed M, et al. Skin cancer incidence among children irradiated for ringworm of the scalp. *Radiat Res*. 1984;100:192–204.
224. Ron E, Modan B, Preston D, et al. Radiation-induced skin carcinomas of the head and neck. *Radiat Res*. 1991;125:318–325.

225. Perkins JL, Liu Y, Mitby PA, et al. Nonmelanoma skin cancer in survivors of childhood and adolescent cancer: a report from the childhood cancer survivor study. *J Clin Oncol.* 2005;23:3733–3741.
226. Levi F, Moeckli R, Randimbison L, et al. Skin cancer in survivors of childhood and adolescent cancer. *Eur J Cancer.* 2006;42:656–659.
227. Armstrong BK, Kricker A. The epidemiology of UV induced skin cancer. *J Photochem Photobiol.* 2001;63:8–18.
228. Hildreth NG, Shore RE, Hempelmann LH, et al. Risk of extrathyroid tumors following radiation treatment in infancy for thymic enlargement. *Radiat Res.* 1985;102:378–391.
229. Shore RE. Overview of radiation-induced skin cancer in humans. *Int J Radiat Biol.* 1990;57:809–827.
230. Marin-Gutzke M, Sanchez-Olaso A, Berenguer B, et al. Basal cell carcinoma in childhood after radiation therapy: case report and review. *Ann Plastic Surg.* 2004;53:593–595.
231. Dinehart SM, Anthony JL, Pollack SV. Basal cell carcinoma in young patients after irradiation for childhood malignancy. *Med Pediatr Oncol.* 1991;19:508–510.
232. Euvrard S, Kanitakis J, Claudy A. Skin cancers after organ transplantation. *N Engl J Med.* 2003;348:1681–1691.
233. Swerdlow AJ, English J, MacKie RM, et al. Benign melanocytic naevi as a risk factor for malignant melanoma. *BMJ* (Clin Res) ed. 1986;292:1555–1559.
234. Kraehn GM, Schartl M, Peter RU. Human malignant melanoma. A genetic disease? *Cancer.* 1995;75:1228–1237.
235. Gorlin RJ. Nevoid basal cell carcinoma (Gorlin) syndrome. *Genet Med.* 2004;6:530–539.
236. Traboulsi EI, Zimmerman LE, Manz HJ. Cutaneous malignant melanoma in survivors of heritable retinoblastoma. *Arch Ophthalmol.* 1988;106:1059–1061.
237. Bataille V, Hiles R, Bishop JA. Retinoblastoma, melanoma and the atypical mole syndrome. *Br J Dermatol.* 1995;132:134–138.
238. Albert LS, Sober AJ, Rhodes AR. Cutaneous melanoma and bilateral retinoblastoma. *J Am Acad Dermatol.* 1990;23:1001–1004.
239. Belt PJ, Smithers M, Elston T. The triad of bilateral retinoblastoma, dysplastic naevus syndrome and multiple cutaneous malignant melanomas: a case report and review of the literature. *Melanoma Res.* 2002;12:179–182.
240. Yoshihara T, Ikuta H, Hibi S, et al. Second cutaneous neoplasms after acute lymphoblastic leukemia in childhood. *Int J Hematol.* 1993;59:67–71.
241. Guerin S, Dupuy A, Anderson H, et al. Radiation dose as a risk factor for malignant melanoma following childhood cancer. *Eur J Cancer.* 2003;39:2379–2386.
242. Dickerman JD. The late effects of childhood cancer therapy. *Pediatrics.* 2007;119:554–568.
243. Benton E, Tidman M. Cutaneous complications. In: Wallace WaG, DM, ed. *Late Effects of Childhood Cancer.* London, UK: Arnold; 2004:321–331.
244. Moll AC, Imhof SM, Bouter LM, et al. Second primary tumors in patients with hereditary retinoblastoma: a register-based follow-up study, 1945–1994. *Int J Cancer.* 1996;67:515–519.
245. Green A, Smith P, McWhirter W, et al. Melanocytic naevi and melanoma in survivors of childhood cancer. *Br J Cancer.* 1993;67:1053–1057.
246. Baird EA, McHenry PM, MacKie RM. Effect of maintenance chemotherapy in childhood on numbers of melanocytic naevi. *BMJ* (Clin Res) ed. 1992;305:799–801.
247. de Wit PE, de Vaan GA, de Boo TM, et al. Prevalence of naevocytic naevi after chemotherapy for childhood cancer. *Med Pediatr Oncol.* 1990;18:336–338.
248. Karagas MR, McDonald JA, Greenberg ER, et al. Risk of basal cell and squamous cell skin cancers after ionizing radiation therapy. For The Skin Cancer Prevention Study Group. *J Natl Cancer Inst.* 1996;88:1848–1853.
249. Lichter MD, Karagas MR, Mott LA, et al. Therapeutic ionizing radiation and the incidence of basal cell carcinoma and squamous cell carcinoma. The New Hampshire Skin Cancer Study Group. *Arch Dermatol.* 2000;136:1007–1011.

250. Cutuli B, Borel C, Dhermain F, et al. Breast cancer occurred after treatment for Hodgkin's disease: analysis of 133 cases. *Radiother Oncol.* 2001;59:247–255.

251. Preston DL, Mattsson A, Holmberg E, et al. Radiation effects on breast cancer risk: a pooled analysis of eight cohorts. *Radiat Res.* 2002;158:220–235.

252. Broeks A, Russell NS, Floore AN, et al. Increased risk of breast cancer following irradiation for Hodgkin's disease is not a result of ATM germline mutations. *Int J Radiat Biol.* 2000;76:693–698.

253. Nichols KE, Heath JA, Friedman D, et al. TP53, BRCA1, and BRCA2 tumor suppressor genes are not commonly mutated in survivors of Hodgkin's disease with second primary neoplasms. *J Clin Oncol.* 2003;21:4505–4509.

254. Nichols KE, Levitz S, Shannon KE, et al. Heterozygous germline ATM mutations do not contribute to radiation-associated malignancies after Hodgkin's disease. *J Clin Oncol.* 1999;17:1259.

255. Cutuli B. In regard to Gaffney et al., IJROBP. 2001;49:539–546. *Int J Radiat Oncol Biol Phys.* 2002;52:272–274.

256. Gaffney DK, Hemmersmeier J, Holden J, et al. Breast cancer after mantle irradiation for Hodgkin's disease: correlation of clinical, pathologic, and molecular features including loss of heterozygosity at BRCA1 and BRCA2. *Int J Radiat Oncol Biol Phys.* 2001;49: 539–546.

257. Travis LB, Hill D, Dores GM, et al. Cumulative absolute breast cancer risk for young women treated for Hodgkin lymphoma. *J Natl Cancer Inst.* 2005;97:1428–1437.

258. Cutuli B. Radiation-induced breast cancer after treatment for Hodgkin's disease. *J Clin Oncol.* 1998;16:2285–2287.

259. Yasui Y, Liu Y, Neglia JP, et al. A methodological issue in the analysis of second-primary cancer incidence in long-term survivors of childhood cancers. *Am J Epidemiol.* 2003;158:1108–1113.

260. Kaste SC, Hudson MM, Jones DJ, et al. Breast masses in women treated for childhood cancer: incidence and screening guidelines. *Cancer.* 1998;82:784–792.

261. de Vathaire F, Hardiman C, Shamsaldin A, et al. Thyroid carcinomas after irradiation for a first cancer during childhood. *Arch Int Med.* 1999;159:2713–2719.

262. Acharya S, Sarafoglou K, LaQuaglia M, et al. Thyroid neoplasms after therapeutic radiation for malignancies during childhood or adolescence. *Cancer.* 2003;97: 2397–2403.

263. Schlumberger M, Cailleux AF, Suarez HG, et al. Irradiation and second cancers. The thyroid as a case in point. *Comptes rendus de l'Academie des Sciences.* 1999;322:205–213.

264. Black P, Straaten A, Gutjahr P. Secondary thyroid carcinoma after treatment for childhood cancer. *Med Pediatr Oncol.* 1998;31:91–95.

265. Bhatia S, Ramsay NK, Bantle JP, et al. Thyroid Abnormalities after Therapy for Hodgkin's Disease in Childhood. *Oncologist.* 1996;1:62–67.

266. Agartan CA, Ustundag N, Gurleyik G, et al. Secondary thyroid carcinoma after treatment of yolk sac tumor. *J Pediatr Hematol Oncol.* 2004;26:77.

267. Fugazzola L, Pilotti S, Pinchera A, et al. Oncogenic rearrangements of the RET proto-oncogene in papillary thyroid carcinomas from children exposed to the Chernobyl nuclear accident. *Cancer Res.* 1995;55:5617–5620.

268. Ito T, Seyama T, Iwamoto KS, et al. Activated RET oncogene in thyroid cancers of children from areas contaminated by Chernobyl accident. *Lancet.* 1994;344:259.

269. Klugbauer S, Lengfelder E, Demidchik EP, et al. High prevalence of RET rearrangement in thyroid tumors of children from Belarus after the Chernobyl reactor accident. *Oncogene.* 1995;11:2459–2467.

270. Caudill CM, Zhu Z, Ciampi R, et al. Dose-dependent generation of RET/PTC in human thyroid cells after in vitro exposure to gamma-radiation: a model of carcinogenic chromosomal rearrangement induced by ionizing radiation. *J Clin Endocrinol Metab.* 2005;90:2364–2369.

271. Gray L. Radiation Biology and Cancer. In: Cellular radiation biology: A collection of works presented at the 18th Annual Symposium on Experimental Cancer Research 1964, Baltimore: Williams and Wilkins; 1965:7–25.
272. Ron E. Cancer risks from medical radiation. *Health Phys.* 2003;85:47–59.
273. Whatley WS, Thompson JW, Rao B. Salivary gland tumors in survivors of childhood cancer. *Otolaryngol Head Neck Surg.* 2006;134:385–388.
274. Lorigan P, Radford J, Howell A, et al. Lung cancer after treatment for Hodgkin's lymphoma: a systematic review. *Lancet Oncol.* 2005;6:773–779.
275. Kleinerman RA, Tarone RE, Abramson DH, et al. Hereditary retinoblastoma and risk of lung cancer. *J Natl Cancer Inst.* 2000;92:2037–2039.
276. Horowitz JM, Park SH, Bogenmann E, et al. Frequent inactivation of the retinoblastoma anti-oncogene is restricted to a subset of human tumor cells. *Proc Natl Acad Sci USA.* 1990;87:2775–2779.
277. Xu HJ, Hu SX, Cagle PT, et al. Absence of retinoblastoma protein expression in primary non-small cell lung carcinomas. *Cancer Res.* 1991;51:2735–2739.
278. Cance WG, Brennan MF, Dudas ME, et al. Altered expression of the retinoblastoma gene product in human sarcomas. *N Engl J Med.* 1990;323:1457–1462.
279. Shearer P, Kapoor G, Beckwith JB, et al. Secondary acute myelogenous leukemia in patients previously treated for childhood renal tumors: a report from the National Wilms Tumor Study Group. *J Pediatr Hematol Oncol.* 2001;23:109–111.
280. Thirman MJ, Larson RA. Therapy-related myeloid leukemia. *Hematol/Oncol Clinics North America.* 1996;10:293–320.
281. Kaldor JM, Day NE, Clarke EA, et al. Leukemia following Hodgkin's disease. *N Engl J Med.* 1990;322:7–13.
282. Bhatia S, Krailo MD, Chen Z, et al. Therapy-related myelodysplasia and acute myeloid leukemia after Ewing sarcoma and primitive neuroectodermal tumor of bone: A report from the Children's Oncology Group. *Blood.* 2007;109:46–51.
283. Sandoval C, Pui CH, Bowman LC, et al. Secondary acute myeloid leukemia in children previously treated with alkylating agents, intercalating topoisomerase II inhibitors, and irradiation. *J Clin Oncol.* 1993;11:1039–1045.
284. Kantarjian HM, Keating MJ. Therapy-related leukemia and myelodysplastic syndrome. *Semin Oncol.* 1987;14:435–443.
285. Casteels K, Renard M, Van Gool S, et al. Secondary acute lymphoblastic leukemia in a child three years after treatment for medulloblastoma. *Med Pediatr Oncol.* 2001;36: 390–391.
286. Latagliata R, Petti MC, Fenu S, et al. Therapy-related myelodysplastic syndrome-acute myelogenous leukemia in patients treated for acute promyelocytic leukemia: an emerging problem. *Blood.* 2002;99:822–824.
287. Rubin CM, Le Beau MM. Cytogenetic abnormalities in childhood acute lymphoblastic leukemia. *Am J Pediatr Hematol/Oncol.* 1991;13:202–216.
288. Su YW, Chang MC, Chiang MF, et al. Treatment-related myelodysplastic syndrome after temozolomide for recurrent high-grade glioma. *J Neuro-oncol.* 2005;71:315–318.
289. Pedersen-Bjergaard J, Andersen MK, Johansson B. Balanced chromosome aberrations in leukemias following chemotherapy with DNA-topoisomerase II inhibitors. *J Clin Oncol.* 1998;16:1897–1898.
290. Smith G, Stanley LA, Sim E, et al. Metabolic polymorphisms and cancer susceptibility. *Cancer Surv.* 1995;25:27–65.
291. Raunio H, Husgafvel-Pursiainen K, Anttila S, et al. Diagnosis of polymorphisms in carcinogen-activating and inactivating enzymes and cancer susceptibility – a review. *Gene.* 1995;159:113–121.
292. Pedersen-Bjergaard J, Pedersen M, Roulston D, et al. Different genetic pathways in leukemogenesis for patients presenting with therapy-related myelodysplasia and therapy-related acute myeloid leukemia. *Blood.* 1995;86:3542–3552.

293. Pedersen-Bjergaard J, Andersen MK. Secondary or therapy-related MDS and AML and their chromosome aberrations: important to study but difficult to establish causality. *Haematologica.* 1998;83:481–482.
294. Mistry AR, Felix CA, Whitmarsh RJ, et al. DNA topoisomerase II in therapy-related acute promyelocytic leukemia. *N Engl J Med.* 2005;352:1529–1538.
295. Pui CH, Ribeiro RC, Hancock ML, et al. Acute myeloid leukemia in children treated with epipodophyllotoxins for acute lymphoblastic leukemia. *N Engl J Med.* 1991;325: 1682–1687.
296. Pui CH, Relling MV, Rivera GK, et al. Epipodophyllotoxin-related acute myeloid leukemia: a study of 35 cases. *Leukemia.* 1995;9:1990–1996.
297. Fisher PG. Rethinking brain tumors in babies and more. *Ann Neurol.* 1998;44:300–302.
298. Estey EH. Prognosis and therapy of secondary myelodysplastic syndromes. *Haematologica.* 1998;83:543–549.
299. Leith CP, Kopecky KJ, Godwin J, et al. Acute myeloid leukemia in the elderly: assessment of multidrug resistance (MDR1) and cytogenetics distinguishes biologic subgroups with remarkably distinct responses to standard chemotherapy. A Southwest Oncology Group study. *Blood.* 1997;89:3323–3329.
300. Slovak ML, Kopecky KJ, Cassileth PA, et al. Karyotypic analysis predicts outcome of preremission and postremission therapy in adult acute myeloid leukemia: a Southwest Oncology Group/Eastern Cooperative Oncology Group Study. *Blood.* 2000;96: 4075–4083.
301. Anderson JE, Gooley TA, Schoch G, et al. Stem cell transplantation for secondary acute myeloid leukemia: evaluation of transplantation as initial therapy or following induction chemotherapy. *Blood.* 1997;89:2578–2585.
302. Witherspoon RP, Deeg HJ. Allogeneic bone marrow transplantation for secondary leukemia or myelodysplasia. *Haematologica.* 1999;84:1085–1087.
303. Zuna J, Cave H, Eckert C, et al. Childhood secondary ALL after ALL treatment. *Leukemia.* 2007;21:1431–1435.
304. Lehrnbecher T, Deinlein F, Marx A, et al. Mediastinal T-cell lymphoma in a boy 7 years after treatment of supratentorial primitive neuroectodermal tumor. *J Pediatr Hematol Oncol.* 2003;25:657–659.

Part III
Psychosocial Implications of Brain Tumor Survivorship

Chapter 17
Neuropsychological Impact of Treatment of Brain Tumors

Cinzia R. De Luca, Rowena Conroy, Maria C. McCarthy, Vicki A. Anderson, and David M. Ashley

Introduction

Advances in treatments for brain tumors have seen a significant increase in survival rates over the past few decades. This increase has been particularly dramatic in the pediatric population; for example, long-term (>5 years) survival rates for medulloblastoma, the most common primary malignant brain tumor of childhood, are now between 70 and 85%.[1] The figures for adults are less heartening, but nonetheless show a considerable improvement from previous decades when most treatment was considered palliative. As the number of survivors continues to increase, attention has increasingly focused on the late effects of treatment. Neurotoxicity is a widely acknowledged side effect of those treatments most successful at achieving 'cure'. Thus, risk-adapted modifications are currently being made to achieve an acceptable balance between effectiveness and toxicity.

In this chapter, we discuss the neuropsychological impact of treating brain tumors in children and adults. We begin with a review of the major research findings regarding the neurocognitive effects of radiation, chemotherapy, and surgery, and describe some of the factors that are important in determining the severity of these deficits. We then discuss the mechanisms by which treatments may influence neurocognitive outcome and review the few psychological interventions that have been conducted to assist those survivors with cognitive sequelae. Finally, we consider factors that warrant further attention in future efforts to better understand the neuropsychological profile of late effects.

Cognitive Sequelae of Brain Tumor Treatments

Brain tumors are treated according to their pathophysiology, size, and location, with a number of factors such as age, comorbid medical conditions, and impact on quality of life, also considered in treatment planning. Typically, treatment

C.R. De Luca (✉)
Children's Cancer Centre, Royal Children's Hospital, Melbourne, VIC, Australia
e-mail: cinzia.deluca@rch.org.au

S. Goldman, C.D. Turner (eds.), *Late Effects of Treatment for Brain Tumors*, Cancer Treatment and Research 150, DOI 10.1007/b109924_17, © Springer Science+Business Media, LLC 2009

includes a combination of surgery, chemotherapy, and radiation. Low-grade tumors that are able to be fully resected usually require little further treatment, whereas chemotherapy and radiation are used for more aggressive tumors that have the potential to recur or metastasize. The majority of studies examining the impact of brain tumor treatment on neuropsychological functioning have been with children and adolescents. We will describe this literature first, followed by a review of the smaller body of research investigating neurocognitive outcomes in adults.

Children and Adolescents

Most research examining neuropsychological outcomes of childhood brain tumors has focused on survivors of medulloblastoma. Treatment of these tumors typically involves radical surgery along with radiation and chemotherapy. As most studies have not assessed the baseline functioning of participants before treatment, and due to the multimodal nature of these treatments, disentangling the influence of the illness and each specific treatment component is challenging. However, the tumor, hydrocephalus, radiation, chemotherapy, and surgery have all been shown to have both independent and additive effects on neurocognitive functioning.

Radiation

Where cranial irradiation therapy (CRT) has been used in children and adolescents (in addition to other treatments) it has been shown to be associated with impairments in IQ. This finding has been seen in both cross-sectional and longitudinal studies.[2–5] Most studies have focused on patients who have received whole-brain radiation, for example those with medulloblastoma in doses in excess of 24–36 Gy. In these patients, longitudinal research has documented a progressive decline in IQ of approximately 2–4 points per year.[6–10] These impairments are typically not evident immediately following treatment, but emerge around 12–24 months after completion of CRT.[6] This decline is initially quite rapid, but slows over time.[1,12] In fact, a recent study by Stargatt and colleagues[13] suggests that, following an initial decline in performance over the first treatment year, patients experience an improvement in cognitive abilities over the next 12 months, before a more insidious CRT-related decline commences. Outcome beyond the first 10 years post-CRT is unclear due to the paucity of studies following survivors beyond this time.

Studies of IQ have consistently reported nonverbal abilities to be more vulnerable to the effects of CRT than language skills.[3,14,15] There is, however, evidence that both domains are affected, but that the trajectory of impairment is disparate, with visuospatial deficits emerging at an earlier stage.[5] Impaired performance in academic domains has also been found, and has been shown to be independent of intellectual decline.[7,14,16]

These observed impairments in intellectual and academic functions likely reflect the slowed acquisition of new skills which are due to come online during development, rather than a functional decline.[6] For example, Palmer and colleagues (2003) showed that survivors' raw IQ scores improved with increasing time post-irradiation, but when compared against same-aged peers their standardized scores declined because these raw scores had not increased at the rate that would be expected for their age.

It has more recently been proposed that underlying this slowed learning are deficits in key processing skills. Although most studies have focused on IQ and academic achievement as indicators of cognitive functioning, deficits in these areas are likely to reflect underlying disruption in more fundamental processing domains, such as attention, processing speed, and working memory.[14,17–21] Impairment of these information processing abilities limits a child's access to learning opportunities, resulting in the reduced acquisition of cognitive and academic skills. Over time this influences the amount and integrity of stored knowledge and will impact both IQ and academic test results.

A number of factors have been found to be associated with the severity of cognitive late effects post-irradiation. Most significantly, children who are younger at the time of treatment, and those who receive greater volumes and higher doses of CRT have consistently been shown to have more severe cognitive deficits.[5,22] Furthermore, as described earlier, over time skills fail to emerge at key developmental stages; thus greater time since treatment is also associated with poorer neuropsychological outcomes.[8,23]

Importantly, it should also be restated that most of this research has documented outcomes for children receiving whole-brain cranial radiation in relatively high doses of 24–36 Gy and above. The impact of more focused CRT in smaller volumes is currently under investigation, and limited studies suggest that these methods result in fewer long-term neurocognitive effects.[24–26]

Chemotherapy

Although radiation is a neurotoxic treatment modality, there is also some evidence that chemotherapeutic drugs may lead to neurocognitive impairment. Much of the evidence implicating chemotherapy agents in cognitive impairment comes from other cancer populations, particularly children with Acute Lymphoblastic Leukaemia (ALL), as these drugs are rarely used without CRT in the treatment of brain tumors. The drug that has attracted the greatest interest is methotrexate (MTX), which is typically used in high doses as prophylatic treatment for ALL. MTX has been introduced as a substitute to whole-brain radiation in CNS-directed therapy in an effort to overcome the neurocognitive impact of radiation. It is usually administered intrathecally, often in conjunction with systemic (i.e., intravenous) administration.

Research findings in this area are inconsistent, and the independent contribution of MTX remains controversial. A number of studies have found no significant neurocognitive effect from chemotherapy (including

MTX) alone.[27–32] However, a recent review found that two-thirds of studies report a decline in one or more aspects of cognition following intrathecal MTX.[33]

In ALL, it is well established that when paired with CRT, MTX can result in significant neurocognitive impairment. For example, Bleyer and colleagues[34] found that CRT patients who received concomitant intrathecal MTX as part of their treatment scored around 11 points lower in IQ than those children who received CRT alone. Young females appear most vulnerable to the neurocognitive effects of MTX when it is paired with CRT.[34,35] The greatest cognitive impact of this combination therapy is usually reported for nonverbal functions,[27,28,36,37] although it has been suggested that this relationship is mediated by age, with children under the age of five at the time of treatment showing greater verbal deficits.[38]

In children receiving chemotherapy (including MTX) alone, deficits in spatial functions and visuomotor integration have been observed, although these are milder than those seen following CRT.[39–41] A related deficit in academic performance in all domains, but most notably in arithmetic, has also been reported in a number of studies.[29,42,43] As with radiation, MTX is thought to induce changes in fundamental learning skills, including attention, processing speed and memory.[2,8,33,44,45]

Factors associated with poorer neurocognitive outcomes following MTX include a younger age at treatment, increased time since treatment, and female gender (although the latter is found only for very young children undergoing treatment).[40,44,46] In addition, higher doses of MTX administered either intrathecally or intravenously have been shown to be associated with poorer neurocognitive functioning than lower doses.[44,47,48] It is still unclear whether these deficits progress over time, due to a paucity of longitudinal studies.

Although most research on the unique impact of chemotherapy on cognitive functioning has been with children with ALL, Rutkowski et al.[49] recently reported that postoperative chemotherapy containing high-dose intravenous and intrathecal methotrexate is a promising treatment for medulloblastoma in young children without metastases. However, concerns were raised regarding the neurotoxicity of MTX in this regimen as the mean IQ of the surviving group remained significantly lower than that of healthy, age-matched controls.

Surgery

Surgical resection of brain tumors can also have a significant impact on neurocognitive functioning. The type of impairment seen is associated with the location of the lesion in the infratentorium or supratentorium, with the relative risk considered higher when the tumor has infiltrated normal tissue. Surgery to remove tumors in the cortical mantle will logically affect functions coordinated by that area.[50] It is now also recognized that removing infratentorial tumors can contribute to neurocognitive dysfunction, with documented impairments in working memory, sustained, selective and divided attention, organization and planning, and emotional control in children undergoing surgery alone for low-grade posterior fossa tumors.[51–54]

Interesting findings regarding the impact of surgery and/or a tumor on cognitive functioning in infants come from the recently completed COG study P9934 of infants with medulloblastoma (David M. Ashley, personal communication). This study represents the first comprehensive analysis of the neurodevelopmental progress of this group prior to, during, and after treatment (including surgery). On the basis of parent interviews and formal neuropsychological assessments, these children were found to be delayed following surgery, but prior to commencement of chemotherapy and radiation. No significant declines were evident in either cognitive or motor functioning following chemotherapy or focal conformal radiation. However, while these children continued to make developmental gains in all areas, their progress remained slower than that of same-aged peers posttreatment. This study provides supporting evidence for the impact of surgery and/or a tumor on the cognitive development of this population of children, and highlights the need for a greater emphasis on early assessment.

The impact of potential peri- and postoperative factors (i.e., seizures, infections, bleeds and edema) is also relevant to neurocognitive outcomes following surgery. A greater number of perioperative events is associated with a more pronounced decline in IQ postsurgery,[55] with shunt insertion to treat hydrocephalus linked to impaired attention and slowed processing.[18,56,57] Associations have been reported between younger age at diagnosis and neurocognitive deficits following surgery, because younger children are more likely to present with hydrocephalus and undergo more aggressive surgery than older children in order to delay further treatment.[55,58,59]

Adults

There has been less research into the neurocognitive side effects of brain tumor treatments in adults than in pediatrics, where investigation has been driven by the increasing appreciation of the vulnerability of the developing brain to toxic disruption. While there is now a growing body of literature in the adult population, the etiology of brain tumors in patients over 20 years of age is sufficiently different from that in children, making direct comparisons between the two populations problematic. Crucial to this distinction is the higher occurrence of aggressive cortical tumors in adults (i.e., glioblastoma multiforme), which are more often incurable. The growth characteristics of tumors in adults also differ from those in children,[60] while there is more of a disease-specific focus in the adult literature, which precludes a general analysis of treatment effects per se.

Neurocognitive outcomes from treatment with radiation and chemotherapy are, therefore, less clear in adults than in children. The majority of studies with adults have assessed patients soon after completion of treatment. While findings are inconsistent, there is evidence of an impact of radiation on memory.[61] Similar to the pediatric literature, there are also reports of declines in attention, executive abilities, motor functioning, language, visuospatial, and general intellectual skills posttreatment.[62] These neurocognitive sequelae have been divided into early- and late-delayed phases to differentiate transient versus irreversible side effects of radiation.[63] Early-delayed effects appear to be specific to memory (arguably retrieval of verbal material) and are seen 6–12 weeks posttreatment,[64] and these resolve over time.[65] Late-delayed effects may present anywhere from one to several years post-radiation, and may worsen with time since treatment. Older patients (>60 years) are most vulnerable due to the compounding influence of radiation toxicity on normal age-related decline.[64] However, even younger adults can be affected, and the consideration of factors such as dose, volume of exposed tissue, and fraction size, is important in explaining some of this variance.[43,66]

The research on chemotherapy-related cognitive deficits in adults is particularly difficult to interpret as findings are confounded by the use of combination treatments with heterogeneous dose schedules. Based on findings for lymphoma and breast cancer populations it appears that, in high doses, MTX, cytarabine, cisplatin and the combination of cyclophosphamide, thiotepa and carboplatin may cause cognitive deficits similar to the profile described above for radiation.[63] The relevance to brain tumor groups remains uncertain. Many of these reported effects are thought to be transient, and there is some evidence that patients may show white matter changes related to MTX encephalopathy without any cognitive sequelae.[67,68]

The adult literature is better developed than the pediatric literature in the area of surgical outcomes, with studies showing that location may play a role in predicting the specific nature of neurocognitive dysfunction.[69] It is, therefore, likely that a significant proportion of tumor patients suffer specific cognitive impairment prior to chemotherapy or radiation,[70] and that perioperative factors also contribute to cognitive outcome.[64,71]

In summary, while cognitive dysfunction following treatment for brain tumors in adulthood is documented, it is difficult to estimate the prevalence and course of treatment-related deficits given the high rates of tumor recurrence and the tendency to use follow-up periods that do not cover the length of time required for late effects to emerge.

Mechanisms Underlying Neurocognitive Outcomes

While group-based studies have frequently documented the presence of neurotoxic effects posttreatment, there is remarkable variance in outcome at an individual level, with some survivors functioning normally and others experiencing severe disability. In the next section, we explore the relationship of several patient- and treatment-related factors that may be particularly important in predicting risk and resilience for individuals with brain tumors.

Treatment Factors

Brain tumor treatments impact all cerebral tissue. White matter injury appears to be the principal common anatomical pathway for the induction of treatment-related late effects.[72] Myelin is selectively damaged, disrupting its role in promoting efficient transmission of nerve impulses.[73] Imaging studies identify white matter hyperintensities, although some studies have reported the resolution of these lesions over time.[74] The degree of damage has been determined by quantifying the volume of "Normal Appearing White Matter" (NAWM) in the brain. Children with medulloblastoma undergoing radiation have been found to have less NAWM than healthy children, with volume loss correlated with deficits in attention and IQ.[47,75,76] More recently, diffusion tensor imaging has been employed to assess the integrity of the existing white matter, with results suggesting damage to insulating fibers.[77] Importantly, greater damage to white matter structures is seen in younger children, as well as those receiving higher doses of radiation,[47,78,79] and is associated with poorer cognitive outcome in many instances.

Radiation-induced white matter compromise is generally presented as either the end result of damage to glial cells, or the vascular system. The first pathophysiologic model highlights the sensitivity of oligodendrocytes to radiation.[80] Their destruction is thought to lead to the inefficient remyelination of damaged fibers and, with time, the loss of healthy tissue. The latter model refers mainly to adults who, through age, are more susceptible to vascular damage.[64] Animal studies suggest microangiopathy and capillary loss following radiation exposure, which eventually results in reduced vessel density and white matter necrosis.[63,81,82] Interestingly, findings for MTX suggest the same underlying vascular damage through hypothesized disruption to the folate pathway.[83] As an anti-folate, MTX has the potential to disrupt DNA and RNA synthesis, gene regulation and myelin maintenance.[33] As a result there is demyelination, occlusive vascular disease and microangiopathy leading to cognitive late effects. It has recently been acknowledged that impairment of neurogenesis in the hippocampus may provide another model to explain deficits in learning following treatment for a brain tumor.[84] Specifically, the deficit in cell proliferation impacts memory systems, and can occur without any evidence of damage on imaging.[85] Since there is evidence to support each of these models, it would appear that the mechanism of damage is complex and likely involves disruption to all of these systems.

Dosage

Most study findings support a dose-response relationship for radiation and MTX with regard to neuropathology.[22,44,86] It is unclear whether there is a minimum threshold or 'safe' dose for either treatment that carries no risk of cognitive late effects. As a result contemporary protocols are geared towards limiting doses using risk-adapted regimes. Radiation has again received the greatest focus in this area, given its known toxicity. Standard doses in children with malignant tumors are set around 24–40 Gy, and this level is known to place children at significant risk of long-term neurocognitive deficits.[3,6] The more recent use of reduced-dose regimes (20–35 Gy) has shown promise in decreasing rates of cognitive morbidity, but some children, namely those who are younger at the time of treatment, are vulnerable even at doses as low as 18 Gy.[27,87] While analyses of dose relationships have not commonly been undertaken in the adult field, it does appear that the same relationship applies, with very high doses (70 Gy) posing some risk for cognitive delayed effects, while moderate doses hold very low risk (50 Gy).[66]

For chemotherapy, dosage effects are less clear, with a number of nonsignificant findings reported.[30,32] There is evidence that deficits are only seen with high-dose regimens, a high infusion rate, or a greater number of injections.[88,89] A threshold effect also appears most likely for MTX as the drug is considered more toxic as the cumulative dose increases.[39]

Administration Method and Timing

The volume of healthy tissue exposed to radiation is closely related to the modality in which the beams are delivered. Whole-brain or craniospinal techniques are used with malignant tumors that have the potential to metastasize within the CNS. These methods place healthy brain tissue at risk, and can result in generalized dysfunction when given at high doses. An inverse relationship exists between the amount of brain volume irradiated and the level of intellectual functioning.[4,6,22] For this reason whole-brain radiation dosage is often kept to a minimum, while providing the tumor site with a higher dose boost. This has been achieved through technological advances in the form of conformal techniques and stereotactically guided administration.

Unlike radiation, chemotherapy works at a systemic level. For MTX, the administration method has been shown to be related to effectiveness, with intrathecal and intravenous administration providing the most direct route to tumor cells. The intrathecal method allows the drug access to healthy developing brain tissue and, particularly when used together with intravenous administration, appears to increase the risk of toxicity.[33] Of particular significance to the brain tumor population is the finding that intrathecal MTX appears most toxic when administered in close succession to radiation.[34,35] The synergistic effect of the two treatments is thought to be explained through the weakening of the brain's natural defense (the blood-brain barrier) by radiation, which then allows MTX to cross this protective membrane and come into direct contact with nerve cells.[90]

Developmental Factors

Cognitive dysfunction is a symptom of structural damage or disruption to a neural system. When considering treatment-related effects it must be acknowledged that the brain is constantly undergoing change and is different in both structure and function throughout the lifespan. To truly appreciate the consistent finding of age at treatment as a strong predictor of outcome, treatment effects must be considered within a developmental context of normal maturation.

Normal Maturational Trajectory

The brain develops rapidly during gestation, with brain cells reaching their cortical destination by the 24th week of gestation, after which they begin to differentiate into unique cell types.[91] Various anatomical processes (e.g., synaptogenesis, dendritic branching) lead to a major expansion of the cortex over the first four years of life, initially in primary areas such as the visual cortex and later in tertiary areas such as the prefrontal cortex.[92] Programmed cell death then takes over as the major force shaping and refining gray matter structure over adolescence and early adulthood.[93] This results in a decrease in gray matter volume, which is offset by a corresponding expansion in white matter.[94]

Proliferation and differentiation of oligodendrocytes occurs at the tail end of maturation, and continues to follow a delayed maturational trajectory, with those white matter structures that are particularly vulnerable to CRT and MTX reaching adult levels only in the late 20s.[95,96] Parietal and frontal structures are the last areas to complete myelination and are, therefore, most susceptible to damage in childhood and adolescence.[96] If these normal developmental processes are disrupted by factors such as CRT or MTX, they have the potential to cause permanent alteration in the wiring of brain circuitry. Disruption to connectivity between cortical areas, in turn, leads to deficits in cognitive skills such as information processing, attentional control, and memory. Normal age-related degeneration occurs later in life around age 50, with a progressive decrease in the efficiency of information transfer.[97] White matter structures in the prefrontal areas show a preferential loss of tissue.[98] Disruption to circuits during this time will further compound the cognitive effects of this normal decay.

Age at Treatment

Age is a convenient proxy for structural and, therefore, functional development. In parallel with the trajectory described above, damage resulting from radiation and chemotherapy treatments in the first few years of life will likely impact the amount and integrity of both white and gray matter. Children under four years of age, and in particular infants, are therefore at greatest risk.[4,99] Deficits in this group are seen across all cognitive domains, with devastating results. It has become common practice not to use radiation treatment with children under three years and, whenever possible, chemotherapy is used to delay the need for radiation in the young child.

Damage after this time would be expected to target myelin production more specifically. An inverse relationship between age at treatment and cognitive performance is generally reported for children below 7–8 years of age,[87] while some studies argue for a broader age range at increased risk (e.g., 5- to 10-year-olds).[52] The deficits in learning that occur through damage to white matter structures result in a failure to acquire skills at an age-appropriate rate, which is evidenced as a drop in IQ scores over time.[10] For the older child and adolescent, with their greater skill base and experience, this decrease in intellectual ability may not be seen, as the skills they have already mastered are retained.[64] Instead, deficits occur in skills that they are yet to acquire such as mathematics and executive functions.

The adult brain is better able to deal with the side effects of radiation and chemotherapeutic drugs because of its relatively stable state. Even if subtle processing or memory deficits occur, this is unlikely to result in the same type, or degree, of functional impairment as that seen in children, given that most adults have acquired all the skills necessary to work and live independently. However, the degree of functional impairment will again increase in the older adult population, as individuals in their late 60s who are already experiencing normal age-related cerebral atrophy are less able to compensate, both neurologically and cognitively, for a further insult to the brain.

Age at Assessment

Another important factor to consider in defining the structural and functional development of a patient is age at assessment. Consistent with a developmental framework, individuals of different ages can be expected to show different levels of competence in unique cognitive domains. Therefore, deficits in functions will not become evident until the time that they are due to come 'on-line'. For example, a child who has received high-dose cranial radiation for a frontal lobe tumor at five years of age may not show significant deficits until assessed at the age of 10 years when they have failed to develop competence in working memory and organizational skills. This pattern has been described in the pediatric literature as "growing into deficits"[100] and highlights the need for long-term follow-up of brain tumor survivors.

Genetics – Epigenetics

It is likely that genes have a role in determining the vulnerability of individual patients to these risk and resilience factors. In particular, differences in the patient's genetic background known as polymorphisms in key pathways are likely to contribute significantly to the observed variability. Toxicities that occur after chemotherapy represent useful paradigms for identifying genetic polymorphisms in enzyme systems that modulate local and systemic responses to stress during therapy. Ongoing studies in this area are providing clues to the prevention of adverse clinical outcomes based on the genetic milieu. A review of studies that explore genetic risk factors for treatment complications indicates that significant progress is being made in this rapidly evolving area. However, further large scale sophisticated clinical and translational studies are needed before genomic screening can be widely used to individualize treatment.[101–105]

Environmental Factors

Neurocognitive outcomes following treatment for brain tumors may also be influenced by environmental factors.[106] Although little research has directly investigated the impact of such factors on neurocognitive outcomes in brain tumor survivors, evidence pointing to the potential importance of environmental variables comes from research with other brain injured populations. In children who have sustained traumatic brain injuries, for example, characteristics of the family environment, such as socioeconomic status and family functioning, have been shown to contribute to neurocognitive outcomes.[107–110] That these environmental factors interact with developmental and injury-related factors in producing neurocognitive outcomes following traumatic brain injury has also been emphasized.[108,111] An important direction for future research with brain tumor survivors will be to investigate the impact of environmental factors on neurocognitive outcomes, and to understand how these factors interact with developmental and illness-related factors to predict outcomes.

Interventions

Despite the well-documented neurocognitive late effects of childhood cancer treatments, there is little published research examining the effectiveness of interventions to address these deficits.[106] A notable exception is the work of Butler and Copeland,[112] who implemented a cognitive remediation program with childhood cancer survivors with attentional difficulties. Their intervention involved 40 hours of treatment over six months, comprising mainly individual sessions with an interventionist, and incorporated massed practice drills aimed at directly improving attentional skills as well as training in metacognitive and cognitive-behavioral strategies. Six-month pilot data showed significant improvement in vigilance, attention, and concentration for the intervention group ($N=20$; 4 brain tumor survivors), relative to a no-treatment control group.

Further support for cognitive remediation with brain tumor survivors comes from research by van't Hooft and colleagues,[113] who implemented a cognitive retraining program with nine- to 17-year-olds experiencing attention and memory difficulties following a variety of brain injuries, including brain tumors. Teachers or parents encouraged participants to complete exercises targeting attentional and metacognitive skills every day (30 min) for 17 weeks. Participants also attended weekly hospital-based sessions where they discussed their cognitive, emotional, and behavioral experiences. Post-training, the intervention group (N=20; 4 brain tumor survivors), relative to a no-treatment group, showed improved attention and memory.

These studies provide preliminary evidence supporting the use of cognitive remediation to address cognitive deficits in brain tumor survivors. Clearly, however, intervention research with this population is in its infancy, and further research is needed to establish how best to address these deficits. A number of factors warrant consideration. To develop maximally efficient interventions, it will be important to disentangle which specific components of the multimodal and time-intensive intervention programs just described are most effective. Further, these intervention studies involved pediatric populations with heterogeneous diagnoses; it will, therefore, be important in future research to establish the extent to which survivors of brain tumors, specifically, benefit from cognitive remediation, as well as whether adults can benefit from these types of interventions.

Developing methods for early identification of patients most likely to require intervention, as well as those most likely to respond to different forms of intervention, will also facilitate the delivery of targeted programs. Investigating the optimal timing for interventions is also important; for example, "prophylactic" cognitive interventions may be more beneficial than those implemented after deficits have emerged.[8,106] Related to this, a developmental approach to remediation is critical since, as we discussed earlier, some cognitive deficits will only become evident as emerging skills are due to come "on line" at specific developmental stages. Intervention approaches that involve tracking patients over time and intervening at key developmental and recovery time-points may, therefore, be most effective.[114]

In addition, there have recently been calls for multimodal, ecologically valid, environmentally based intervention approaches with brain tumor survivors; that is, interventions that do not target cognitive deficits in isolation, but address the multiple environmental factors that may contribute to neurocognitive outcomes.[10,20] Indeed, growing support for the effectiveness of such interventions in the traumatic brain injury population[114] underscores the importance of determining and targeting environmental factors that may influence neurocognitive outcomes in brain tumor survivors. Assessing the impact of interventions on functional outcomes should also be a priority, in view of the poor educational and occupational outcomes that have been documented in a significant proportion of brain tumor survivors.[115]

Other promising data regarding the remediation of cognitive deficits in pediatric cancer survivors comes from research examining pharmacological interventions such as methylphenidate.[116,117] A detailed description of this research is beyond the scope of this chapter, but the reader is referred to Chapter 20 in this volume for more on this topic.

Limitations and Future Directions

This chapter has focused upon the major trends in the literature on the neuropsychological impact of treating brain tumors. However, there is still much contention regarding the type, degree, and mechanism of cognitive impairment seen in survivors. These mixed findings are a reflection of the inherent difficulty in conducting research into rare diseases. Sample sizes are often small, patient characteristics diverse, tumor types heterogeneous, age ranges and time since treatment disparate, and treatment regimes multimodal. Differentiating the contribution of individual treatments and treatment components to neurocognitive outcome is, therefore, extremely difficult, and subtle effects may be overlooked because of the amount of variance in the samples. This is particularly relevant for older patients who are often on polytherapy for other medical conditions (e.g., cerebrovascular disease, diabetes) which may make them more vulnerable to tumor treatments.

While the impact of the tumor (hydrocephalus, seizures, mass effect) and perioperative complications (bleeds, edema, infection) on neurocognitive outcome have recently been acknowledged, pretreatment baseline assessments of cognitive functioning are rarely obtained due to the urgency with which these patients undergo treatment.[18,56,57] Follow-up assessments are then often performed soon after completing treatment (within the first 12 months) without further tracking of patient progress. Late effects are, therefore, potentially overlooked as the emergence of deficits occurs at a later stage, peaking around the 24-month mark. Most studies that have attempted a longer follow-up have used retrospective, cross-sectional samples of patients, which limits the analysis of the trajectory of deficits and the relationship between treatment and patient factors. More prospective, longitudinal studies that track individual patients over time, while taking into account preexisting and surgery-related deficits, and accounting for chemotherapy regimes, are much needed and will help to elucidate the complex algorithm for risk of treatment-related decline.

Furthermore, a more refined approach in the measurement of cognitive deficits is crucial to further research on neuropsychological outcomes. Traditionally, and particularly with adults, tests of IQ have been used, but these provide only a relatively crude assessment of neuropsychological capacity. Such tests mainly sample acquired knowledge with little emphasis on learning ability, or 'fluid' intelligence, which are the skills that appear most affected by tumor treatments. Learning or processing deficits will only be reflected in IQ over time as they impact the rate of skill and knowledge acquisition. This is consistent with a delayed picture of impairment in IQ scores, and highlights the possibility that attentional and working memory deficits occur earlier in the treatment phase. Therefore, a more targeted approach, based on a theoretical model of white matter damage and normal maturational trajectories, needs to be implemented, with specific measurement of these abilities over time. Neuropsychological assessment could then be paired with structural and functional imaging to better understand the anatomical correlates of cognitive impairment. Such studies would provide valuable information to guide the development and implementation of appropriate strategies to stem the decline in knowledge attainment, particularly for children.

Finally, further research is clearly needed to establish effective and targeted interventions to address the neurocognitive deficits that are now well-documented in brain tumor survivors. Ultimately, the goal is to develop interventions that will not only improve neuropsychological outcomes, but that will also yield improvements in related functional outcomes, such as educational and vocational functioning, which have the potential, in turn, to enhance survivors' quality of life.

References

1. Gajjar A, Chintagumpala M, Ashley D, et al. Risk-adapted craniospinal radiotherapy followed by high-dose chemotherapy and stem-cell rescue in children with newly diagnosed medulloblastoma (St. Jude Medulloblastoma-96): long-term results from a prospective, multicentre trial. *Lancet Oncol.*2006;7:813–820.
2. Garcia-Perez A, Narbona-Garcia J, Sierrasesumaga L, Aguirre-Ventallo M, Calvo-Manuel F. Neuropsychological outcome of children after radiotherapy for intracranial tumours. *Dev Med Child Neurol.* 1993;35:139–148.
3. Maddrey AM, Bergeron JA, Lombardo ER, et al. Neuropsychological performance and quality of life of 10 year survivors of childhood medulloblastoma. *J Neurooncol.* 2005;72:245–253.
4. Mulhern RK, Hancock J, Fairclough D, Kun L. Neuropsychological status of children treated for brain tumors: A critical review and integrative analysis. *Med Pediatr Oncol.* 1992;20:181–191.
5. Roman DD, Sperduto PW. Neuropsychological effects of cranial radiation: current knowledge and future directions. *Int J Radiat Biol Phys.*1995;31:983–998.
6. Palmer SL, Gajjar A, Reddick WE, et al. Predicting Intellectual Outcome Among Children Treated With 35– 40 Gy Craniospinal Irradiation for Medulloblastoma. *Neuropsychology.* 2003;17:548–555.
7. Ris MD, Packer R, Goldwein J, Jones-Wallace D, Boyett JM. Intellectual outcome after reduced-dose radiation therapy plus adjuvant chemotherapy for medulloblastoma: a Children's Cancer Group study. *J Clin Oncol.* 2001;19:3470–3476.
8. Moore BD. Neurocognitive outcomes in survivors of childhood cancer. *J Pediatr Psychol.* 2005;30:51–63.
9. Mulhern RK, Merchant TE, Gajjar A, Reddick WE, Kun LE. Late neurocognitive sequelae in survivors of brain tumours in childhood. *Lancet Oncol.* 2004;5:339–408.
10. Palmer SL, Reddick, WE, Gajjar, A. Understanding the cognitive impact on children who are treated for medulloblastoma. *J Pediatr Psychol.* 2007;32:1040–1049.
11. Kieffer-Renaux V, Viguier D, Raquin M-A, et al. Therapeutic schedules influence the pattern of intellectual decline after irradiation of posterior fossa tumors. *Pediatr Blood Cancer.* 2005;45:814–819.
12. Spiegler BJ, Bouffet E, Greenberg ML, Rukta JT, Mabbott DJ. Change in neurocognitive functioning after treatment with cranial radiation in childhood. *J Clin Oncol.* 2004;22:706–713.
13. Stargatt R, Rosenfeld JV, Maixner W, Ashley D. Multiple factors contribute to neuropsychological outcome in children with posterior fossa tumors. *Dev Neuropsychol.* 2007;32:729–748.

14. Mulhern RK, Kepner JL, Thomas PR, Armstrong FD, Friedman HS, Kun LE. Neuropsychologic functioning of survivors of childhood medulloblastoma randomized to receive conventional or reduced-dose craniospinal irradiation: a Pediatric Oncology Group study. *J Clin Oncol.* 1998;16:1723–1728.
15. Riva D, Milani N, Pantaleoni C, Ballerini E, Giorgi C. Combined treatment modality for medulloblastoma in childhood: effects on neuropsychological functioning. *Neuropediatrics.* 1991;22:36–42.
16. Mabbott DJ, Spiegler BJ, Greenberg ML, Rutka JT, Hyder DJ, Bouffet E. Serial Evaluation of Academic and Behavioral Outcome After Treatment With Cranial Radiation in Childhood. *J Clin Oncol.* 2005;23:2256–2263.
17. Copeland DR, deMoor C, Moore BD, 3rd, Ater JL. Neurocognitive development of children after a cerebellar tumor in infancy: A longitudinal study. *J Clin Oncol.* 1999;17:3476–3486.
18. Reimers TS, Mortensen EL, Schmiegelow K. Memory deficits in long-term survivors of childhood brain tumors may primarily reflect general cognitive dysfunctions. *Pediatr Blood Cancer.* 2007;48:205–212.
19. Schatz J, Kramer JH, Ablin A, Matthay KK. Processing speed, working memory, and IQ: a developmental model of cognitive deficits following cranial radiation therapy. *Neuropsychology.* 2000;14:189–200.
20. Mulhern RK, Butler RW. Neurocognitive sequelae of childhood cancers and their treatments. *Pediatr Rehabil.* 2004;7:1–14.
21. Butler RW, Haser JK. Neurocognitive effects of treatment for childhood cancer. *Ment Retard Dev Disabil Res Rev.* 2006;12:184–191.
22. Merchant TE, Kiehna EN, Li C-S, Xiong X, Mulhern RK. Radiation dosimetry predicts IQ after conformal radiation therapy in pediatric patients with localized ependymoma. *Int J Radiat Biol Phys.* 2005;63:1546–1554.
23. Dennis M, Spiegler BJ, Hetherington CR, Greenberg ML. Neuropsychological sequelae of the treatment of children with medulloblastoma. *J Neurooncol.* 1996;29:91–101.
24. Kiehna EN, Mulhern RK, Li C, Xiong X, Merchant TE. Changes in attentional performance of children and young adults with localized primary brain tumors after conformal radiation therapy. *J Clin Oncol.* 2006;24:5283–5290.
25. Fouladi M, Gilger E, Kocak M, et al. Intellectual and functional outcome of children 3 years old or younger who have CNS malignancies. *J Clin Oncol.* 2005;23:7152–7160.
26. Merchant TE, Mulhern RK, Krasin MJ, et al. Preliminary results from a phase II trial of conformal radiation therapy and evaluation of radiation-related CNS effects for pediatric patients with localized ependymoma. *J Clin Oncol.* 2004;22:3156–3162.
27. Anderson VA, Godber T, Smibert E, Weiskop S, Ekert H. Cognitive and academic outcome following cranial irradiation and chemotherapy in children: a longitudinal study. *Br J Cancer.* 2000;82:25–62.
28. Butler RW, Hill JM, Steinherz PG, Meyers PA, Finlay JL. Neuropsychological effects of cranial irradiation, intrathecal methotrexate and systemic methotrexate in childhood cancer. *J Clin Oncol.* 1994;12:2621–2629.
29. Copeland DR, Moore BDI, Francis DJ, Jaffe N, Culbert SJ. Neuropsychologic effects of chemotherapy on children with cancer: a longitudinal study. *J Clin Oncol.* 1996;14:2826–2835.
30. Nathan PC, Whitcomb T, Wolters PL, et al. Very high-dose methotrexate (33.6 g/m2) as central nervous system preventive therapy for childhood acute lymphoblastic leukemia: results of National Cancer Institute/Children's Cancer Group trials CCG-191P, CCG-134P and CCG-144P. *Leuk Lymphoma.* 2006;47:248–504.
31. Smibert E, Anderson VA, Godber T, Ekert H. Risk factors for intellectual and educational sequelae of cranial irradiation in childhood acute lymphoblastic leukaemia. *Br J Cancer.* 1996;73:825–830.

32. Spiegler BJ, Kennedy K, Maze R, et al. Comparison of long-term neurocognitive outcome in young children with acute lymphoblastic leukemia treated with cranial radiation or high-dose or very high-dose intravenous methotrexate. *J Clin Oncol*. 2006;24:3858–3864.
33. Moleski M. Neuropsychological, neuroanatomical, and neurophysiological consequences of CNS chemotherapy for acute lymphoblastic leukemia. *Arch Clin Neuropsychol*. 2000;15: 603–630.
34. Bleyer WA, Fallavollita J, Robison L, et al. Influence of age, sex and concurrent intrathecal methotrexate therapy on intellectual function after cranial irradiation during childhood: a report from the Children's Cancer Study Group. *Pediatr Hematol Oncol*. 1990;7:329–338.
35. Waber DP, Tarbell NJ, Fairclough D, et al. Cognitive sequelae of treatment in childhood acute lymphoblastic leukemia: cranial radiation requires an accomplice. *J Clin Oncol*. 1995;13:3490–3496.
36. Campbell LK, Scaduto M, Sharp W, et al. A meta-analysis of the neurocognitive sequelae of treatment for childhood acute lymphocytic leukemia. *Pediatr Blood Cancer*. 2007;49: 65–73.
37. Riva D, Giorgi C, Nichelli F, et al. Intrathecal methotrexate affects cognitive function in children with medulloblastoma. *Neurology*. 2002;59:48–53.
38. Anderson V, Godber T, Smibert E, Ekert H. Neurobehavioural sequelae following cranial irradiation and chemotherapy in children: an analysis of risk factors. *Pediatr Rehabil*. 1997;1:63–76.
39. Montour-Proulx I, Kuehn SM, Keene DL, et al. Cognitive changes in children treated for acute lymphoblastic leukemia with chemotherapy only according to the Pediatric Oncology Group 9605 protocol. *J Child Neurol*. 2005;20:129–133.
40. Brown RT, Madan-Swain A, Walco GA, et al. Cognitive and academic late effects among children previously treated for acute lymphocytic leukemia receiving chemotherapy as CNS prophylaxis. *J Pediatr Psychol*. 1998;23:3–40.
41. von der Weid N, Mosimann I, Hirt A, et al. Intellectual outcome in children and adolescents with acute lymphoblastic leukaemia treated with chemotherapy alone: age- and sex-related differences. *Eur J Cancer*. 2003;39:359–365.
42. Raymond-Speden E, Tripp G, Lawrence B, Holdaway D. Intellectual, Neuropsychological, and Academic Functioning in Long-Term Survivors of Leukemia. *J Pediatr Psychol*. 2000; 25:59–68.
43. Crossen JR, Garwood D, Glatstein E, Neuwelt EA. Neurobehavioral sequelae of cranial irradiation in adults: a review of radiation-induced encephalopathy. *J Clin Oncol*. 1994; 12:627–642.
44. Buizer AI, de Sonneville LMJ, van den Heuvel-Eibrink MM, Veerman AJP. Chemotherapy and attentional dysfunction in survivors of childhood acute lymphoblastic leukemia: effect of treatment intensity. *Pediatr Blood Cancer*. 2005;45:281–290.
45. Mennes M, Stiers P, Vandenbussche E, et al. Attention and information processing in survivors of childhood acute lymphoblastic leukemia treated with chemotherapy only. *Pediatr Blood Cancer*. 2005;44:478–486.
46. Espy KA, Moore IM, Kaufmann PM, Kramer JH, Matthay KK, Hutter JJ. Chemotherapeutic CNS prophylaxis and neuropsychologic change in children with acute lymphoblastic leukemia: a prospective study. *J Pediatr Psychol*. 2001;26:1–9.
47. Reddick WE, Glass JO, Palmer SL, et al. Atypical white matter volume development in children following craniospinal irradiation. Neuro-Oncology. 2005;7:12–19.
48. Shapiro WR, Allen JC, Horten BC. Chronic methotrexate toxicity to the central nervous system. *Clin Bull*. 1980;10:49–52.
49. Rutkowski S, Bode U, Deinlein F, et al. Treatment of early childhood medulloblastoma by postoperative chemotherapy alone. *N Engl J Med*. 2005;352:978–986.
50. Anderson V, Northam E, Hendy J, Wrennall J. *Developmental Neuropsychology*. UK: Psychology Press Ltd; 2001.

51. Gottwald B, Wilde B, Mihajlovic Z, Mehdorn HM. Evidence for distinct cognitive deficits after focal cerebellar lesions. *J Neurol Neurosurg Psychiatry*. 2004;75:1524–1531.
52. Steinlin M, Imfeld S, Zulauf P, et al. Neuropsychological long-term sequelae after posterior fossa tumour resection during childhood. *Brain*. 2003;126:1998–2008.
53. Gottwald B, Mihajlovic Z, Wilde B, Mehdorn HM. Does the cerebellum contribute to specific aspects of attention? *Neuropsychologia*. 2003;41:1452–1460.
54. Stargatt R, Anderson V, Rosenfeld JV. Neuropsychological Outcome of Children Treated for Posterior Fossa Tumours: A Review. *Brain Impairment*. 2002;3:92–104.
55. Kao GD, Goldwein JW, Schultz DJ, Radcliffe J, Sutton L, Lange B. The impact of perioperative factors on subsequent intelligence quotient deficits in children treated for medulloblastoma/posterior fossa primitive neuroectodermal tumors. *Cancer*. 1994;74: 965–971.
56. Merchant TE, Lee H, Zhu J, et al. The effects of hydrocephalus on intelligence quotient in children with localized infratentorial ependymoma before and after focal radiation therapy. *J Neurosurg*. 2004;101:159–168.
57. Merchant TE, Kiehna EN, Miles MA, Zhu J, Xiong X, Mulhern RK. Acute effects of irradiation on cognition: changes in attention on a computerized continuous performance test during radiotherapy in pediatric patients with localized primary brain tumors. *Int J Radiat Biol Phys*. 2002;53:1271–1278
58. Chapman CA, Waber DP, Bernstein JH, et al. Neurobehavioral and neurologic outcome in long-term survivors of posterior fossa brain tumors: role of age and perioperative factors. *J Child Neurol*. 1995;10:209–212.
59. Packer RJ, Sposto R, Atkins TE, et al. Quality of life in children with primitive neuroectodermal tumors (medulloblastoma) of the posterior fossa. *Pediatr Neurosci*. 1987;13:169–175.
60. Sarkar C, Pramanik P, Karak AK, et al. Are childhood and adult medulloblastomas different? A comparative study of clinicopathological features, proliferation index and apoptotic index. *J Neurooncol*. 2002;59:49–61.
61. Armstrong CL, Stern CH, Corn BW. Memory performance used to detect radiation effects on cognitive functioning. *Appl Neuropsychol*. 2001;8:129–139.
62. Welzel G, Steinvorth S, Wenz F. Cognitive effects of chemotherapy and/or cranial irradiation in adults. *Strahlenther Onkol*. 2004;181:141–156.
63. Taphoorn MJB, Klein M. Cognitive deficits in adult patients with brain tumours. *Lancet Neurol*. 2004;3:159–168.
64. Armstrong CL, Gyato K, Awadalla AW, Lustig R, Tochner ZA. A critical review of the clinical effects of therapeutic irradiation damage to the brain: the roots of controversy. *Neuropsychol Rev*. 2004;14:65–86.
65. Torres IJ, Mundt AJ, Sweeney PJ, et al. A longitudinal neuropsychological study of partial brain radiation in adults with brain tumors. *Neurology*. 2003;60:1113–1118.
66. Laack NN, Brown PD. Cognitive sequelae of brain irradiation in adults. *Semin Oncol*. 2004;31:702–713.
67. Neuwelt EA, Guastadisegni PE, Varallyay P, Doolittle ND. Imaging changes and cognitive outcome in primary CNS lymphoma after enhanced chemotherapy delivery. *AJNR*. 2005; 26:258–265.
68. Fliessbach K, Urbach H, Helmstaedter C, et al. Cognitive performance and magnetic resonance imaging findings after high-dose systemic and intraventricular chemotherapy for primary central nervous system lymphoma. *Arch Neurol*. 2003;60:563–568.
69. Brown PD, Buckner JC, Uhm JH, Shaw EG. The neurocognitive effects of radiation in adult low-grade glioma patients. Neuro-Oncology. 2003;5:161–167.
70. Tucha O, Smely C, Preier M, Lange K. Cognitive deficits before treatment among patients with brain tumors. *Neurosurgery*. 2000;47:324–334.
71. Klein M, Heimans JJ, Aaronsen NK, et al. Effect of radiotherapy and other treatment-related factors on mid-term to long-term cognitive sequelae in low-grade gliomas: a comparative study. *The Lancet*. 2002;360:1361–1368.

72. Steen RG, Spence D, Shengjie W, Xiong X, Kun LE, Merchant TE. Effect of therapeutic ionizing radiation on the human brain. *Ann Neurol.* 2001;50:787–795.

73. Fletcher JM, Copeland DR. Neurobehavioural effects of central nervous system prophylactic treatment of cancer in children. *J Clin Exp Neuropsychol.* 1988;10:495–537.

74. Fouladi M, Chintagumpala M, Laningham FH, et al. White matter lesions detected by magnetic resonance imaging after radiotherapy and high-dose chemotherapy in children with medulloblastoma or primitive neuroectodermal tumor. *J Clin Oncol.* 2004;22:4551–4560.

75. Reddick WE, White HA, Glass JO, et al. Developmental model relating white matter volume to neurocognitive deficits in pediatric brain tumor survivors. *Cancer.* 2003;97: 2512–2519.

76. Reddick WE, Shan ZY, Glass JO, et al. Smaller white-matter volumes are associated with larger deficits in attention and learning among long-term survivors of acute lymphoblastic leukemia. *Cancer.* 2006;106:941–949.

77. Khong PL, Leung LH, Chan GC, et al. White matter anisotropy in childhood medulloblastoma survivors: association with neurotoxicity risk factors. *Radiology.* 2005;236: 647–652.

78. Khong PL, Leung LH, Fung AS, et al. White matter anisotropy in post-treatment childhood cancer survivors: preliminary evidence of association with neurocognitive function. *J Clin Oncol.* 2006;24:884–890.

79. Qiu D, Leung LH, Kwong DL, Chan GC, Khong PL. Mapping radiation dose distribution on the fractional anisotropy map: applications in the assessment of treatment-induced white matter injury. *Neuroimage.* 2006;31:109–115.

80. Perry A, Schmidt RE. Cancer therapy-associated CNS neuropathology: an update and review of the literature. *Acta Neuropathol.* 2006;111:197–212.

81. Brown WR, Thore CR, Moody DM, Robbins ME, Wheeler KT. Vascular damage after fractionated whole-brain irradiation in rats. *Radiat Res.* 2005;164:662–668.

82. Brown WR, Blair RM, Moody DM, et al. Capillary loss precedes the cognitive impairment induced by fractionated whole-brain irradiation: a potential rat model of vascular dementia. *J Neurol Sci.* 2007;257:67–71.

83. Cole PD, Kamen BA. Delayed neurotoxicity associated with therapy for children with acute lymphoblastic leukemia. *Ment Retard Dev Dis.* 2006;12:174–183.

84. Rola R, Raber J, Rizk A, et al. Radiation-induced impairment of hippocampal neurogenesis is associated with cognitive deficits in young mice. *Exp Neurol.* 2004;188:316–330.

85. Monje ML, Palmer T. Radiation injury and neurogenesis. *Curr Opin Neurol.* 2003;16: 129–134.

86. Grill J, Renaux VK, Bulteau C, et al. Long-term intellectual outcome in children with posterior fossa tumors according to radiation doses and volumes. *Int J Radiat Biol Phys.* 1999;45:137–145.

87. Mulhern RK, Palmer SL, Merchant TE, et al. Neurocognitive consequences of risk-adapted therapy for childhood medulloblastoma. *J Clin Oncol.* 2005;23:551–559.

88. Carey ME, Hockenberry MJ, Moore IM, et al. Effect of intravenous methotrexate dose and infusion rate on neuropsychological function one year after diagnosis of acute lymphoblastic leukemia. *J Pediatr Psychol.* 2007;32:189–193.

89. Iuvone L, Mariotti P, Colosimo C, Guzzetta F, Ruggiero A, Riccardi R. Long-term cognitive outcome, brain computed tomography scan, and magnetic resonance imaging in children cured for acute lymphoblastic leukemia. *Cancer.* 2002;95:2562–2670.

90. Storm AJ, van der Kogel AJ, Nooter K. Effect of X-irradiation on the pharmacokinetics of methotrexate in rats: alteration of the blood-brain barrier. *Eur J Cancer Clin Oncol.* 1985;21:759–764.

91. Lagercrantz H, Ringstedt T. Epigenetic and functional organization of the neuronal circuits in the CNS during development. In: Levene MI, Chervenak FA, Whittle M, Bennett MJ, Punt J, eds. *Fetal and Neonatal Neurology and Neurosurgery.* 3rd ed. London: Churchill Livingstone; 2001:3–9.

92. Huttenlocher PR. Morphometric study of human cerebral cortex development. In: Johnson MH, ed. *Brain Development and Cognition*. Cambridge, USA: Blackwell Publishers; 1993: 112–124.
93. Erecinska M, Cherian S, Silver IA. Energy metabolism in mammalian brain during development. *Prog Neurobiol*. 2004;73:392–445.
94. Giedd JN. Brain development during childhood and adolescence: a longitudinal MRI study. *Nat Neurosci*. 1999;2:861–863.
95. Benes FM, Turtle M, Farol P. Myelination of a key relay zone in the hippocampal formation occurs in the human brain during childhood, adolescence, and adulthood. *Arch Gen Psychiatry*. 1994;51:47–84.
96. Yakovlev PI, Lecours AR. The myelogenetic cycles of regional maturation of the brain. In: Minokowski A, ed. Regional development of the brain in early life. Philadelphia: Blackwell; 1967:3–70.
97. Brickman AM, Zimmerman ME, Paul RH, et al. Regional white matter and neuropsychological functioning across the adult lifespan. *Biol Psychiatry*. 2006;60:4–53.
98. Salat DH, Tuch DS, Greve DN, et al. Age-related alterations in white matter microstructure measured by diffusion tensor imaging. *Neurobiol Aging*. 2005;26:1215–1227.
99. Fouladi M, Gilger E, Kocak M, et al. Intellectual and functional outcome of children 3 years old or younger who have CNS malignancies. *J Clin Oncol*. 2005;23:7152–160.
100. Hebb DO. *The Organization of Behavior*. New York: McGraw-Hill; 1949.
101. Andreassen CN, Alsner J, Overgaard J. Does variability in normal tissue reactions after radiotherapy have a genetic basis-where and how to look for it? *Radiother Oncol*. 2002; 64:131–140.
102. Andreassen CN, Alsner J, Overgaard J, et al. TGFB1 polymorphisms are associated with risk of late normal tissue complications in the breast after radiotherapy for early breast cancer. *Radiother Oncol*. 2005;75:18–21.
103. De Ruyck K, Wilding CS, Van Eijkeren M, Morthier R, Tawn EJ, Thierens H. Microsatellite polymorphisms in DNA repair genes XRCC1, XRCC3 and XRCC5 in patients with gynecological tumors: association with late clinical radiosensitivity and cancer incidence. *Radiat Res*. 2005; 164:237–244.
104. Hall EJ, Schiff PB, Hanks GE, et al. A preliminary report: frequency of A-T heterozygotes among prostate cancer patients with severe late responses to radiation therapy. *Cancer J Sci Am*. 1998;4:385–389.
105. Hendry JH. Genomic instability: potential contributions to tumour and normal tissue response, and second tumours, after radiotherapy. *Radiother Oncol*. 2001;59:117–126.
106. Butler RW, Mulhern RK. Neurocognitive Interventions for Children and Adolescents Surviving Cancer. *J Pediatr Psychol*.2005, 30(1): 65–78.
107. Kinsella GJ, Prior M, Sawyer M, et al. Predictors and indicators of academic outcome in children 2 years following traumatic brain injury. *J Int Neuropsychol Soc*. 1997;3: 608–616.
108. Taylor H. Research on outcomes of pediatric traumatic brain injury: current advances and future directions. *Dev Neuropsychol*. 2004;25:19–225.
109. Taylor H, Yeates KO, Wade SL, Drotar D, Klein SK, Stancin T. Influences on first-year recovery from traumatic brain injury in children. *Neuropsychology*. 1999;13:76–89.
110. Yeates KO, Taylor H, Drotar D, et al. Preinjury family environment as a determinant of recovery from traumatic brain injuries in school-age children. *J Int Neuropsychol Soc*. 1997;3:617–630.
111. Taylor H, Yeates KO, Wade SL, Drotar D, Stancin T, Burant C. Bidirectional child-family influences on outcomes of traumatic brain injury in children. *J Int Neuropsychol Soc*. 2001;7:75–67.
112. Butler RW, Copeland DR. Attentional processes and their remediation in children treated for cancer: a literature review and the development of a therapeutic approach. *J Int Neuropsychol Soc*. 2002;8:115–124.

113. van' t Hooft I, Andersson K, Bergman B, Sejersen T, Von Wendt L, Bartfai A. Beneficial effect from a cognitive training programme on children with acquired brain injuries demonstrated in a controlled study. *Brain Inj.* 2005;19:51– 58.
114. Anderson V, Catroppa C. Advances in postacute rehabilitation after childhood-acquired brain injury: a focus on cognitive, behavioral, and social domains. *Am J Phys Med Rehabil.* 2006;85:767–778.
115. Mitby PA, Robison LL, Whitton JA, et al. Utilization of special education services and educational attainment among long-term survivors of childhood cancer: a report from the Childhood Cancer Survivor Study. *Cancer.* 2003;97:1115–1126.
116. Conklin HM, Khan RB, Reddick WE, et al. Acute neurocognitive response to methylphenidate among survivors of childhood cancer: a randomized, double-blind, cross-over trial. *J Pediatr Psychol.* 2007;32: 1127– 1139.
117. Thompson SJ, Leigh L, Christensen R, et al. Immediate neurocognitive effects of methylphenidate on learning-impaired survivors of childhood cancer. *J Clin Oncol.* 2001;19:1802–1808.

Chapter 18
Psychological and Social Impact of Being a Pediatric Brain Tumor Survivor

Stephen A. Sands and Keith P. Pasichow

Introduction

Advances in imaging and neurosurgical technologies, as well as the development of targeted radiation therapy using three-dimensional imaging and more potent chemotherapies, have led to a steady rise in pediatric neuro-oncology survival rates since the 1970s. Consequently, pediatric oncologists, nurses, psychologists and researchers have increasingly focused on issues concerning the health-related quality of life (QoL) of brain tumor patients, both during and after treatment. This increased focus on patient QoL has led to the understanding that QoL is related to both the physical and emotional status of the patient, as well as the perceived effect both of these domains have on the patient's life.[1,2]

The emotional effects of cancer upon a patient vary depending on the diagnosis, the location of the tumor and the treatment type, and on the patient's family dynamics and preexisting psychological conditions.[3] The vast majority of studies to date indicate that survivors of pediatric cancer are generally at no greater risk for long-term emotional sequelae than one would expect to see in a healthy population.[3-9] It is important to note, however, that these studies often do not include brain tumor patients, mainly because of the physical effects that brain tumors and their treatments have on the central nervous system (CNS)[5,7,10,11] and the apparent difficulty in separating organic and psychological causes of discrepancies in patient QoL. Of those studies that do include brain tumor patients, approximately half conclude that these patients are at no greater risk than the healthy controls, whereas the other half find that they are at greater risk. For example, according to Patenaude and Kupst, survivors of pediatric brain tumors, as opposed to survivors of other forms of pediatric malignancy, were at greater risk for long-term psychosocial sequelae,[5] echoing

S.A. Sands (✉)
Departments of Pediatrics and Psychiatry, Columbia University Medical Center,
161 Fort Washington Avenue, New York, NY 10032, USA
e-mail: ss2341@columbia.edu

S. Goldman, C.D. Turner (eds.), *Late Effects of Treatment for Brain Tumors*,
Cancer Treatment and Research 150, DOI 10.1007/b109924_18,
© Springer Science+Business Media, LLC 2009

Vannatta, Gartestein and Noll's earlier finding that survivors of pediatric brain tumors were more likely than the general population to have social deficits.[12] In contrast, a review article by Fuemmeler, Elkin and Mullins demonstrated that brain tumor survivors were at no greater risk for psychosocial deficits than the normal ("healthy") population,[13] a conclusion similar to that of Carpentieri et al. who determined, based on self-reports, that survivors were at no greater risk than the general population.[8] However, in the same Carpentieri study, reports by parents and teachers contradicted this finding,[8] suggesting that those studies that rely primarily on parents' reports of their children's QoL, which had been the standard for much of the early QoL research, may not be sufficient to ascertain true incidence levels. Thus, while information about brain tumor patients' QoL continues to emerge, there does appear to be an increased risk for deficit in certain domains of physical and psychosocial functioning specific to brain tumor survivors.

Relationship of Physical Sequelae to QoL

Physical sequelae of brain tumor treatment may influence QoL in survivors even though many studies have shown no direct link.[2,14–16] Looking at tumors for which cranial irradiation is used, specifically brain tumors and previous treatment regimens for acute lymphoblastic leukemia (ALL), researchers have found that cranially irradiated patients have endocrine deficiencies more often than nonirradiated patients.[17] These deficiencies, especially insufficient growth hormone (GH), may impact a patient's physical abilities. In many patients with low GH levels, osteopenia may result in gait disturbances or frequent fracture[18] that limit a survivor's ability to participate in recreational physical activities with his or her peers. This may lead peers to taunt the survivor or otherwise result in his or her social isolation, decreasing the survivor's overall health-related QoL. Additionally, many brain tumor survivors develop epileptic seizures because of either the tumor or its treatment. A literature review has found epilepsy rates of between 15 and 40% for survivors, a percentage significantly higher than for the healthy population.[17] Such seizures may also limit the survivor's ability to participate in social activities and, thus, further increase his or her isolation from peers. Such isolation is one possible cause of the social deficits of brain tumor survivors, and will be discussed in more detail later in this chapter.

Psychological Distress

Psychological distress is one of the more extensively studied sequelae in CNS tumor survivors. The definition of psychological distress is somewhat different in each study reviewed, but it typically includes internalizing behaviors such as depression and anxiety, as well as externalizing behaviors such as conduct problems.[3,4,19] Meyer and Kieran, who investigated the prevalence of depression among brain tumor survivors treated with surgery only, found the rates of psychological distress among the survivors to be significantly higher than the expected normative values in the general population[20] whereas, in an examination of brain tumor patients from a variety of treatment regimens, Carpentieri et al. found no difference between the rates of distress in the patients and in the general population.[8] It is important to note that Meyer and Keiran's study employed semi-structured interviews with parents, and sometimes with the patients themselves, to identify those patients who were at risk for psychological adjustment problems stemming from depression.[20] Alternately, Carpentieri et al.'s study employed a standardized questionnaire with three different formats – a parent report form, a patient self-report form and a teacher report form – and then used the three responses for each patient to determine the individual's risk for psychosocial sequelae, compared to standardized normative values.[8]

The two above-mentioned studies appear to present contradictory results; however, there is a salient difference in their research designs: interviews of any kind (structured or unstructured) generally indicate a higher level of psychopathology than do standardized questionnaires.[13] The use of standardized questionnaires may raise debates about the control groups selected for comparison to cancer patients, about responder bias in non-self-reports and about a questionnaire's ability to accurately reflect a patient's overall QoL. Nevertheless, compared to standardized questionnaires, structured and unstructured interviews show a higher variability in rates of clinically significant distress and find higher levels of distress in general, according to a study by Eiser and Jenny.[13,21] Possibly, it is a lack of uniformity in interview-based assessments that causes the variation between interview and standardized questionnaire results; however, it is also possible that questionnaires are simply not as sensitive as interviews are in picking up on subclinical levels of distress.[22] Trained interviewers may elicit more candid responses from patients, or they may ask patients questions that are more probing than those found on paper-and-pencil surveys, leading to a higher rate of diagnosis.

In addition to the varied results seen in studies utilizing various interview formats, studies selecting different control groups also show discordant rates of psychosocial sequelae. For example, comparing the rates of clinical depression among hematologic cancer patients and their matched siblings, one study using standardized questionnaires found that the patients' depression rates were within the population's expected values.[3] However, when the patients were compared directly to their siblings, the rates of depression were 1.6–1.7 times higher among the survivors. These results indicate that even though overall depression rates among cancer survivors are reportedly no higher than those in the healthy population, there may be an increased risk of depressive symptoms in cancer survivors as a direct result of the diagnosis and treatment process. This determination illustrates the difficulty of selecting control groups for use in this research. In the previously mentioned study, had the patients been compared only to population norms, and not to their siblings, there would be no indication of any increased risk for depression among cancer survivors. The difference in depression rates between survivors and their siblings indicates a greater need to focus upon patient risk as siblings tend to control for family history and risk factors prior to diagnosis.

Social-Emotional Sequelae

Social-emotional sequelae of cancer affect a variety of patients' personal and social characteristics, including leadership ability, self-esteem, intimacy with peers and being withdrawn versus being outgoing. Studies of patients with non-CNS tumors have found no significant difference in the social behaviors of those patients when compared to healthy matched peer controls.[7] Similarly, studies that examined the social-emotional and behavioral functioning of brain tumor survivors have also found those survivors to be functioning, on average, within normal limits, although brain tumor survivors tend to exhibit somatization behaviors, as well as often lowered leadership skills.[8,11,13] Although it is reasonable to expect that brain tumor survivors, who have had a range of illnesses and treatments, may experience more physical pain posttreatment than other cancer patients. An examination of the specific somatic concerns reported may illustrate which complaints are normal for this group, and which may be a manifestation of their emotional state. For example, sequelae such as headaches, pain and dizziness are understandable given the insult to the central nervous system caused by surgery, radiation or simply by the tumor itself. Other symptoms that are commonly endorsed, such as being cold or hot, having shortness of breath or having stomach problems, may represent physical manifestations of emotional or psychosocial concerns, such as anxiety. Of interest is the discrepancy between CNS and non-CNS tumor survivors, suggesting that tumor location and physical damage caused by treatment may play a role in the psychosocial deficits seen in brain tumor survivors.

In addition to the organic influence of brain tumors on long-term effects, as seen above, a variety of emotional factors may also play a part in sequelae development. Social isolation has been an inevitable side effect of oncology treatment, and may be one factor in the development of social deficits among survivors. Brain tumor patients may be isolated by their peers' reactions to their physical or neurocognitive differences, or they may choose to isolate themselves because of their personal perception that they are too different from their peers. *It has been demonstrated that brain tumor patients exhibit higher rates of internalizing behaviors than non-CNS tumor survivors,*[13] and that their teachers and peers perceived them as being less well medically and more isolated.[12] Thus, evidence suggests that self-imposed social isolation plays some role in the social deficits seen among brain tumor survivors, but that peer- and possibly even teacher-imposed social isolation may also be involved. Interestingly, research on patient-rated levels of social enjoyment has indicated that brain tumor survivors tend to experience "less joy"[12] from their social interactions than their healthy peers, supporting the idea that much of the survivors' isolation is self-imposed. Multimodal treatment for brain tumors is intensive and often involves patients' prolonged isolation from their peers for both medical reasons (i.e., somnolence, immune deficiency, infection, nausea and vomiting) and social/organizational reasons (friends may be unable to visit the patient because of their school schedules or distance from the hospital, patients may be too fatigued or physically compromised to have visitors, either the patient or the friend may feel awkward because of physical changes in the patient resulting from the cancer or its treatment). Current child development theory points to positive peer relations as being central to the healthy social and emotional growth of children.[12] *If pediatric cancer patients are indeed suffering from their isolation during treatment, then focusing on intervention geared toward reducing and overcoming the social isolation inherent in oncology treatment may help to minimize the social deficits for which brain tumor survivors are at increased risk.*

Relationship to Age at Diagnosis

As evidence of the intertwining of organic and emotional causes of survivors' social deficits, recent studies have shown that an older age at time of both diagnosis and radiation treatment is protective with regard to social and emotional sequelae,[13] suggesting that the physical development of the CNS and the protective qualities of emotional maturity may be important factors in preserving healthy psychosocial functioning. In contrast to the impact of older age on patient depression, *young age at diagnosis and treatment appears to be a protective factor against post-traumatic stress.*[3,23] This condition is a relatively new area of inquiry in the field of pediatric oncology, in which research has shown that cancer patients who are diagnosed and treated as young adults have a higher prevalence of clinically significant symptoms than do those treated as younger children.[5] Given the varied experiences that pediatric brain tumor patients go through, it seems reasonable to expect a percentage of survivors to exhibit symptoms of post-traumatic stress. Furthermore, while it appears that only a small minority of cancer patients overall will experience enough symptoms to warrant a clinical diagnosis of post-traumatic stress disorder (PTSD) as defined by the DSM IV, studies have shown that anywhere between 5 and 20% of these patients report clinically significant levels of post-traumatic stress symptoms (PTSS) – a subclinical level of distress related to PTSD – making PTSS a significant long-term psychosocial sequelae that may arise within this population.[23] In families of brain tumor survivors, PTSS generally appears to impact one family member who may serve as the resonating emotional chord in the family system, and it affects parents more often than it does patients or their siblings.[23] Currently, there are no studies that look specifically at methods of preventing PTSS in brain tumor survivors and their families, but the propensity of PTSS to primarily affect only one member of a patient's family suggests that interventions targeting the immediate family of pediatric cancer patients may be effective in diminishing the symptoms of post-traumatic stress. Finally, as with depression, patients are at increased risk of experiencing stress symptoms as compared to their siblings.[24] Siblings control for a patient's baseline risk, so that the increased incidence of symptoms in comparison to siblings suggests that the diagnosis of and treatment for brain tumors is in itself a major risk factor for developing psychosocial difficulties.

Overall Quality of Life

Studies have found that pediatric brain tumor patients consistently score lower in the domains of psychosocial health and of physical health than do other, non-CNS tumor patients.[25] Tumors of the CNS are particularly nefarious as the QoL of patients with these tumors does not regularly improve with time from treatment as it does in patients with non-CNS tumors.[26] In particular, CNS tumor survivors have a lower marriage rate than do either healthy controls or non-CNS tumor survivors,[27] as well as a higher incidence of both visual and emotional disturbances. As with all patients having tumors that require radiation to the CNS, they also have higher rates of IQ deficits.[13,26] According to data from the Childhood Cancer Survivors Study, survivors at particular risk for low QoL ratings are those who are unemployed, those who have not completed or never attended college and those who are members of the lower socioeconomic classes. Interestingly, these risk factors hold true regardless of initial diagnosis or treatment modality or intensity.[28]

While it is highly recommended that QoL data be gathered from multiple informants in order to gain an in-depth understanding of patients' overall level of functioning, younger children (those 2–8 years of age) are often unable to complete the surveys currently available.[29,30] In particular, younger children may not be intellectually mature enough to understand the emotions and the physical sensations that they are experiencing. For example, a young child who feels pain may not be able to adequately verbalize that feeling and, therefore, may be unable to accurately answer a survey question about the sensation.[21] Consequently, many researchers and clinicians rely on parent-proxy reports to evaluate the health-related QoL of young patients.[21,22] Such proxy evaluation of patient QoL raises important issues for researchers, however, because proxies tend to agree more often with patient ratings in objective areas (externalizing behaviors, conduct disorders, aggression) than they do in subjective ones (internalizing behaviors such as anxiety and depression), and they tend to rate QoL lower, and anxiety higher, than do the patients themselves.[30–33] Evidence of, and possible explanations for, such inaccuracy appears in studies that look at proxy–patient response correlations. Creemens, Eiser and Blades found that parents' own QoL and their ratings of their child's QoL were positively correlated,[32] suggesting that the answers parents give on questionnaires may reflect their own feelings projected onto their child, rather than be an accurate representation of their child's QoL.[10] One explanation for this finding may be that parents are more likely to focus on the limitations of their children who are cancer patients when compared to healthy peers and siblings,[10] so that their ratings of patient QoL are hypersensitive to these deficits. Along these lines, researchers have found that parent reports of QoL, social-emotional functioning and internalizing and externalizing behaviors tend to rate survivors lower than do the survivors' self-reports.[8,13,25] *Compared to cancer survivors across all tumor types, parents of brain tumor survivors tend to rate their children's QoL lower than the ratings for QoL in these domains of survivors of non-CNS tumors.*[25] Noll et al. compared parental distress ratings in families with children undergoing treatment for cancer to the ratings in families with healthy children and found that parental distress levels directly affected the development and emotional adaptability of the young patient.[34] They also found that parental distress can lead to a diminished self-concept for the patient, a result that may persist even after treatment is completed. *Additionally, studies have found that discrepancies between patient self-reports and parent-proxy reports are greater between cancer patients and their parents than between healthy peers and their parents.*[10] This finding supports the theory that parents project some of their own anxiety and perception of illness onto their children, and that they rate their children's QoL based on these observations rather than on an objective view of their child's true feelings.[10,21]

The same areas of discrepancy that exist between patient reports and parent-proxy reports of patient QoL commonly crop up between patient reports and physician reports. *Studies comparing these reports have concluded that physicians tend to overestimate the importance of physical symptoms* (e.g., quantified pain ratings, lab results, radiological studies, etc.) in assessing their patients' QoL.[14,35] Supporting these studies is the finding that sequelae traditionally attributed solely to physical symptoms may more accurately be attributed to the interaction between physical symptoms and emotional responses based on the developmental stage of the patient.[5] This interaction can help explain why there is a greater degree of agreement between proxies and patients in areas that are objectively evaluated (i.e., physical disability), and greater discordance in subjective domains (e.g., internalizing symptoms). In short, patient experience and proxy interpretation exhibit differences in personal perception.[36]

Researchers have found that many standardized questionnaires rely too heavily on the link between the patient's physical symptoms and his or her psychological distress, just as they may rely too much on proxy responders.[16,24] Although it may seem logical that patient QoL be correlated with physical and neurocognitive impairment, many studies have demonstrated no link between the two.[15] Discrepancies between the results of varying measures of QoL may be attributed, in part, to the extent that they are based upon this correlation.[37] One possible explanation for the differences between the patient's experience of QoL and the way that proxies and QoL questionnaires evaluate it is that patients with a physical limitation may reduce their quality of life expectations to below those of the healthy population and then evaluate their psychosocial QoL as normal. It may also be that their intellectual or neurocognitive impairments prevent these patients from fully appreciating their limitations; thereby decreasing the effect those limitations have on their self-reported QoL. Finally, cancer survivors may compare their current QoL to the deadly prospect that faced them prior to treatment and choose to diminish their posttreatment physical and intellectual needs, negating the feelings of dissatisfaction that otherwise healthy individuals with the same physical limitations might experience. In other words, the patients may simply have decided to accept the consequences of what they went through. The fact that parents, physicians and nurses tend to rate children's QoL lower than the children do themselve.[10,15,33] would suggest that proxies may not fully understand the coping mechanisms being used by the patient.

Future Directions

It is important to determine the physical and psychosocial domains necessary to accurately assess a pediatric patient's quality of life, taking into account the weight a patient places on each domain measured. In addition, future researchers must choose against which comparison group the patients' health-related QoL should be compared in order to give health care providers the truest indication of how their patients are doing and what interventions may be necessary. Whereas the effective selection of controls is critical to any research project, such selection is even more challenging in cancer QoL studies because consensus about the appropriate control group is lacking. Although to control for socioeconomic status, educational opportunities, parenting and family dynamics some researchers have used siblings as the comparison group in QoL and psychosocial studies. While the merits of this approach are clear, it is likely that siblings are affected by the diagnosis of cancer in their brother or sister and by the treatment of the disease, diminishing the siblings' utility as an unaffected healthy control group.[5]

Current research focuses upon determining which adjustment and coping strategies are most effective for long-term pediatric cancer survivors; however, no single strategy has proven to be effective for all patients.[5] Researchers must find new ways to identify risk factors in patients and to evaluate those factors in light of patient histories, family coping mechanisms and existing patient psychopathology so that interventions may be tailored to meet patient needs and to develop a holistic approach to preventing psychological sequelae in long-term survivors of brain tumors. As our understanding of the relationship between physical trauma and psychological manifestations improves, it will be easier to predict the specific long-term deficits that particular patients will be at risk for because of tumor location, and to monitor patients for changes in their level of overall functioning both during and after treatment. Taking into account the various risk factors that have been studied to date, clinicians hope to be able to use the age of the patient, the type and location of the tumor and the kind of treatment required to predict the patient's relative risk for psychological sequelae, and to initiate interventions early in the treatment process to help mitigate late effects. Future research needs to concentrate on the prevention of psychological sequelae in cancer patients and on their early treatment through psychopharmacological management, individual therapy, group and family therapy, social skills education and school reentry programs to diminish psychosocial sequelae in pediatric brain tumor survivors, as well as on the early initiation of physical and occupational therapy to reduce the morbidity associated with physical sequelae. Through early identification and intervention, survivors can achieve the highest possible levels of health-related QoL.

The authors offer their appreciation to Susan Greenberg for editing this chapter.

References

1. Eiser C, Morse R. The measurement of quality of life in children: past and future perspectives. *Dev Behav Pediatr.* 2001;22:248–256.
2. Varni JW, Katz ER, Seid M, et al. The pediatric cancer quality of life inventory (PCQL). I. Instrument development, descriptive statistics, and cross-informant variance. *J Behav Med.* 1998;21:179–204.
3. Marsland AL, Ewing LJ, Thompson A. Psychological and social effects of surviving childhood cancer. In: Brown RT, ed. *Comprehensive Handbook of Childhood Cancer and Sickle Cell Disease.* Oxford: Oxford University Press; 2006:237–261.
4. Elkin TD, Phipps S, Mulhern RK, et al. Psychological functioning of adolescent and young adult survivors of pediatric malignancy. *Med Pediatr Oncol.* 1997;29:582–588.
5. Patenaude AF, Kupst MJ. Psychosocial functioning in pediatric cancer. *J Pediatr Psychol.* 2005;30:9–27.
6. Noll RB, Gartstein MA, Vannatta K, et al. Social, emotional, and behavioral functioning of children with cancer. *Pediatrics.* 1999;103:71–78.
7. Reiter-Purtill J, Vannatta K, Gerhardt CA, et al. A controlled longitudinal study of the social functioning of children who completed treatment of cancer. *J Pediatr Hematol/Oncol.* 2003;25:467–473.
8. Carpentieri SC, Meyer EA, Delaney BL, et al. Psychosocial and behavioral functioning among pediatric brain tumor survivors. *J Neuro-Oncol.* 2003;63:279–287.
9. Holmquist LA, Scott J. Treatment, age, and time-related predictors of behavioral outcome in pediatric brain tumor survivors. *J Clin Psychol Med Settings.* 2002;9:315–321.
10. Levi RB, Drotar D. Health-related quality of life in childhood cancer: discrepancy in parent-child reports. *Int J Cancer.* 1999;22:58–64.
11. Newby WL, Brown RT, Pawletko TM, et al. Social skills and psychological adjustment of child and adolescent cancer survivors. *Psycho-Oncology.* 2000;9:113–126.
12. Vannatta K, Gartstein MA, Noll RB. Peer relationships of children surviving brain tumors. *J Pediatr Psychol.* 1998;23:279–288.
13. Fuemmeler BF, Elkin TD, Mullins LL. Survivors of childhood brain tumors: behavioral, emotional, and social adjustment. *Clin Psychol Rev.* 2002;22:547–585.

14. Loonen HJ, Derkx BHHF, Griffiths AM. Pediatricians overestimate importance of physical symptoms upon children's health concerns. *Med Care*. 2002;40:996–1001.
15. Koot HM, Wallander JL. Challenges in child and adolescent quality of life research. In: Koot HM, Wallander JL, eds. *Quality of life in children and adolescents: Concepts, methods, and findings*. London, UK: Harwood Academic Publishers; 2002:431–456.
16. Koot HM. Challenges in child and adolescent quality of life research. *Acta Paediatr*. 2002;91:265–266.
17. Benesch M, Lackner H, Sovinz P, et al. Late sequela after treatment of childhood low-grade gliomas: a retrospective analysis of 69 long-term survivors treated between 1983 and 2003. *J Neuro-Oncol*. 2006;78:199–205.
18. Odame I, Duckworth J, Talsma D, et al. Osteopenia, physical activity and health-related quality of life in survivors of brain tumors treated in childhood. *Pediatr Blood Cancer*. 2006;46:357–362.
19. Maddrey AM, Bergeron JA, Lombardo ER, et al. Neuropsychological performance and quality of life of 10 year survivors of childhood medulloblastoma. *J Neuro-Oncol*. 2005;72:245–253.
20. Meyer EA, Kieran MW. Psychological adjustment of 'surgery-only' pediatric neuro-oncology patients: a retrospective analysis. *Psycho-Oncology*. 2002;11:74–79.
21. Eiser C, Jenny MEM. Measuring symptomatic benefit and quality of life in pediatric oncology. *Br J Cancer*. 1996;73:1313–1316.
22. Landgraf JM. Measuring health-related quality of life in pediatric oncology patients: a brief commentary on the state of the art of measurement and application (discussion). *Int J Cancer*. 1999;12:147–150.
23. Kazak AE, Alderfer M, Rourke MT, et al. Posttraumatic stress disorder (PTSD) and posttraumatic stress symptoms (PTSS) in families of adolescent childhood cancer survivors. *J Pediatr Psychol*. 2004;29:211–219.
24. Zebrack BJ, Gurney JG, Oeffinger K, et al. Psychological outcomes in long-term survivors of childhood brain cancer: a report from the childhood cancer survivors study. *J Clin Oncol*. 2004;22:999–1006.
25. Meeske K, Katz ER, Palmer SN, et al. Parent proxy-reported health-related quality of life and fatigue in pediatric patients diagnosed with brain tumors and acute lymphoblastic leukemia. *Cancer*. 2004;101:2116–2125.
26. Bhat SR, Goodwin TL, Burwinkle TM, et al. Profile of daily life in children with brain tumors: an assessment of health-related quality of life. *J Clin Oncol*. 2005;23: 5493–5499.
27. Rauck AM, Green DM, Yasui Y, et al. Marriage in the survivors of childhood cancer: a preliminary description from the childhood cancer survivors study. *Med Pediatr Oncol*. 1999;33:60–63.
28. Nathan PC, Ness KK, Greenberg ML, et al. Health-related quality of life in adult survivors of childhood Wilms' tumor or neuroblastoma: a report from the childhood cancer survivors study. *Pediatr Blood Cancer*. 2007;49(5):704–715.
29. Palmer SN, Meeske KA, Katz ER, et al. The PedsQLTM brain tumor module: initial reliability and validity. *Pediatr Blood Cancer*. 2007;49(3):287–293.
30. Varni JW, Burwinkle T, Katz ER, et al. The PedsQL^{TM} in Pediatric Cancer Reliability and Validity of the Pediatric Quality of Life Inventory^{TM} Generic Core Scales, multi-dimensional fatigue scale, and cancer module. *Cancer*. 2002;94:2090–2106.
31. Raat H, Botterweck AM, Landgraf JM, et al. Reliability and validity of the short form of the child health questionnaire for parents (CHQ-PF28) in large random school based and general population samples. *J Epidemiol Commun Health*. 2005;59:75–82.
32. Cremeens J, Eiser C, Blades M. Factors influencing agreement between child self-report and parent proxy-reports on the Pediatric Quality of Life Inventory^{TM} 4.0 (PedsQL^{TM}) generic core scales. *Health and Quality of Life Outcomes*. 2006;4.

33. Coen RF. Individual quality of life and assessment by carers or 'proxy' respondents. In: Joyce CRB, McGee HMM, eds. *Individual Quality of Life: Approaches to Conceptualisation and Assessment*. Amsterdam: Harwood Academic Publishers; 1999:185–196.
34. Noll RB, Gartstein MA, Hawkins A, et al. Comparing parental distress for families with children who have cancer and matched comparison families without children with cancer. *Family Syst Med*. 1995;13:11–27.
35. Janse AJ, Sinnema G, Uiterwaal CSPM, et al. Quality of life in chronic illness: perceptions of parents and paediatricians. *Arch Dis Children*. 2005;90:486–491.
36. Janse AJ, Uiterwaal CSPM, Gemke RJBJ, et al. A difference in perception of quality of life in chronically ill children was found between parents and pediatricians. *J Clin Epidemiol*. 2005;58:495–502.
37. Sung L, Greenberg ML, Doyle JJ, et al. Construct validation of the Health Utilities Index and the Child Health Questionnaire in children undergoing cancer chemotherapy. *Br J Cancer*. 2003;88:1185–1190.

Chapter 19
Psychological and Social Impact of Being a Brain Tumor Survivor: Adult Issues

R.D. Calhoun-Eagan

Introduction

The broad application of cancer survivorship research offers excellent templates for psychosocial assessment and intervention in the specialized population of adult neuro-oncology. However, by exclusively utilizing a cancer model of survivorship, clinicians might overlook vital, relevant work in the field of neurology. Preference for a cancer lens in survivorship programming is understandable given that most neuro-oncology workers identify the field of oncology as their foundation for care. To counteract this trend, a summary of relevant research in related populations (stroke, brain injury) is offered with the premise that consideration of similarities across populations has much to offer.

Lessons from Stroke Survivors

A recent case study describes a stroke survivor whose loss of work identity, reassignment to easier tasks and feelings of being half a man mirrors experiences of many brain tumor survivors.[1] Common issues among the two populations include uncertain prognosis,[2] cognitive deficits,[3] disruption in mood,[3] clinical depression,[4] and loss of familiar identity and self-image.[5] These issues are further complicated by limited insight,[6] social isolation,[4] frustration directed towards significant others,[6] and an unlikely return to baseline functioning.[2] It may take two years post-stroke before survivors begin to relinquish the treasured goal of resuming normal life. The loss of this dream is associated with anguish and depression. In essence, the process of coming to terms with a stroke takes years.[2]

R.D. Calhoun-Eagan (✉)
Canandaigua VA Medical Center, 400 Fort Hill Avenue, Canandaigua, NY 14424, USA
e-mail: roberta.calhoun-eagan@va.gov

S. Goldman, C.D. Turner (eds.), *Late Effects of Treatment for Brain Tumors*,
Cancer Treatment and Research 150, DOI 10.1007/b109924_19,
© Springer Science+Business Media, LLC 2009

Thirty years ago, stroke professionals' pessimism regarding rehabilitation[7] limited referrals for services. Improved outcomes have promoted greater focus on life well after stroke,[6] with one study reaching the 14-year mark.[8]

Lessons from Brain Injury Survivors

Compared to stroke, 78% of patients now survive brain injury and face varying degrees of impairment that are usually lifelong.[9] Substantial cognitive loss may occur even with mild brain injury.[10] Subtle or fluctuating symptoms may remain undetected for months or more, well after treatment has ended. *Intensive treatment typically ends before families realize the extent to which life has changed. As caregivers grow less tolerant and optimistic about recovery, professional support has dwindled.*[11] *Therefore, a program of routine, proactive follow-up that includes cognitive evaluation is recommended.*[12]

Adjusting to brain injury takes years, yet only one-fourth of survivors receive post-acute rehabilitation.[13] Many patients face a "disruption in continuity" in development that requires them to reconstruct identity.[14] As self-image is closely tied to work, any employment short of former standards may be viewed as a loss. Coming to terms with even mild injury may be a long process.[15] The best rehabilitation includes strategies that rebuild self-efficacy and self-confidence.[16]

Brain Tumor Survivors

Unlike brain injury and stroke, brain tumors reflect an uncommon diagnosis. It is so rare to survive a glioblastoma multiforme (GBM) that when the tumor fails to progress after a few years, the diagnosis itself may undergo review, resulting in reclassifications of as many as half of these tumors.[17] In a 1996 discussion of statistics and prognosis entitled *Odds and Ends*, Jordan Fieldman, M.D. recalled reading in 1988 that five-year survival for his tumor was nonexistent, as recurrences were "invariable."[18] As recently as 2003, the three-year point after diagnosis was characterized as an "unusually long" survival time for GBM .[19]

Individuals surviving cancers this rare have a particular need to find peers who understand and validate their situation.[20] While accessed by patients, the research literature rarely meets this need, nor is it likely to explore concerns such as the existential experiences of survivors whose GBM has been reclassified. For now, peer groups remain elusive. Several states have no brain tumor support groups; others offer only one. Survivors relay that those who are newly diagnosed approach them for advice and reassurance, but they don't know how to respond. They ask, what worked for me? How—and why—did I survive?

Survivor Guilt

While patients express guilt upon the deaths of peers with similar diagnoses, the cancer literature has said little about survivor guilt.[21] Characteristics of survivor guilt include feelings of responsibility for the deaths of others as well as a compelling need to "make things right" by striving, often through hard work, to "justify" survival. Case studies from a treatment setting suggest that close identification with peers may intensify these feelings.[22] In adult neuro-oncology, where long-term survivors remain scarce, survivor guilt may be particularly acute.

Survivor guilt in the clinic is implied by expressions of remorse about interrupting staff with substantial concerns—because they are not life-threatening. Patients may also restate they are lucky to be alive. A strong professional focus on survival may subtly reinforce patient behaviors that appear heroic or inspirational.

Projecting Wellness

Families relay that patients strain to appear well, especially in clinic. With energy already compromised, much is expended on the struggle to maintain normal appearances. The work of projecting wellness, while simultaneously hiding the struggle, takes a sizeable toll. When these efforts succeed, survivors may paradoxically increase their isolation by blocking opportunities for acknowledgement and validation of the permanent changes in their lives.

The quest to resume former life[23] ***tends to persist until some grieving has occurred***. In survivor groups, unresolved grief is suggested by superficiality and avoidance of negative focus. Some survivors keep earlier trauma at arm's length, or respond to bad news by withdrawal. Limited emotional awareness and loss of psychological insight represent additional factors that impact coping; these symptoms of brain injury should be distinguished from classic denial.[16,24–26]

During intensive treatment, patients cannot identify acute versus long-term symptoms; they must adapt to impairments that are still evolving.[27] Losses become more apparent after therapy;[28] therefore, grief may be delayed or prolonged. Cultural views of grief as dwelling on the past, failing to let go or wallowing in negativity are reinforced by the depiction of cancer survival as a milestone or event (such as the five-year mark) rather than as a process.

Long-Term Psychosocial Issues

Depression and Anxiety

In a report of coping 6–12 months after diagnosis of stroke, brain injury, Parkinson's disease and brain cancer, all patients used minimization and wishful thinking to a degree. While not statistically significant, brain tumor patients had the highest scores for depressive coping.[29] Clinical depression has been observed in 38–41% of brain tumor patients.[30–32] In a study that included survivors, depressive symptoms did not correlate with time since diagnosis.[30] *Prior or concurrent medical illness, single status, female gender, a lower educational level and a lower grade tumor have been associated with depression and/or anxiety.*[31]

In a Scottish study of five-year brain tumor survivors who received whole-brain irradiation, all reported cognitive impairments, mood disturbance, and reduced quality of life. Community involvement was limited by physical impairment, and reduced self-confidence attributed to altered appearance and seizures.[33] In low-grade glioma survivors 16 years post-diagnosis, sources of isolation included loss of ability to drive, memory impairment, seizures, and dependence on family.[34]

Physical and Mental Slowing

Symptoms such as slowed thinking, forgetfulness, impaired multitasking and fatigue persist even among high functioning survivors. Follow-up is routinely available to neuro-oncology patients who received chemotherapy, while survivors of low-grade tumors whose treatment ended with surgery or radiation receive less surveillance. Most report that they manage well until employers adopt novel procedures or tools, as new learning can be difficult. Task management may be so draining that there is no energy left over to face job-related stress. Recommended workplace accommodations (for both cancer and brain injury) include added rest periods and a quieter work area that minimizes interruptions and distractions.

Families observe that work consumes all energy, leaving no reserve for help around the house. Children may exploit parental exhaustion. Families coping with brain injury report that personality and behavior changes pose far greater management challenges than physical impairments.[14,35] Cognitive deficits may be so subtle[36] that few relatives or friends realize the survivor's actual limits.

While reduced stamina may be lifelong, brain tumor-specific guidance regarding energy management is not routinely accessed. Survivors grapple with slowed processing speed in an increasingly fast-paced world. They find that recovery from mistakes takes longer. Vital skills such as self-pacing may be undermined by guilt about setting limits or fears of burdening others.

Challenges of Treatment and Resource Utilization

To optimize coping, survivors need skills of self-pacing, energy conservation, revised expectations and external reminders.[16] Preliminary evidence exists for the efficacy of an outpatient rehabilitation program using cognitive approaches adapted from a traumatic brain injury (TBI) program. Average cost and length of stay were significantly lower than that for TBI survivors using the same model.[36]

However, brain tumor patients are infrequently referred for rehabilitation.[36,37] With an overwhelming focus on survival, rehabilitation may come up as an afterthought rather than a routine step in treatment. Admission to inpatient rehabilitation requires a demonstrated need for more than one modality, documentation of continued progress, the ability to tolerate three or more hours of therapy per day, sustained motivation, and a feasible discharge plan.[27] While timely postoperative intervention places acute rehabilitation alongside irradiation therapy, physical and cognitive gains similar to those observed in TBI can still occur.[26]

The 1980s are recalled as a golden age for rehabilitation, as patients could access therapies for extended periods. Funding has plummeted to the extent that rehab stays now last days or weeks rather than months. Some insurance carriers limit coverage to the few techniques supported by research.[24,38]

One might anticipate that cancer patient organizations and agencies covering neurological disorders would collaborate to offer assistance—but as suggested by the following examples, help may come from neither:

- A national cancer organization declines to fund medical equipment with the rationale that brain cancer-related disability is neurological in nature
- A mobility professional denies a visually impaired survivor access to resources based on an assessment that occurred during radiation therapy
- A large number of brain injury organizations omit brain cancer as an eligible diagnosis
- Many adult day care centers exclude brain tumor patients

These scenarios reflect current realities at the intersection of cancer and neurology. Neurology professionals' lack of oncology exposure often isolates survivors from resources and services. Typically admitted to TBI or stroke rehab programs,[39,40] survivors encounter therapists well versed in neurological disorders who have never worked with a brain tumor patient. Patients matched with stroke survivors by lesion location and size experience fewer deficits than their stroke counterparts.[41] Brain tumor survivors hear they are "doing great"—and they are, compared to their comrades in therapy, but not compared to their own baseline. Goals are not adjusted accordingly; all too often, one size fits all.[24]

Insurance coverage may terminate before therapy has ended with little or no warning, with few plans to maintain gains. Some patients manage limited resources by rationing visits or choosing which therapy to pursue. The uneven process of recovery makes the small number of covered visits critical.

Impact of Medical Issues

Seizures

It is not uncommon for individuals who experience seizures to have substantial setbacks at work and depletion of insurance benefits.[42] Epilepsy affects 30–60%

of patients with high-grade gliomas, and over 80% with low-grade gliomas.[43] Focus on survival overshadows epilepsy as a concurrent diagnosis. Common use of the term "seizure disorder" among brain tumor professionals may delay access to resources offered by epilepsy groups. Adults with epilepsy value information about the condition, but tend not to seek it until the second or third year after diagnosis.[44] In people whose epilepsy is unrelated to a brain tumor diagnosis, attention deficits, common even among people with focal seizures, respond to cognitive therapy.[45] Anticonvulsant use is associated with impairments in nearly all cognitive domains;[46] in one small study, a decline in neurocognitive functioning at tumor recurrence was attributable to use of antiepileptic drugs.[47] During rehabilitation for adults with epilepsy, lost confidence requires as much focus as skill building.[42]

Sexuality and Sexual Dysfunction

Research on sexuality has centered on cancers involving sexual organs; tumors that affect sexuality less directly are rarely highlighted.[48] Deficits associated with frontal lobe tumors involving expression of affection, the ability to "read" emotions, social insensitivity, and demanding behavior are likely to have substantial impact. Even minor changes in body image affect self-esteem.[49] Coping varies widely, from dwelling on former appearance, to destroying old photos, to the liberal use of humor. Some patients go unrecognized by colleagues or friends.[50] Support groups can provide a vital first step in social reintegration.

Feeling ever more out of sync as time passes, survivors may limit interactions to contacts found within Internet chat rooms. Little is known about how survivors reorganize self-image.[14] and rebuild confidence. Small steps may best allow them to stretch skills slowly. A vital focus of cognitive therapy is practice in managing "internal distractions" such as self-doubt and negative self talk.[16]

Conclusion

Given the small and diverse adult brain tumor survivoship population, it will take years to complete robust studies of survivorship. In the interim, our shared clinical knowledge can guide colleagues in neurology, general oncology, rehabilitation, social services and education as they respond to the needs of this unique group.

References

1. Davis W. Ethical conflicts in the vocational rehabilitation of stroke survivors. *Top Stroke Rehabil.* 2002;9:57–60.
2. Becker G, Kaufman SR. Managing an uncertain illness trajectory in old age: patients' and physicians' views of stroke. *Med Anthropol Quar.* 1995;9:165–187.

3. Teasdale TW, Engberg AW. Psychosocial consequences of stroke: a long-term population-based follow-up. *Brain Inj.* 2005;19:1049–1058.
4. Astrom M, Asplund K, Astrom T. Psychosocial function and life satisfaction after stroke. Stroke. *J Cerebral Circ.* 1992;23:527–531.
5. Flick CL. Stroke rehabilitation. 4. Stroke outcome and psychosocial consequences. *Arch Phys Med Rehabil.* 1999;80:S21–S26.
6. Glass TA, Dym B, Greenberg S, et al. Psychosocial intervention in stroke: Families in Recovery from Stroke Trial (FIRST). *Am J Orthopsychiatry.* 2000;70:169–181.
7. Smolkin C, Cohen BS. Socioeconomic factors affecting the vocational success of stroke patients. *Arch Phys Med Rehabil.* 1974;55:269–271.
8. Tuomilehto J, Nuottimaki T, Salmi K, et al. Psychosocial and health status in stroke survivors after 14 years. Stroke. *J Cerebral Circ.* 1995;26:971–975.
9. Vandiver VL, Johnson J, Christofero-Snider C. Supporting employment for adults with acquired brain injury: a conceptual model. *J Head Trauma Rehabil.* 2003;18:457–463.
10. Turner-Stokes L, Wade D. Rehabilitation following acquired brain injury: concise guidance. *Clin Med* (London, England). 2004;4:61–65.
11. Webster G, Daisley A, King N. Relationship and family breakdown following acquired brain injury: the role of the rehabilitation team. *Brain Inj.* 1999;13:593–603.
12. Turner-Stokes L, Disler PB, Nair A, et al. Multi-disciplinary rehabilitation for acquired brain injury in adults of working age. Cochrane Database Syst Rev (Online). 2005:CD004170.
13. Eriksson G, Tham K, Borg J. Occupational gaps in everyday life 1–4 years after acquired brain injury. *J Rehabil Med.* 2006;38:159–165.
14. Florian V, Katz S, Lahav V. Impact of traumatic brain damage on family dynamics and functioning: a review. *Brain Inj.* 1989;3:219–233.
15. Johansson U, Tham K. The meaning of work after acquired brain injury. *Am J Occup Ther.* 2006;60:60–69.
16. Mateer CA, Sira CS. Cognitive and emotional consequences of TBI: Intervention strategies for vocational rehabilitation. *Neuro Rehabil.* 2006;21:315–326.
17. Scott JN, Rewcastle NB, Brasher PM, et al. Which glioblastoma multiforme patient will become a long-term survivor? A population-based study. *Ann Neurol.* 1999;46:183–188.
18. Fieldman J. Odds and Ends (Closing keynote speech). In: *Making Headlines: A Brain Tumor Conference.* NYU Medical Center, New York, NY: The Brain Tumor Society; 1996.
19. Senger D, Cairncross JG, Forsyth PA. Long-term survivors of glioblastoma: statistical aberration or important unrecognized molecular subtype? *Cancer J* (Sudbury, Mass). 2003;9:214–221.
20. Calhoun RD. Practice guidelines for patients with rare cancers. *Cancer Prac.* 1998;6:247–250.
21. Maxwell T, Aldredge-Clanton J. Survivor guilt in cancer patients: a pastoral perspective. *J Pastoral Care.* 1994;48:25–31.
22. Vamos M. Survivor guilt and chronic illness. *Aust N Z J Psychiatry.* 1997;31:592–596.
23. Salander P, Bergenheim AT, Henriksson R. How was life after treatment of a malignant brain tumour? *Soc Sci Med.* (1982). 2000;51:589–598.
24. Morris J. Cognitive rehabilitation: where we are and what is on the horizon. *Phys Med Rehabil Clin N Am.* 2007;18:27–42, v–vi.
25. Meyers CA, Hess KR, Yung WK, et al. Cognitive function as a predictor of survival in patients with recurrent malignant glioma. *J Clin Oncol.* 2000;18:646–650.
26. Schmidinger M, Linzmayer L, Becherer A, et al. Psychometric- and quality-of-life assessment in long-term glioblastoma survivors. *J Neuro-oncol.* 2003;63:55–61.
27. Huang ME, Wartella J, Kreutzer J, et al. Functional outcomes and quality of life in patients with brain tumours: a review of the literature. *Brain Inj.* 2001;15:843–856.

28. Giovagnoli AR. Quality of life in patients with stable disease after surgery, radiotherapy, and chemotherapy for malignant brain tumour. *J Neurol Neurosurg Psychiatry*. 1999;67:358–363.
29. Herrmann M, Curio N, Petz T, et al. Coping with illness after brain diseases – a comparison between patients with malignant brain tumors, stroke, Parkinson's disease and traumatic brain injury. *Disability Rehabil*. 2000;22:539–546.
30. Pelletier G, Verhoef MJ, Khatri N, et al. Quality of life in brain tumor patients: the relative contributions of depression, fatigue, emotional distress, and existential issues. *J Neuro-oncol*. 2002;57:41–49.
31. ArnoldSD, Forman LM, Brigidi BD, et al. Evaluation and characterization of anxiety and depression in patients with primary brain tumors. *Neuro Oncol*. 2008;10(2):171–181.
32. Wellisch DK, Kaleita TA, Freeman D, et al. Predicting major depression in brain tumor patients. *Psycho-oncology*. 2002;11:230–238.
33. Awwad S, Cull A, Gregor A. Long-term survival in adult hemispheric glioma: prognostic factors and quality of outcome. *Clin Oncol* (Royal College of Radiologists (Great Britain)). 1990;2:343–346.
34. Edvardsson T, Ahlstrom G. Illness-related problems and coping among persons with low-grade glioma. *Psycho-oncology*. 2005;14:728–737.
35. Draper BM, Poulos CJ, Cole AM, et al. A comparison of caregivers for elderly stroke and dementia victims. *J Am Geriatr Soc*. 1992;40:896–901.
36. Sherer M, Meyers CA, Bergloff P. Efficacy of postacute brain injury rehabilitation for patients with primary malignant brain tumors. *Cancer*. 1997;80:250–257.
37. Davies E, Hall S, Clarke C. Two year survival after malignant cerebral glioma: patient and relative reports of handicap, psychiatric symptoms and rehabilitation. *Disability Rehabil*. 2003;25:259–266.
38. McCabe P, Lippert C, Weiser M, et al. Community reintegration following acquired brain injury. *Brain Inj*. 2007;21:231–257.
39. O'Dell MW, Barr K, Spanier D, et al. Functional outcome of inpatient rehabilitation in persons with brain tumors. *Arch Phys Med Rehabil*. 1998;79:1530–1534.
40. Huang ME, Cifu DX, Keyser-Marcus L. Functional outcome after brain tumor and acute stroke: a comparative analysis. *Arch Phys Med Rehabil*. 1998;79:1386–1390.
41. Anderson SW, Damasio H, Tranel D. Neuropsychological impairments associated with lesions caused by tumor or stroke. *Arch Neurol*. 1990;47:397–405.
42. Ponds RW, Hendriks M. Cognitive rehabilitation of memory problems in patients with epilepsy. *Seizure*. 2006;15:267–273.
43. Hildebrand J, Lecaille C, Perennes J, et al. Epileptic seizures during follow-up of patients treated for primary brain tumors. *Neurology*. 2005;65:212–215.
44. Chaplin JE, Wester A, Tomson T. The perceived rehabilitation needs of a hospital-based outpatient sample of people with epilepsy. *Seizure*. 1998;7:329–335.
45. Engelberts NH, Klein M, Ader HJ, et al. The effectiveness of cognitive rehabilitation for attention deficits in focal seizures: a randomized controlled study. *Epilepsia*. 2002;43:587–595.
46. Klein M, Engelberts NH, van der Ploeg HM, et al. Epilepsy in low-grade gliomas: the impact on cognitive function and quality of life. *Ann Neurol*. 2003;54:514–520.
47. Bosma I, Vos MJ, Heimans JJ, et al. The course of neurocognitive functioning in high-grade glioma patients. *Neuro-oncology*. 2007;9:53–62.
48. Schover LR. Sexual dysfunction. In: Holland JC, ed. *Psycho-oncology*. New York: Oxford University Press; 1998:494–499.
49. Howes HF, Edwards S, Benton D. Female body image following acquired brain injury. *Brain Inj*. 2005;19:403–415.
50. Libutti RL. *That's Unacceptable. Surviving a Brain Tumor: My Personal Story*. Martinsville, NJ: Krystal Publishing; 1997.

Chapter 20
Academic Issues: Special Education and Related Interventions

Frank A.J. Zelko and Lisa G. Sorensen

Introduction

As demonstrated in Chapter 17, pediatric brain tumor survivors are at increased risk for neurocognitive deficits. The educational setting is a critical one within which to consider their impact. The school environment places tremendous demands upon students for efficient information acquisition, demands that increase with age. Recent models of late effects suggest that the cognitive substrate of efficient information acquisition (e.g., attention, executive skills, processing speed) is highly vulnerable in cancer survivors, particularly those who have undergone cranial radiation.[1] The educational setting provides a sensitive context for monitoring cognitive effects, serving as a continuous "proving ground" within which neurocognitive deficits are likely to be first observed.

An even more important role of the educational setting, however, is as a context for neurocognitive intervention. Schools serve as the de facto primary setting of long-term cognitive intervention for many if not most pediatric cancer survivors. Because such interventions are often provided within the framework of the special education system, a brief introduction to that system in the United States is presented.

The provision of special education services in the United States is governed by a series of federal laws dating back to 1969 which allocate funds to state and local public education agencies. The laws also outline rights and regulations for the process by which a student is determined to be eligible for special education services, and how those services are to be provided and monitored. Despite the pivotal role of federal legislation, the special education process is implemented largely at state and local levels, with interpretation of federal statutes that vary from one school district to another. While it is possible to present common features of this process, it is essential for parents and clinicians to access specific

F.A.J. Zelko (✉)
Pediatric Neuropsychology, Children's Memorial Hospital, Chicago, IL, USA
e-mail: fzelko@childrensmemorial.org

S. Goldman, C.D. Turner (eds.), *Late Effects of Treatment for Brain Tumors,*
Cancer Treatment and Research 150, DOI 10.1007/b109924_20,
© Springer Science+Business Media, LLC 2009

local information, particularly state educational resources when seeking assistance for a specific student.

The latest refinement of U.S. special education law is the *Individuals with Disabilities Education Improvement Act of 2004,* often referred to as IDEA 04 (P.L. 108–446). IDEA 04 and the laws preceding it stipulate that all students with educational handicaps shall be identified and provided a free and appropriate public education in the least restrictive environment possible. These statutes determine categories of educational handicap, the process by which they are formally identified, and how interventions for handicaps are to be designed.

Key Elements of the Special Education Process

In order to receive special education services, a multidisciplinary *Case Study Evaluation* is typically conducted to determine whether a student meets eligibility criteria for one or more of 13 federally mandated categories of disability. The disability must be shown to have a handicapping impact upon the student's education. A case study is typically comprised of multiple evaluation components, which may include, but are not limited to, reviews of social and health factors, psychological, educational and speech/language evaluations, occupational or physical therapy evaluations, and a classroom observation. Evaluation results are discussed at a multidisciplinary meeting with the parents and educational staff in order to determine the student's eligibility for services.

After one or more categories of special education eligibility has been established, a proposal for services called an *Individual Educational Plan (IEP)* is written at a similar multidisciplinary meeting (often the two meetings are combined). In order to be implemented, the student's parents must agree to the IEP. Parents are expected to be active participants in this process, and have "veto power" over the implementation of a service program. Once initiated, the program must be reviewed at least annually and the student's eligibility for services reconsidered at least every three years.

Accessing Special Education Services

The process for accessing services under IDEA is carefully structured. Though details vary slightly among school districts, the following steps are common:

1. A *request* is made to the school principal or special education coordinator for an evaluation to determine the student's eligibility for services. This request is typically made by a parent, but may also be initiated by an educator or other clinician working with the student. It is advisable to make the request in writing.

2. In response to the request, the school district may provide *pre-referral assistance* (accommodations or modifications in a regular classroom environment) rather than pursuing a full case study. Some students benefit from this approach, which minimizes segregation within a special education environment and avoids the cumbersome and resource-intensive case study process.
3. If pre-referral assistance has already been given and found inadequate, or is not appropriate, the school district may conduct a *Case Study Evaluation*, as described above. Though the specific makeup of such evaluations varies with the student and the issues involved, they are intended to be a multidisciplinary process soliciting input from parents, educators, and other specialists involved in a student's life. The outcome of the case study should be a determination of the student's eligibility for services under the federally mandated categories.
4. If criteria for one or more of the categories are met, a multidisciplinary team collaborates in the preparation of an *Individual Educational Plan (IEP)* which indicates the types of services that will be provided, specific service goals, and any necessary adjustments of the learning environment.
5. If a parent disagrees with the findings of the case study evaluation or the IEP, appeals at various levels are possible. An initial approach might be to request further discussion by the case study team, with consideration of new or additional information if it is available. As a method of last resort, parents may file for *due process*, a formal legal hearing before an impartial judge or hearing officer. Various forms of negotiation and mediation are also possible between these two extremes.

Other Considerations

Other Health Impairment

The handicap designation of *Other Heath Impairment (OHI)* is of particular relevance to cancer survivors. OHI describes health conditions that do not fall under other special education designations, but which have an adverse impact upon academic functioning. Many cancer late effects fall under this category, as do adverse effects of other conditions such as epilepsy, hydrocephalus, and Attention-Deficit Hyperactivity Disorder (ADHD).

Section 504

Services and adjustments may also be provided under a statute of the Rehabilitation Act of 1973 (P.L. 93–112) called *Section 504*. Support provided under Section 504 need not follow the formal special education process outlined above, and can vary greatly among school settings. 504 services do not require a case study evaluation, though the student must demonstrate a physical or mental handicap that interferes with school activities. Section 504 also differs from the formal special education process in that it is not federally funded. Many cancer survivors are served effectively by "504 plans", which also have the advantage that they can be implemented quickly and with relatively little administrative overhead.

Americans with Disabilities Act (ADA)

The *Americans with Disabilities Act of 1990* (ADA; P.L. 101–336) is a civil rights law that protects individuals with real or perceived disabilities, or a history of disability (e.g., cancer survivorship), from discrimination in academic and employment settings. Modifications that allow cancer survivors to participate in educational and extracurricular activities are supported by this statute. ADA also holds, however, that a disabled individual may decline services or program adjustments that are offered.

Response to Intervention (RTI)

Until recently, special education assistance under the designation of a *learning disability* has typically required a lengthy and costly process of evaluations and multidisciplinary meetings. Learning disability diagnostic criteria have often been based on a *discrepancy model* by which the student's academic skills in reading, math, or writing are demonstrated to be significantly weaker than his intelligence. However, research over the past decade has led to the conclusion that discrepancy-based approaches to defining learning disabilities are problematic.[2] A key tenet of IDEA 04 is that such discrepancies no longer need to be demonstrated in order for special education services to be provided.

An alternate approach to special education called *Response to Intervention (RTI)* is gaining in popularity.[3] Under RTI, a student with poor achievement (regardless of intelligence) may be placed directly into an intervention program without an extensive evaluation. In RTI models, the focus of assessment is upon how the student's academic skills respond to educational intervention. RTI models are varied and currently evolving. Some still provide for traditional multidisciplinary evaluations and IEPs for students who fail to make gains within the RTI framework.[4]

Private Schools

Private schools do not receive federal special education funds and are, therefore, not compelled to provide services under IDEA 04. However, cancer survivors in private school settings are entitled to seek special education assistance through their local public school district. The same case study/IEP process outlined above may be used to access services, often at a student's neighborhood public school, to supplement private school participation. For example, arrangements might allow a qualifying student to receive speech therapy at the neighborhood public school while continuing to receive the majority of her instruction at a private school.

Private school settings are, however, subject to the statutes of ADA. The extent to which private and post-secondary education settings are compelled to provide adjustments and services under ADA has not yet been fully established, and is under scrutiny within the legal arena. While the focus of ADA-related litigation in the past has been mostly upon physical disabilities, an additional focus is emerging upon the question of adjustments for cognitive handicaps under ADA.

High School

High school poses a particular challenge for many cancer survivors, due to demands upon organization skills, work speed, and efficiency that are greater than those of the elementary years. Special education support in high school is also different in that it typically involves less emphasis upon remediation of basic academic skills, and an increased reliance upon the initiative of the student in intervention efforts. As a result, transitions to high school special education programs must be carefully planned.

High school is also a critical period for exploring potential career paths, via coursework and extracurricular activities. Close work with a guidance counselor is important, to insure that the high school years are effectively used not only to develop academic skills, but also to begin charting a career path. Special education statutes provide for the creation of a *transition plan* at age 16 to help students prepare for life after high school, considering options such as college, career education, and employment. Students with educational handicaps remain eligible for services through their local school district until age 22 or high school graduation, whichever comes first. For some handicapped students, formal graduation is not necessarily the best endpoint of schooling, if it would curtail further special education efforts prior to age 22.

College and Post-secondary Education

Federal special education laws do not apply in post-secondary environments such as college and career education settings. However, 504 and ADA statutes continue to protect students beyond high school against discrimination on the basis of disability. Academic adjustments may be necessary in this period to insure that a student is not discriminated against due to a disability. However, after high school, the responsibility for documenting the presence of a disability rests with the student and not the educational institution. Adjustments at the post-secondary level can be broad ranging, involving modifications of learning materials, work requirements, and even housing.

School-Based Interventions

Because the rate of cancer is low relative to other educational handicapping conditions, schools often have little experience with the neurocognitive effects of cancer and its treatment. For this reason, private neuropsychological evaluation can be particularly helpful in assessing the survivor's neurocognitive functioning and informing educational interventions. For example, attention and executive functioning, critical processes impacted by brain tumor diagnosis and treatment, are often not adequately addressed within school-based evaluations. Similarly, parameters of learning, memory, and language versus visuospatial processing may not be assessed in depth and in the context of the survivor's medical history.

The efficacy of special education interventions in childhood cancer survivors has not been examined in depth. However, in a cohort of 12,430 survivors of pediatric cancer, Mitby et al.[5] found that **CNS tumor survivors are nearly three times less likely than their siblings to complete high school**. Interestingly, this gap was smaller (only twice the risk) for survivors who had received special education services compared to siblings with a history of special education.

Common Academic Adjustments

Effective interventions for cancer survivors often depend as much on academic adjustments as they do special classroom placements and out-of-classroom therapies. Academic adjustments are often referred to as *accommodations* or *modifications,* the definitions of which vary from setting to setting and often overlap. The key to academic adjustments is that they involve modifications of activities or work environments that are designed to minimize the impact of a disability upon a student's learning and academic performance. Table 20.1 presents examples of adjustments that can be particularly helpful to brain tumor survivors.

Resource Services

When a student's deficits are not adequately managed by adjustments alone within the regular classroom, direct special education support may be necessary. Assistance may be provided, still within the regular classroom, under an

Table 20.1 Common academic adjustments for brain tumor survivors

Area of vulnerability	Adjustments
Attention and executive functioning (weaknesses in study skills, organization, and planning; forgetfulness; reduced processing speed/efficiency)	Preferential Seating (near teacher, front of class)
	Frequent/subtle cueing to re-engage attention
	Repeat/verify comprehension of instructions
	Test-taking in a quiet room
	Extra set of books for home
	Extra time to complete assignments and tests
	Reduced volume/redundancy of work
	Grading based on material completed – no penalty for uncompleted work
	Break down complex tasks; assist with planning long-term assignments
	Provide study guides
	Regular check-ins regarding assignment instructions, materials, and turning in completed tasks.
Fine motor / Visuomotor skills	Word processor or keyboard communication device for writing
	Oral dictation/transcription software
	Peer note taker; audio/videotape lectures; provide copies of teacher notes/outline
	Provide printed instructions/assignments – minimize copying from the blackboard
	Extra time on writing tasks
	Do not penalize for poor handwriting
	Reduce repetitive writing demands
Visuospatial skills	Reduce density of material on texts/worksheets
	Use alternative to Scantron forms
	Supplement visual information (graphs, maps, pictures, diagrams) with verbal explanation
Language skills	Use simple, concrete instructions/explanation
	Avoid multistep instructions
	Supplement verbal instructions with visual aids such as demonstration, pictures, diagrams, manipulatives
	Verify comprehension by having student repeat back concept/instruction or complete a sample item
Learning / Memory skills	Reduce volume of material to be learned; break down information into manageable "chunks"
	Use teaching strategies that favor child's strengths/preference for verbal or visual learning

Table 20.1 (continued)

Area of vulnerability	Adjustments
	Use multiple choice tests rather than open-ended response formats
	Provide word bank
	Emphasize repetition/practice of material
Arithmetic	Encourage use of calculator
	Multimodal instruction (verbal explanation along with manipulatives/visuals)
	Use graph paper to assist with alignment of numbers
	Provide a table of math facts for reference
	Group similar problems together
Written expression (especially essays/expository writing)	Use word processor or keyboard communication device for writing
	Encourage use of software to assist in spelling, grammar, punctuation, and style
	Use graphic organizers
Reading	Use books on CD / audiotape
	Provide assistance in reading test items
	Provide both oral and written instructions
	Provide summaries of chapters
	Provide books with similar content at an easier level
	Encourage efficient outlining/note taking as a study strategy
	Allow use of highlighter/underlining
Fatigue	Allow/schedule rest breaks during school day
	Preferential scheduling of key subjects in morning, when student is most alert
	Avoid scheduling several effortful subjects in succession, intersperse with easier subjects
	Reduced homework load
	Reduced course load
	Study hall to allow extra time for completion of assignments at school

inclusion model. Alternatively, the student may be "pulled-out" of the regular class for a portion of the day into a smaller, specialized class with other disabled students. Separate "resource" classes place the student with specially trained educators at a lower student–to-teacher ratio, allowing more individualized pacing and instruction, and substantial modification to curricula as needed. Resource support may be provided in circumscribed academic areas such as math or language arts, or can be more general, as with a resource study hall. The latter option can be especially valuable for survivors at the middle and high school levels, when students often struggle due to limitations of executive functioning. This can serve several purposes: providing extra time and support to complete homework, the opportunity to reinforce concepts/skills, explicit instruction in organizational and study strategies, and a liaison with other teachers to help the student advocate for his needs across subjects.

Self-contained Classroom Placement

When a student's deficits are severe and pervasive, such as with a severe learning disability or mental retardation, it may be necessary to provide primary instruction in a *self-contained* setting. This more restrictive placement offers specialized instruction for most or all core academic areas, but may include the option of student participation with non-handicapped peers in non-core academic experiences such as lunch, physical education, music, and art. High school programming for self-contained classroom students should include a special emphasis upon preparation for the transition to post-secondary work and life activities.

Ancillary Services

Additional services may also be included in the student's IEP, to supplement and support primary academic instruction. For example, *speech/language* services may be appropriate if the student has a deficit in speech (articulation) and/or language (receptive or expressive communication). *Physical* and *occupational* therapies can address issues related to pain, sensory-motor weakness, and motor coordination (e.g., impact on handwriting). *Social work* services can provide support for socio-emotional concerns that affect school functioning (e.g., mood lability resulting in peer conflicts, anxiety/low self-esteem about schoolwork).

Making Adjustments over Time

Over time, there are likely to be more frequent changes in the brain tumor survivor's educational needs than for other special education students. During active treatment, school attendance may be sporadic, and a home- or hospital-bound teacher may be needed to minimize academic disruption. If, following treatment and acute recovery, full-time school attendance is not possible, a plan should be developed that focuses on key subjects and does not overburden the student with homework. With return to full-time school attendance, an updated assessment of programming needs is often appropriate. Some pediatric centers offer reentry support with direct consultation to school staff to facilitate a patient's reintegration. While those programs would seem to hold promise for the comprehensive care of the survivor, their efficacy has not been adequately explored.[6]

As academic demands increase, the survivor needs close monitoring to ensure that academic supports are appropriately meeting her needs. In addition to more frequent assessment of academic mastery and cognitive abilities, frequent communication between educators and parents is crucial. If the student spends an inordinate amount of time and effort on homework, or requires excessive assistance from parents, his work products may not accurately reflect the amount of difficulty he is experiencing. Educators may mistakenly expect more from a student than is realistic, and fail to provide needed supports such as adjustments to homework load or reinforcement of concepts.

Monitoring is particularly important around periods of academic transition, when learning demands increase dramatically and weaknesses may become more evident. For example, educational demands increase significantly from the primary years, when the emphasis is on basic skills (e.g., "learning to read"), to later elementary years, when fluency in those skills is essential to efficient information acquisition (e.g., "reading to learn"). The transition to middle school entails increased organizational demands as well as an emphasis on abstract thinking and higher level language skills. Transitions to high school and college present even greater demands with regard to independent thinking, problem solving, completion of long-term projects, higher level essay writing, and more efficient study and notetaking strategies. Productivity and "load" (complexity or amount of material) requirements also increase dramatically over time.

Interventions Outside of School

Interventions outside of the formal educational setting can also have a significant impact upon the academic functioning of the brain tumor survivor. While IEP and 504 plans are intended to minimize the adverse impact of educational handicaps upon learning, their goal is not universally seen as eliciting a student's optimal performance. Though the distinction between these aims is open to interpretation, it is clear that many handicapped students stand to benefit from additional interventions outside of school. Furthermore, some interventions (e.g., medication management) are not feasible or appropriate for delivery within the school setting.

Ancillary Therapies and Tutoring

Speech-language services and physical and occupational therapies may be provided privately to supplement school-based services and to address concerns outside the school setting. In addition, survivors may benefit from private tutoring in specific subject areas (e.g., math, writing) or in "metacognitive" study and organizational strategies. Metacognitive tutoring can be especially helpful in the middle and high school years, as it provides students with tools and strategies they can apply to compensate for executive/organizational weaknesses.

Very little empirical research has examined the benefits of formal educational interventions for late effects of childhood cancer. The only published study to date was done by Moore and colleagues.[7] They examined a math intervention consisting of a skill-based approach providing 40 to 50 hours of tutoring to eight children with a history of leukemia. The intervention was found to have a moderate to large beneficial effect on arithmetic skills, compared to seven control patients who did not receive the intervention. Though promising, the small sample size, lack of randomization, and singular nature of this study urge caution in interpreting its results.

Cognitive Rehabilitation

Interest is growing in the promise of cognitive rehabilitation, defined as "a systematic effort to assist brain damaged individuals in developing ways to compensate for cognitive deficits".[8,9] Research on cognitive rehabilitation has most often examined deficits of attention, memory, and executive functioning following traumatic brain injury (TBI) and other central nervous system (CNS) insults. While initial studies focused on massed practice interventions, recent models are emerging which emphasize a multicomponent, holistic approach targeting school, family, peer relations, self-awareness, and cognitive-behavioral modification.[9,10,11]

The efficacy of cognitive rehabilitation following CNS insult in children is not yet established, although research is ongoing in this area.[12] Butler[9] describes a positive, but modest effect of cognitive remediation in a sample of childhood cancer survivors participating in a Phase III randomized clinical trial. Interventions in that study, described below, were associated with improved academic functioning and parent/teacher reports of improved attention.

In the above study, Butler and colleagues used the Cognitive Remediation Program (CRP), which has been comprehensively described in several papers.[1,9,13] The CRP is described as programmatic (i.e., all participants are expected to meet certain goals over the 20-week therapy period) and individualized (i.e., goals are set according to the specific needs of the participant). CRP draws upon brain injury rehabilitation techniques, but adds instruction in metacognitive strategies and clinical psychological techniques in the form of cognitive-behavioral therapy. The program utilizes a team approach involving the therapist, parents, school, and other relevant personnel working with the student. A key aspect of the program is its attempt to promote generalization to the real world by teaching the student specific metacognitive strategies and how, why, and when they are to be used. Parents are expected to reinforce concepts with the student and to communicate with educators so the strategies can also be applied within the classroom.

Initial research into the field of cognitive remediation is encouraging. However, a word of caution is in order. While some cognitive rehabilitation techniques are currently being marketed to the public for treating brain injury in children, outcome research on their efficacy and generalizability remains inconclusive.

Stimulant Medication

Declines of IQ and academic achievement indices in pediatric brain tumor survivors are partly mediated by impairments of attention.[14] This finding, and the common finding of deficient attention in cancer survivors, suggests that attention skills are a particularly important target of intervention in this population. Given the demonstrated efficacy of stimulant medication for Attention-Deficit Hyperactivity Disorder (ADHD),[15] this treatment has also been explored with cancer survivors. Initial studies yielded variable results, but suggested positive short-term effects with both adults and children.[16] However, those studies were limited by methodology and sample size. A randomized, double-blind crossover trial of methylphenidate (MPH) has recently been completed with 122 pediatric cancer survivors,[17] indicating a significant advantage of MPH over placebo on indices of attention, processing speed, and cognitive flexibility.

It has been suggested that effective stimulant doses for cancer survivors may be lower than in patients with uncomplicated ADHD.[9] Little information is available, however, to guide the physician with respect to treatment levels. Similarly, the question of increased risk among survivors for stimulant side effects has been raised, though Conklin et al.[17] monitored such effects and did not find them to be greater for MPH than for placebo.

Summary

The special education system is a critical resource for pediatric brain tumor survivors, and one of the most important contexts for life skills rehabilitation. However, educators often have limited experience with the challenges that survivors face, and they stand to benefit from assistance in developing appropriate academic support programs. With age, students face increased academic demands, and the impact of adverse cognitive effects becomes more apparent. As a result, it is important to closely monitor the survivor's academic progress and implement services and adjustments as they are needed. High school and post-secondary education settings present special challenges for survivors, but they should also be seen as unique opportunities for adaptive growth in the transition to independent work and life activities.

Adjustments to mainstream academic requirements and work activities are often as important as specialized educational placements in meeting the needs of the cancer survivor. Effective adjustments reduce the impact of cognitive disabilities, such as impaired attention and vulnerability to mental fatigue, upon the survivor's learning and academic performance. Students are entitled to seek assistance through the high school years under special education statutes. Rehabilitation and disability laws also apply to educational activities throughout the lifespan.

Surprisingly little research has addressed the educational impact of brain tumor therapies, and educational interventions for survivors. One noteworthy exception is the recent study of a multi-component cognitive remediation intervention, with outcome data now emerging. Pharmacologic approaches targeting attention deficits are also being studied, with promising results.

Further research is needed to establish an empirical foundation for educational and rehabilitation interventions with brain tumor survivors. It will also be important to explore variables outside the formal educational environment, such as familial and social factors, that influence academic outcomes. Pharmacologic treatments for cognitive late effects deserve particular attention, given the promise they hold for enhancing the survivor's response to educational intervention efforts. Studies of long-term stimulant efficacy considering dose levels and side effects are necessary, as are studies of alternate attention medications such as atomoxetine.

References

1. Butler RW, Mulhern RK. Neurocognitive interventions for children and adolescents surviving cancer. *J Pediatr Psychol*. 2005; 30:65–78.
2. Fletcher JM, Foorman BR, Boudousquie A, et al. Assessment of reading and learning disabilities: a research-based intervention-oriented approach. *J Sch Psychol*. 2002; 40:27–63.
3. Fletcher JM, Lyon GR, Fuchs LS, et al. *Learning Disabilities: from Identification to Intervention*. New York: Guilford Press, 2007.
4. Hale JB, Kaufman A, Naglieri JA, et al. Implementation of IDEA: integrating response to intervention and cognitive assessment methods. *Psychol Sch*. 2006; 43:753–770.
5. Mitby PA, Robison LL, Whitton JA, et al. Utilization of special education services and educational attainment among long-term survivors of childhood cancer. *Cancer*. 2003; 97:1115–1126.
6. Nortz MJ, Hemme-Phillips JM, Ris MD. Neuropsychological sequelae in children treated for cancer. In: Hunter SJ, Donders J, eds. *Pediatric Neuropsychological Intervention: A Critical Review of Science and Practice*. Cambridge: Cambridge University Press, 2007:112–132.
7. Moore IM, Espy KA, Kaufmann P, et al. Cognitive consequences and central nervous system injury following treatment for childhood leukemia. *Semin Oncol Nurs*. 2000; 16:279–290.
8. Brett AW, Laatsch L. Cognitive rehabilitation therapy of brain-injured students in a public high school setting. *Pediatr Rehabil*. 1998; 2:27–31.

9. Butler RW. Cognitive rehabilitation. In: Hunter SJ, Donders J, eds. *Pediatric Neuropsychological Intervention: A Critical Review of Science and Practice*. Cambridge: Cambridge University Press, 2007:444–464.

10. Ylvisaker M. *Traumatic Brain Injury: Children and Adolescents*. 2nd ed. Boston: Butterworth-Heinemann Publishing, 1998.

11. Ylvisaker M, Adelson PD, Braga LW, et al. Rehabilitation and ongoing support after pediatric TBI: twenty years of progress. *J Head Trauma Rehabil*. 2005; 20:95–109.

12. Limond J, Leeke R. Practitioner review: cognitive rehabilitation for children with acquired brain injury. *J Child Psychol Psychiatry*. 2005; 46:339–352.

13. Butler RW, Copeland DR. Attentional processes and their remediation in children treated for cancer: a literature review and the development of a therapeutic approach. *J Int Neuropsychol Soc*. 2002; 8:115–124.

14. Reddick WE, White HA, Glass JO, et al. Developmental model relating white matter volume to neurocognitive deficits in pediatric brain tumor survivors. *Cancer*. 2003; 97:2512–2519.

15. Brown RT, Amler RW, Freeman WS, et al. Treatment of attention-deficit/hyperactivity disorder: overview of the evidence. *Pediatrics* 2005; 115:749–757.

16. Daly BP, Brown RT. Scholarly literature review: management of neurocognitive late effects with stimulant medication. *J Pediatr Psychol*. 2007; 32:1111–1126.

17. ConklinHM, Khan RB, Reddick WE, et al. Acute neurocognitive response to methylphenidate among survivors of childhood cancer: a randomized, double-blind, cross-over trial. *J Pediatr Psychol*. 2007; 32:1127–1139.

General Resources on Educational Handicaps and Services

Internet Sites

Greatschools.Net: An excellent source of online information about educational handicaps, interventions, and advocacy. http://www.greatschools.net/content/specialNeeds.page

Parent Advocacy Center for Educational Rights (PACER): This is a parent training and information center for families of youth with disabilities. www.pacer.org

United States Department of Education: State contacts and educational information. http://www.ed.gov/about/contacts/state/index.html

Educational Advocacy Information

Anderson W, Chitwood S, Hayden D. *Negotiating the Special Education Maze: A Guide for Parents & Teachers*. 3rd ed. Bethesda, MD: Woodbine House, 1997.

Siegel LM. *The Complete IEP Guide: How to advocate for your special ed child*. 3rd ed. Berkeley, CA: Nolo. 2004

Chapter 21
Caregiver and Family Issues for Brain Tumor Survivors

Tracy Moore and Stacia Wagner

Introduction

In the context of an oncology setting, a psychosocial assessment exploring family strengths, beliefs, coping mechanisms, socioeconomic status and disease understanding can play an important role in a family-centered care approach.[1] Since each diagnosis and treatment represents a unique pathway for the patient and family, premorbid family functioning should be fully assessed at the time of diagnosis. When a family has continued involvement with the hospital, utilizing the initial assessment and reassessing throughout treatment and into survivorship can aid the health care team in developing a plan to improve and support family resilience and competency.

Some survivors may have severe and long-term medical late effects leaving their future independence in question.[2] Additionally, brain tumors and their treatments may cause moderate to severe neurocognitive effects. Such effects will also impact the survivors' long-term abilities, goals, and quality of life. Similar to the unique path that diagnosis and treatment bring a family, each survivor will adapt differently. Consequently, some survivors have the emotional scars of fear, stress and isolation, while others may experience cognitive growth, maturity and increased empathy.[3–5]

The direct implications of a brain tumor will also impact each family system in a unique way. This impact does not stop at the completion of treatment and the effect will last throughout the lives of patients, as well as parents and siblings of pediatric survivors, spouses and children of adult survivors. Therefore, it is critical to recognize the impact a brain tumor diagnosis has not only on the patient, but also the entire family unit. Each developmental milestone brings the possibility of family challenges and the opportunity for intervention. Clinicians' use of psychoeducation and interviews focusing on each member's perception

T. Moore (✉)
Director of Social Work, North Shore University Hospital, 300 Community Drive, Manhassett, NY 11030, USA
e-mail: tmoore2@nshs.edu

S. Goldman, C.D. Turner (eds.), *Late Effects of Treatment for Brain Tumors*,
Cancer Treatment and Research 150, DOI 10.1007/b109924_21,
© Springer Science+Business Media, LLC 2009

of the disease and disease impact have proven a successful model for minimizing the difficulties a brain tumor can have within the family.[6-11] In addition, strengthening support systems and developing advocacy tools as a means to increase family coping and resiliency have also proven successful.

Finally, the end of treatment can also bring a significant decrease in support from the medical and social community. As the oncology community continues to work nationally to develop standards of care for brain tumor survivors, the impact of the late effects on the family system need to be included within the development of a standard of care. The remainder of this chapter will focus on certain important factors for a survivor's long-term care.

Caregiver

Since families come in all shapes and sizes, it is important to identify who fills the caregiver role within the family. In order to accurately access the possible impact of late effects on the family, each individual responsible for the patient's care and upbringing needs to be evaluated. Evidence shows that clinical assessment of the caregiver's individual attributes, strengths and beliefs plays an important role in evaluating their position within the family and their potential effectiveness in providing late effects care.

Knowledge of the caregiver's family history of cancer, understanding of diagnosis and late effects, spiritual and cultural beliefs, community supports, and coping mechanisms need to be acquired.[12] This evaluation should occur well beyond the completion of treatment, including assessment as the survivor enters new developmental stages.

It is also important to establish a baseline of coping. "Past behavior guides present crisis appraisals, resources management, role assignment and expectations of success-or failure. Family histories also define family assumptions about cancer and the prognosis".[13] Therefore, the caregiver's ability to adapt and cope with parenting a long-term brain tumor survivor may be reflective of past coping with stressful occurrences. For instance, a mother whose previous coping mechanisms included alcohol abuse and illicit drug consumption will probably fare far worse than the parent who relied on a strong peer and family support system.

Along with the assessment of the individual caregiver, other environmental and family factors that influence caregiver coping and should be evaluated. These considerations include: age and developmental stage at time of diagnosis, siblings, social support, socioeconomic standing, coping mechanisms, impact of a rare disease, cause of the tumor (genetic vs. unknown cause), and the perceived controllability of late effects. These considerations may change as the survivor matures. "As many as 25% of primary care-givers give up or lose their job, one third of families lose all their savings or their major source of income. Sixty percent of the remaining care-takers register a significant loss in income due to absenteeism or a shift to lesser paid work".[13] The financial devastation frequently experienced at time of diagnosis and during treatment may be reduced upon the end of treatment or may continue based on the extent of the survivor's medical needs.

Self-care for the Caregiver

Making oneself a priority is a hard concept for many parents to think about when faced with their child's diagnosis of a brain tumor and the long-term impact that may have on the child and entire family. Many parents or spouses often put the needs of their children, partners, extended families and friends before addressing their own emotional and physical well-being. It is essential to emphasize the importance of self-care in the attempt to protect and bolster the survivor's caregiver. Brain tumor survivorship is a lifelong journey and, to use the metaphor, it is a marathon rather than a sprint. Educating parents, spouses, or other caregivers about their own needs in terms of this marathon will enable them to better meet the needs of their families and better maintain coping throughout. **Compared to parents who experience raising children without complex medical needs**, "significantly more mothers of pediatric cancer survivors were diagnosed with lifetime PTSD".[4] This emphasizes the importance of frequent discussion around taking care of oneself.

Caregiver as a Partner

When a child or spouse is diagnosed with a brain tumor, the marital relationship can be strained and/or strengthened. Caregiver roles and the ability to successfully cope often change and evolve throughout the continuum of care. Individual coping styles, including those who are information seekers versus those who learn what they need in the moment, can directly conflict with each other. Since partners will adapt opposing styles on occasion, conflict with communication and presence within the relationship can occur. The opposite can be true as well. Specifically, couples can practice open communication and acquire healthy coping patterns as a team.

Just as caregivers may have different coping styles, they also may develop differing intimacy needs. Some partners may look for sexual experience as a way to reconnect with their loved one, while others may not have the desire to open up physically or emotionally due to a variety of reasons including caregiver exhaustion. The demands brought on by the needs of the survivor may interfere with sexual intimacy. In some relationships, partners look for small gestures and communication before sexual intimacy. If partners have opposing needs, this may lead to conflict and feelings of rejection.

It is important for clinicians to address couples' communication, possible marital stressors, and encourage partners to seek opportunities to strengthen their relationship by focusing on each other. This is especially apparent because, so often, it is the survivor's needs that are the focus of the family. Lack of communication, financial struggles, and intimacy difficulties are frequently linked to causes of divorce. A brain tumor diagnosis and the long-term effects related to it may directly impact each of these areas. Research indicates that most families maintain or return to generally satisfactory levels in their relationships.[14] As former first lady Barbara Bush told the NCCF in 2003, "Cancer has changed your lives- but it does not define you".[15] When offering support to couples in this arena, it can be helpful to establish this concept within the family system.

Caregiver to the Pediatric Survivor

Some say the ultimate goal of parenting is providing the fundamental tools and foundation to allow a child to achieve independence and reach their highest potential. In dealing with the late effects associated with survivorship, parents are frequently forced to modify and adapt the expectations they had for their child. At time of diagnosis, parents may grieve the loss of the healthy child and, as developmental milestones occur, this grief is often revisited and compounded. Parental relationships with the survivor during diagnosis and treatment may create situations where the parent becomes the survivors' closest relationship and that enmeshment can continue well beyond the completion of treatment. This can compromise both the survivor's ability to reach their fullest potential, as well as the parent's true perception of their child's current status. This may mean parents become overprotective, set unrealistic goals, or minimize the actual capability of the survivor. Ultimately, many caregivers are their child's best advocate during treatment. On the continuum of survivorship, it is important for health care providers to educate parents on the importance of empowering their child to be independent and advocate for themselves.

Caregiver to the Siblings of a Pediatric Survivor

Understandably, parents may need to focus their attention and presence on the needs of their child with a brain tumor. Typically this may be for the period during diagnosis and treatment, but can also extend throughout the maturation of the survivor. Siblings may make assumptions based on their parent's absences as to their own self-worth and role within the family system. As health care providers, it is essential to recognize both patients and siblings throughout all family assessments and conversations. Reinforcing the unique needs of siblings with parents may alleviate their feelings of separation and possible guilt when leaving the patient, thus opening the door to allow them to spend quality time with all of their children individually. Without open lines of communication between the parents and the survivor's siblings, relationships may fracture. Conversely, parents making special time between themselves and the survivor's siblings may improve sibling coping and adjustment to diagnosis through survivorship. Taylor and colleagues found "Better sibling adjustment is associated with higher maternal awareness of their attitudes and perceptions".[16] With this in mind, it is important for parents to routinely discuss a sibling's perception and knowledge of their brother's or sister's disease and late effects, while acknowledging the impact it may have on them, as the sibling. It is still important for the parent to recognize the sibling as an individual rather than defining them through their survivor experiences.

Siblings of Pediatric Survivors

The extent of the late effects a pediatric brain tumor survivor experiences has a direct impact on the sibling as well as the patient. Like the patient, the sibling will be affected throughout the course of the survivorship continuum. The sibling's gender, birth order, and age/developmental stage at the time of their brother's or sister's diagnosis need to be accounted for when evaluating the impact. Sibling relationships are, for many, the longest relationship throughout life. The relationships formed, friendships developed, jealousy created, and power struggles within are innate to all families. The dynamics of the sibling relationship will be impacted forever when a child is diagnosed with a brain tumor.

Caregiver roles within the family may shift, also directly impacting the sibling's experience. Some families may need to utilize friends, extended family, and neighbors to offer direct care to the sibling while they are bedside at the hospital with the child diagnosed with a brain tumor. This may lead to a sibling's feelings of isolation and they may develop their own fantasy about the diagnosis, prognosis and cause of their brother's or sister's brain tumor. Without parental communication and intervention, these effects may be long-term. Siblings may develop behaviors contrary to their previous behavioral path prior to diagnosis, including acting out in school, bullying or becoming the "perfect child." Studies have indicated an increased risk of post-traumatic stress disorder among siblings. On the opposite side of the spectrum, studies have shown siblings are resilient and have demonstrated positive outcomes secondary to their brother's or sister's diagnosis. Many siblings have increased compassion and empathy, choose careers in the health care field and become advocates for their brother or sister as a result of the diagnosis.

There are several key components to increasing coping and quality of life for siblings: analyzing the sibling's views and perception of the long-term outlook for the patient, establishing and enhancing a base level of disease knowledge, creating honest communication within the family system, and increasing empowerment through sibling's participation in treatment and follow-up.[17]

Finally, as families mature, siblings may begin to think about taking over the role of caregiver for their brother or sister, when independent living is not an option. This shift in family dynamics may take place at an early stage in the sibling's life. The dual role of being caregiver to their aging parent and sibling may cause alterations in their career and personal paths.

Tools and Support

Group intervention, networking opportunities including camps and programs designed specifically for sibling's needs, advocacy opportunities, and family communication may improve the sibling quality of life and coping with the issues related to survivorship.

Family System

In order to provide the proper intervention to help the brain tumor survivor, one must have a thorough knowledge of the family in its entirety, including family mores, spiritual beliefs and culture. Although there is minimal research specific to brain tumor late effects as they relate to specific cultures, there is culture-specific information related to the impact on a family when a member has been diagnosed with a chronic or life-threatening illness. These studies demonstrate the importance of including extended family, the respect of spiritual differences, and the demand for cultural sensitivity when intervening with families.

As families find themselves geographically scattered across the country and beyond, there is a growing dependence on peer groups as primary support systems. As health care providers, it is critical to empower families to utilize whatever strengths exist within their lives and community. Assessing the family's own definition of who is important in their life and then incorporating those members within the treatment plan and survivorship continuum may aid in family coping and cohesiveness. This may include grandparents, extended family and close friends. Social support and the perception of social support can be key factors in influencing resiliency, especially in the relatively high risk group of families who have a child with a chronic illness.[18] Possible interventions may include role playing scenarios and advocacy training for the caregivers in hopes they will maximize their support system.

Brain tumors remain a relatively uncommon disease. The Central Brain Tumor Registry of the United States (2006) lists 3,410 pediatric and 43,800 adult diagnoses in the United States each year. Some families report a feeling of isolation due to the unique medical, social and emotional challenges they face. There is, however, a growing population of long-term brain tumor survivors. This population currently totals over 26,000 in the United States. The population allows for opportunities for survivors and other family members to network with others who have had a similar experience. Some program models that connect families impacted by childhood brain tumors include: Parent-to-Parent Network (a program created by CBTF which links trained parent volunteers with others looking for peer support around the diagnosis, treatment and survivor issues), family camps (such as Brain Tumor Week at Camp Sunshine), recreational programs, and family conferences with networking opportunities. Families should remember that information is power and family unity provides a vehicle for raising awareness and advocacy.

With the increased knowledge of brain tumor late effects, many of the former cancer myths have been dispelled. The belief that a brain tumor is a guaranteed death sentence is no longer the norm for many. However, there is still a significant gap in the perception that the end of treatment also signifies the end of challenges faced by survivors and their families. This often creates unnecessary hurdles and obstacles for parents trying to receive critical support within the community and necessary programs to enable maximum independence. For example, many educators lack the knowledge of the neurocognitive late effects related to a brain tumor diagnosis in children and its treatment, leaving the learning challenges to be either misdiagnosed or underdiagnosed completely. Frequently, this creates unnecessary hurdles and may leave parents in an adversarial position with the school system. This is yet another opportunity for the health care team to intervene, providing education and advocacy for the survivor and the family.

Tools and Support

In order to measure the long-term impact of a brain tumor diagnosis on the family, several Quality of Life assessment tools have been developed. Health care professionals may want to utilize these tools in assessing family coping and understanding. Two examples of these tools are Ferrans and Powers Quality of Life Index © Cancer Version III and Minneapolis-Manchester Quality of Life- Youth Form (MMQL-YF).

Additionally, standards of care through long-term follow-up clinics need to be developed. Currently, in the pediatric community, the Children's Oncology Group provides survivorship guidelines (www.survivorshipguidelines.org), which address many of the medical and educational late effects experienced by pediatric brain tumor survivors. However, there is limited information and research regarding the psychosocial impact on the family, especially when considering cultural differences. References within research pertaining to the longevity of the survivor experience and family impact are not widely reported on. There can be some broad influences based on data from populations that may have similar psychosocial experiences, such as survivors of pediatric cancer or families dealing with other chronic illnesses. Yet the unique path brain tumor survivors and their families walk is important and complex. This is an area that deserves attention and focus for future research.

Conclusion

Walsh asserts that "The concept of resilience is being the ability to withstand and rebound from crisis and adversity".[18] Overall, survivors of brain tumors and their families show remarkable resilience. Resilient behavior often results in the family defining a **"new normal"**.[19,20] This may mean new roles within the family, lifestyle modifications, strategies for coping, development of support systems, and newfound advocacy skills. Finding the balance for one's self and each other's needs within the family is key to the family's well-being. In optimal circumstances, survivorship is only one element of how the family defines itself, allowing for healing and hope for the future.

References

1. Rolland JS. Chronic illness and the life cycle: a conceptual framework. *Family Proc.* 1987;26:203–221.
2. Patenaude A, Kupst MJ. Psychosocial functioning in pediatric cancer. *J Pediatr Psychol.* 2005;30:9–27.
3. Hobbie W, Stuber M, Meeske K, et al. Symptoms of posttraumatic stress in young adult survivors of childhood cancer. *J Clin Oncol.* 2000;24:4060–4066.
4. Pelcovitz D, Goldenberg B, Kaplan S, et al. Posttraumatic stress disorder in mothers of pediatric cancer survivors. *Psychosomatics.* 1996;37:116–126.
5. Zebrack B, Chesler MA. Quality of life in childhood cancer survivors. *Psycho-Oncology.* 2002;11(2):132–141.
6. Bohanek J, Marin KA, Fivush R. Family narrative interaction and children's sense of self. *Family Proc.* 2006;45:39–54.
7. Dellve L, Samuelsson L, Tallborn A, et al. Stress and well-being among parents of children with rare diseases: a prospective intervention study. *J Adv Nurs.* 2006;53(4); 392–402.
8. Kazak AE, Simms S., Barakat L, et al. Surviving cancer competently intervention program (SCCIP): a cognitive behavioral and family therapy intervention for adolescent survivors of childhood cancer and their families. *Family Proc.* 1999;38:176–191.
9. Rait DS, Ostroff JS, Smith K, et al. Lives in a balance: Perceived family functioning and the psychosocial adjustment of adolescent cancer survivors. *Family Proc.* 1992; 31: 383–397.
10. Sabbeth B. Understanding the impact of chronic illness on families. *Pediatr Clin North Am.* 1984;31:47–57.
11. Wamboldt MZ, Wamboldt FS. Role of the family in the onset and outcome of childhood disorders: selected research findings. *J Am Acad Child Adolesc Psychiatry.* 2000;39:1212–1219.
12. Lederberg M. "The family of the cancer patient." In: Holland J, ed. *Psycho-Oncology.* New York, NY: Oxford University Press, 1988:981–993.
13. Kupst MJ, Schulman JL, Maurer H, et al. Coping with pediatric leukemia: a two-year follow-up. *J Pediatr Psychol.* 1984;9(2):149–163.

14. Mrs. Bush's remarks at the national childhood cancer foundation gold ribbon days 2003. Washington, D.C. Accessed March, 30, 2007 at http://www.whitehouse.gov/news/releases/2003/09/20030917-12.html.
15. Taylor V, Fuggle P, Charman T. Well sibling psychological adjustment to chronic physical disorder in a sibling: how important is maternal awareness of their illness attitudes and perceptions? *J Child Psychol Psychiatry*. 2001;42:953–962.
16. Gallo AM., Breitmayer BJ, Knafl KA, et al. Mothers' perceptions of sibling adjustment and family life in childhood chronic illness. *J Pediatr Nurs*. 1993;8,318–324.
17. Tak YR, McCubbin M. Family stress, perceived social support and coping following the diagnosis of a child's congenital heart disease. *J Adv Nurs*. 2002;39(2):190–198.
18. Walsh F. The concept of family resilience: crisis and challenge. *Family Proc*. 2002;35: 261–281.
19. Woodgate RL, Degner LF. A substantive theory of keeping the spirit alive: The spirit within children with cancer and their families. *J Pediatr Oncol Nurs*. 2003;20:103–119.
20. Clarke-Steffen L. A model of the family transition to living with childhood cancer. *Cancer Pract*. 1993;1(4):285–292.

Part IV
Additional Topics

Chapter 22
Healthy Lifestyle Choices after Cancer Treatment

Victoria W. Willard, Melanie J. Bonner, and A. Bebe Guill

Introduction

In the general population lifestyle factors such as alcohol and tobacco use, exercise, sun exposure, obesity, and diet are associated with the risk of many health problems, including cancer. In the cancer survivor population this risk may be exacerbated due to the treatments used to control or cure the disease. Indeed, all standard treatment modalities including radiation, chemotherapy, hormone therapy, and surgery can adversely affect the health of survivors long after treatment has ended. Novel use of more toxic cancer treatments in multiple combinations and in high doses has increased survival rates, but has also contributed to increased risks of unwanted late effects. Both standard and novel therapies have been associated with an adverse impact on the long-term health of the cancer survivor, including endocrine and cardiac problems as well as the development of secondary cancers. Given the growing number of cancer survivors, attention is increasingly focused on management and prevention of late effects through interventions that address lifestyle habits, such as diet and weight management, exercise, sun protection, smoking cessation, and careful long-term medical follow-up.

Pediatric Brain Tumor Survivors

In pediatric oncology, long-term survivors are typically those that have been off all treatment with stable disease for greater than two years.[1] While all cancer survivors should avoid certain health damaging or risky behaviors such as smoking or excessive alcohol use, childhood cancer survivors in particular are at an increased risk for health problems due to these behaviors because of the

V.W. Willard (✉)
Department of Psychology and Neuroscience, Duke University, Durham, NC, USA
e-mail: victoria.willard@duke.edu

S. Goldman, C.D. Turner (eds.), *Late Effects of Treatment for Brain Tumors*,   343
Cancer Treatment and Research 150, DOI 10.1007/b109924_22,
© Springer Science+Business Media, LLC 2009

vulnerable age at which they are diagnosed and treated. As such, a focus on prevention, particularly with younger survivors, is paramount.

Central nervous system (CNS)-based cancers account for over 20% of all new cancer diagnoses in children. However, the research with survivors of pediatric brain tumors is almost exclusively focused on the cognitive late effects that plague these children. In contrast to the multitudes of studies that are published each year on their cognitive deficits, few, if any, target other late effects and practices, such as lifestyle behaviors. Indeed, the majority of studies that do focus on lifestyle factors in childhood cancer survivors exclude brain tumor survivors from their samples or are from medical centers that see an underrepresented population of brain tumor diagnoses.[2]

Despite this gap in the literature, the abundance of research on lifestyle factors in survivors of other childhood cancers, particularly with regards to tobacco use, can be somewhat generalized to apply to survivors of pediatric brain tumors, as long as caveats regarding diminished cognitive capacities and their unique medical histories related to endocrine risk are taken into account.[3,4] Of note, the one study that included survivors of pediatric brain tumors found no differences on any lifestyle behavior measured when compared to two other cancer groups, despite significant differences in reported quality of life.[5]

In the earliest report of health-related behaviors in childhood cancer survivors, Mulhern and colleagues[6] surveyed adolescent and young adult survivors using parent- and self-report, respectively. Contrary to expectations based on research with healthy adolescents and young adults, demographic factors were not related to health behaviors, though younger survivors and those a shorter time since therapy considered themselves more vulnerable to later health problems.

In a follow-up, Tyc, Hadley and Crocket[7] surveyed 46 survivors (brain tumor survivors were excluded) about tobacco and alcohol use, as well as protective behaviors such as dental, dietary, seat belt, sleep and exercise habits. Participants were also asked to rate perceived vulnerability, importance of health protection and locus of control. The majority of survivors agreed that they were in more danger of developing health problems than their peers and felt that it was "somewhat" to "a lot" more important to protect their health relative to healthy peers. Additionally, the majority also believed that they could control their health through their behavior choices. In terms of health habits, this sample of childhood cancer survivors reported health habits that were as healthy as their healthy peer group and that they engaged in risky health behaviors at a lower rate than their peers. However, many survivors reported inconsistent engagement in protective health behaviors such as exercising, adequate sleep and following a healthy diet, despite their assessment of greater vulnerability to health problems. Contrary to the Mulhern study,[6] but consistent with the general population, in this sample, the practice of health behaviors was largely accounted for by demographic factors such as age and socioeconomic status (SES). Indeed younger survivors and those from higher SES families reported more health-protective behaviors.[7] Such findings help researchers and clinicians target those survivors that are particularly in need of interventions (e.g., those who are older and of a lower SES).

A study completed with a British group of survivors (again, brain tumors were excluded as they were primarily seen at a different medical center) corroborated these results.[8] Young adult survivors were compared to their siblings and a group of age- and sex-matched healthy peers on a Health Behavior Index which combined responses on factors such as tobacco, alcohol and illicit drug use, diet, exercise and sun protection. Survivors reported lower rates of tobacco, alcohol and drug use – both currently and in the past – than either siblings or matched controls. Generally, survivors were more likely to be single, and reported lower self-esteem and a lower locus of control. Despite this, survivors seemed to be living a healthier life than either their siblings or matched controls. It has been suggested that the lower rates of alcohol, drug and tobacco use in childhood cancer survivors may be indicative of a less active social life, though this has yet to be explored.[8]

Reeves et al.[9] surveyed a small group of Australian survivors of childhood cancer, including 43% who were survivors of pediatric brain tumors. The brain tumor survivors were at greater risk for being overweight, with 67% being overweight as compared to 30% of other childhood cancers. They were also less likely to meet recommended physical activity levels, with only 8% meeting guidelines, as compared to 33% of leukemia survivors.[9] Unfortunately for many pediatric brain tumor survivors, their likelihood to be overweight may be due to tumor-related factors such as damage to the hypothalamus, most frequently seen in craniophyarngiomas. Lustig and colleague[10] surveyed a sample of 148 brain tumor survivors seen at St. Jude Children's Research Hospital. They found that those who were younger and those with hypothalamic tumors were particularly at risk for a high BMI. Furthermore, all brain tumor patients, regardless of tumor location, who received radiation therapy to the hypothalamus were at risk for a high BMI.[10] Such findings suggest that particular attention should be paid to lifestyle habits of patients whose tumors or treatments have affected the hypothalamus. In particular, early and intense intervention may help to prevent high levels of weight gain which would put these patients at high risk for comorbid medical problems such as diabetes and heart disease.

Demark-Wahnefried and colleagues[5] completed a survey of 209 survivors of childhood cancer aged 11–33, 43% of whom were survivors of pediatric brain tumors. They found that while brain tumor survivors reported significantly poorer quality of life than either survivors of leukemia or lymphoma, there were no other differences between diagnoses on any lifestyle factor, and 89% of those surveyed reported their overall health to be good to excellent. Despite this, however, almost half of the survivors were overweight or obese, with young adult survivors more likely to be obese than younger survivors. Moreover, less than half met guidelines for physical activity. This was particularly true for survivors of brain tumors.[5] Additionally, only a small minority followed low-fat diets, and few met dietary guidelines for fruit and vegetable and calcium intake. Low calcium intake is of particular concern, given the risk of bone loss in the general population, and increased risk in the childhood cancer survivor population. Survivors in this study were also surveyed about their intervention interests. Most were interested in interventions targeting exercise. Seventy percent of current smokers endorsed interest in smoking cessation programs.[5] While these findings are concerning regarding the relatively poor health habits of childhood cancer survivors, they do present some optimism in that these survivors report high levels of interest in diet and exercise interventions.

In terms of other health behaviors such as those related to follow-up medical appointments and cancer screenings, a report from the Childhood Cancer Survivors Study (CCSS) revealed that even though cancer survivors are slightly more likely than their siblings to engage in regular cancer screening practices, they are well below the optimal level for both the general population and cancer survivors.[11] Another survey from the CCSS reported that 80% of survivors attended either a general exam or visited a cancer center in the past two years. However, this decreased dramatically as time posttreatment increased, a problematic trend given that the incidence of many late effects increases with age.[12]

To examine why some survivors may engage in risky behaviors and others may not, Hollen and colleagues[13] studied the decision making capabilities of a sample of adolescent cancer survivors, many of whom had received CNS-impacting therapy (e.g., intrathecal methotrexate, cranial radiation therapy). They found a trend for therapy that targeted the central nervous system to predict poor decision making. However, contrary to hypotheses, younger age at diagnosis and low cognitive ability were not significant predictors of poor decision making. When these three factors, along with poor decision making, were used as predictors of risky health behaviors, only poor decision making was a significant predictor. Again, these findings were contrary to hypotheses. Furthermore, this study – which excluded survivors of pediatric brain tumors – would suggest that not only are survivors who receive CNS-targeted treatment at risk for cognitive deficits, they are also at risk for poor decision making which, in turn, predicts their engagement in risky behaviors. Given this, it would seem that survivors of pediatric brain tumors, survivors whose disease and treatments fully target the CNS and are at high risk for cognitive deficits, would be particularly at risk for poor decision making and engagement in risky health behaviors. As such, interventions should specifically target this unique group of survivors, as they would seem to be at risk for increased engagement in risky health behaviors that may impact their long-term health status.[13]

Interventions for Childhood Cancer Survivors

Given the potential detrimental effects that engaging in risky health behaviors would have on the long-term health of childhood cancer survivors, recent interventions have been developed to target these behaviors. Cox et al.[14] and Hudson et al.[15] generated two reports on a study of 267 adolescent survivors randomized to standard of care versus an intervention arm who received a clinic-based preventive health training session with telephone follow-up on several topics ranging from breast and testicular self-exam to smoking cessation. Unfortunately no significant differences between arms were noted with regard to knowledge, awareness and practice of health behaviors, and the program was claimed a "disappointment." Although the results of a secondary analysis were more favorable in terms of knowledge and awareness, no significant differences in diet and exercise behaviors were noted, and the potential inability of survivors and parents to focus on long-term health care issues within the acute care environment was cited as a potential reason for failure.[14,15]

In a much smaller study (N = 48) testing the impact of a single brochure on changing readiness to pursue exercise, a healthy diet and sunscreen use questionnaire was sent home with childhood cancer survivors (mean age = 13). Absolom et al.[16] found a significant change in readiness to exercise and, although promising, it must be noted that only 48% of the youth mailed back the follow-up questionnaire and no measures of actual behaviors were assessed. Emmons et al.[17–19] found that a telephone counseling smoking cessation intervention was significantly more effective than self-help materials in promoting quit rates and maintaining abstinence over a 12-month period among 796 adults survivors of childhood cancers.

While those interventions that have been completed have shown some positive strides in affecting change in the lifestyle habits of childhood cancer survivors, there are a number of changes that can be made to the design that may assist in increasing the success of future interventions. Indeed, in their survey of the diet and exercise habits of childhood cancer survivors, Demark-Wahnefried et al.[5] also asked about their intervention interests. Most were interested in interventions targeting exercise and also indicated that they would be interested in participating in an intervention with someone else, such as a parent or other family member.[5] As such, future interventions should consider including the option of having someone else participate along with the survivor in order to increase interest and compliance.

Other studies have assessed the barriers to change that childhood cancer survivors perceive in their own lives. Arroyave and colleagues[20] completed a mailed survey of adolescent and young adult childhood cancer survivors, including leukemia, lymphoma and brain tumors, to assess barriers to changing dietary and exercise habits. In terms of barriers to starting an exercise program, participants noted that they were too tired, too busy, lacked access to facilities, and would rather do something else (i.e., watch TV, read, be on computer). Moreover, brain tumor survivors were more likely than survivors of leukemia or lymphoma to report concerns regarding physical injury or soreness due to increased exercise. In terms of commencing a healthier diet, the most frequently reported barriers were lack of access and taste aversion for all cancer survivors. The barriers identified were similar to those found in healthy populations of adolescents and young adults, though tiredness was a much more common barrier for cancer survivors. Indeed, other studies suggest that survivors face a long-term battle with fatigue[21] which may have implications for the development of exercise-based interventions.

Studies such as this one reflect the challenges that researchers will face in designing comprehensive lifestyle interventions for childhood cancer survivors. Specifically, given that pediatric brain tumor survivors are particularly concerned about physical injury[20] and suffer from fatigue,[21] new interventions should include information and techniques for injury prevention so as to limit these concerns, and should be careful to work within the disability and fatigue constraints set forth by these survivors.

Future Research into Lifestyle Factors Related to Childhood Cancer Survivors

While much research on the health behaviors of childhood cancer survivors has already been completed, much of the research has yielded somewhat conflicting results, perhaps due to the heterogeneous samples and the measures used. Two review papers[2,22] suggest guidelines for future research, including more research on survivors of CNS tumors, and more information on risk factors by diagnosis.[2] They suggest either larger, more representative samples or restricting samples to small age groups and individual diagnoses so as to identify high-risk groups. Additional suggestions involve the development and use of standard measures, and the use of theoretical models that have been used with healthy populations to investigate predictive factors and/or covariates.[22]

Adult Brain Tumor Survivors

Survivorship in adult cancer is commonly understood to begin at diagnosis and extend to the balance of life. As such, many reports of lifestyle choices and behaviors have surveyed patients that are currently undergoing treatment, as opposed to those that have completed treatment. Unfortunately, research into the lifestyle choices of adult survivors of brain tumors is very limited. Indeed, only one study was identified that examined any sort of lifestyle behavior specifically in adult brain tumor patients.[23] Due to the paucity of information about this unique group of patients, this review was limited primarily to studies that combined cancer types.

Lifestyle Habits of Adult Cancer Survivors

Bellizzi and colleagues[24] examined the lifestyle practices of a large, nationally representative sample of cancer survivors and non-cancer controls who participated in the National Health Interview Survey (minimal brain tumor patients). Results revealed that cancer survivors and non-cancer controls were similar with respect to tobacco habits (about 20% of each group were current smokers).[24] Patterns of alcohol use differed by age and cancer site, though since there are no firm guidelines about alcohol consumption for cancer survivors, no conclusions were drawn on these findings except for the need for increased awareness on behalf of clinicians. In terms of cancer screenings, cancer survivors were more likely to meet recommendations for screenings than non-cancer controls, an expected, though encouraging, finding.[24] In contrast, the majority of cancer survivors were not meeting guidelines for physical activity. While cancer survivors' rates of physical activity were similar to those of non-cancer controls and national trends, it is perhaps more concerning for cancer survivors due to their increased risk of developing additional medical problems.

Studies suggest that many cancer patients use their cancer diagnosis as an opportunity to modify their lifestyle – a "teachable" moment – including increases in physical exercise, a healthier diet (e.g., increased fruit and vegetable intake and decreases in red meat consumption) as well as reduction in tobacco and alcohol use.[25] Others suggest that while these changes occur following the cancer diagnosis, they still fall short of the guidelines suggested for cancer patients and survivors.[25–27] The majority of adult cancer survivors surveyed report high levels of interest in interventions that would target lifestyle change such as diet and fitness and smoking cessation.[26] Unfortunately there are a number of barriers specific to cancer survivors that may impede the success of interventions, including medical or functional disabilities, and distance (many survivors live far away from the medical centers where interventions would ideally take place).[26] Some researchers have attempted to transcend these barriers by tailoring programs to the unique needs of individuals or by developing more convenient home-based interventions that use telephone or mailed contact, rather than face-to-face support. Such interventions, particularly those that are exercise-based, have shown positive results.[28]

Demark-Wahnefried, Pinto and Gritz[27] completed a thorough review of 22 exercise, 11 diet, and 10 smoking cessation intervention studies for adult cancer survivors published from 1966 to 2006. While the authors commend those researchers who have completed these interventions with cancer survivors, they note that there are still a number of "gaps in knowledge" and a strong need for future research. Specific examples of gaps include the impact of dietary changes on cancer prevention and recurrence; the impact of smoking cessation on non-smoking-related cancers; the identification of key time-points for intervention, and the optimal combinations of lifestyle interventions (e.g., should diet and exercise interventions be separate or combined?).[27]

Lifestyle Habits of Adult Brain Tumor Survivors

Jones and colleagues[23] retrospectively assessed the physical activity of a cohort of brain tumor patients before diagnosis, during treatment and after treatment

completion. Surprisingly, the study found that these adult brain tumor patients
were more likely than other adult cancer patients to meet national exercise
guidelines both during and after treatment. Such findings are heartening given
the functional ramifications that often accompany a brain tumor diagnosis
in an adult. Indeed, the aftereffects of surgery, including the use of steroids
to reduce cerebral swelling, as well as the almost immediate commencement of
radiation and/or chemotherapy, can have a significant impact on the functional
capability of these patients. Also encouraging is that, while exercise activity
decreased during treatment, posttreatment exercise levels returned to pre-
diagnosis rates, though at slightly less strenuous levels.[23] While the Jones et al.
study was small, hindered by a low response rate, and limited to a single institution,
it does provide the encouraging finding that lifestyle interventions may be well
received by adult brain tumor patients, and that those patients may be just as
capable of participating in exercise interventions as other cancer patients.

Following this initial study, Jones and colleagues[29] surveyed the exercise
preferences of a group of adult brain tumor patients. Patients noted that they
would be more interested in beginning an exercise program after completing
treatment, rather than during, and they would prefer to complete the program
both with a family member and at home. Additionally, these patients requested
that information about exercise be provided through technology-driven ave-
nues such as websites or a CD-ROM, rather than phone calls or face-to-face
interactions.[29] Such information is important to reducing barriers and to
planning effective exercise interventions for adult brain tumor patients.
Furthermore, this information can also be used for the planning of other
potential lifestyle-based interventions with this unique patient population.

Summary

Finding the means to prevent and ameliorate adverse sequelae and to maintain
optimal health and well-being for cancer survivors, including survivors of brain
tumors, is an important challenge that will require myriad of approaches.
Healthy lifestyle promotion is one promising avenue that is receiving increased
attention among researchers, practitioners, and the survivorship community.
Research activity in the fields of physical exercise, nutrition, and smoking
cessation as therapeutic interventions among cancer survivors is thriving. A
rapidly growing body of evidence points to the positive effects of lifestyle
choices, such as maintenance of a healthy body weight, adequate consumption
of fruits and vegetables, and preservation of fitness and function through
physical activity. Consistent evidence supports the benefits of smoking cessation on cancer treatment outcomes, including survival and prevention of recurrence, as well as development of second cancers and chronic diseases. Reports
of cancer survivorship needs and sweeping recommendations published by the
National Institutes of Health Office of Cancer Survivorship, the Centers for

Disease Control with the Lance Armstrong Foundation, and the Institutes of Medicine outline the need for Survivorship Care Plans that might direct careful long-term follow-up. However, as evidenced by this brief overview, there are vast gaps in the current knowledge and practice base. Much more focused research is needed to determine the optimal strategies for addressing lifestyle changes that can benefit survivors of brain tumors.

Nevertheless, as knowledge evolves, opportunities abound. Cancer survivorship represents a timely opportunity for health promotion intervention. Health care providers are uniquely positioned to address health behaviors as survivors and their families face the burden of rebuilding and rebalancing lives while negotiating the often life-altering effects of treatment and disease. Simply understanding what survivors are currently doing to promote their health and well-being and building on this may be critical to health care professionals' ability to reduce the risk for morbidity and mortality after cancer.

Additional Resources

Guidelines for healthy lifestyle after cancer for survivors, both pediatric and adult, are published by many organizations and can be found at many of the websites and resources listed in Chapter 27.

References

1. Meadows AT. Pediatric cancer survivorship: research and clinical care. *J Clin Oncol.* 2006;24:5160–5165.
2. Clarke S, Eiser C. Health behaviours in childhood cancer survivors: a systematic review. *Euro J Cancer.* 43:1373–1384.
3. Gleeson HK, Shalet SM. The impact of cancer therapy on the endocrine system in survivors of childhood brain tumours. *Endocrine-Related Cancer.* 2004;11:589–602.
4. Anderson DM, Rennie KM, Ziegler RS, et al. Medical and neurocognitive late effects among survivors of childhood central nervous system tumors. *Cancer.* 2001;92:2709–2719.
5. Demark-Wahnefried W, Werner C, Clipp EC, et al. Survivors of childhood cancer and their guardians: current health behaviors and receptivity to health promotion programs. *Cancer.* 2005;103:2171–2180.
6. Mulhern RK, Tyc VL, Phipps S, et al. Health-related behaviors of survivors of childhood cancer. *Med Pediatr Oncol.* 1995;25:159–165.
7. Tyc VL, Hadley W, Crockett G. Prediction of health behaviors in pediatric cancer survivors. *Med Pediatr Oncol.* 2001;37:42–46.
8. Larcombe I, Mott M, Hunt L. Lifestyle behaviours of young adult survivors of childhood cancer. *Br J Cancer.* 2002;87:1294–1209.
9. Reeves M, Eakin E, Lawler S, et al. Health behaviours in survivors of childhood cancer. *Aust Family Physician.* 2007;36:95–96.
10. Lustig RH, Post SR, Srivannaboon K, et al. Risk factors for the development of obesity in children surviving brain tumors. *J Endocrinol Metabolism.* 2003;88:611–616.

11. Yeazel MW, Oeffinger KC, Gurney JG, et al. The cancer screening practices of adult survivors of childhood cancer. *Cancer*. 2004;100:631–640.
12. Oeffinger KC, Mertens AC, Hudson MM, et al. Health care of young adult survivors of childhood cancer: a report from the Childhood Cancer Survivor Study. *Ann Fam Med.* 2004;2:61–70.
13. Hollen PJ, Hobbie WL, Finley S. Cognitive late effect factors related to decision making and risk behaviors of cancer-surviving adolescents. *Cancer Nursing.* 1997;20:305–314.
14. Cox C, McLaughline R, Rai S, et al. Adolescent survivors: a secondary analysis of a clinical trial targeting behavior change. *Pediatric Blood Cancer.* 2005;45:144–154.
15. Hudson MM, Tyc VL, Srivastava DK, et al. Multi-component behavioral intervention to promote health protective behaviors in childhood cancer survivors: the Protect Study. *Med Pediatr Oncol.* 2002;39:2–11.
16. Absolom K, Eiser C, Greco V, et al. Health promotion for survivors of childhood cancer: a minimal intervention. *Patient Educ Counseling.* 2004;55:379–384.
17. Emmons K, Li FP, Whitton J, et al. Predictors of smoking initiation and cessation among childhood cancer survivors: a Report from the Childhood Cancer Survivor Study. *J Clin Oncol.* 2002;20:1608–1616.
18. Emmons KM, Butterfield RM, Puleo E, et al. Smoking among participants in the Childhood Cancer Survivors cohort: the Partnership for Health Study. *J Clin Oncol.* 2003;21:189–196.
19. Emmons KM, Puleo E, Park E, et al. Peer-delivered smoking counseling for childhood cancer survivors increases rate of cessation: the Partnership for Health Study. *J Clin Oncol.* 2005;23:6516–6123.
20. Arroyave WD, Clipp EC, Miller PE, et al. Childhood cancer survivors' perceived barriers to improving exercise and dietary behaviors. *Oncol Nursing Forum.* 2008;35:121–130.
21. Meeske K, Katz ER, Palmer SN, et al. Parent proxy-report health-related quality of life and fatigue in pediatric patients diagnosed with brain tumors and acute lymphoblastic leukemia. *Cancer.* 2004;101:2116–2125.
22. Ford JS, Ostroff JS. Health behaviors of childhood cancer survivors: what we've learned. *J Clin Psychol Med Settings.* 2006;13:151–167.
23. Jones LW, Guill B, Keir ST, et al. Patterns of exercise across the cancer trajectory in brain tumor patients. *Cancer.* 2006;106:2224–2232.
24. Bellizzi KM, Rowland JH, Jeffery DD, et al. Health behaviors of cancer survivors: examining opportunities for cancer control intervention. *J Clin Oncol.* 2005;23:8884–8893.
25. Demark-Wahnefried W, Aziz NM, Rowland JH, et al. Riding the crest of the teachable moment: promoting long-term health after the diagnosis of cancer. *J Clin Oncol.* 2005;23:5814–5830.
26. Stull VB, Snyder DC, Demark-Wahnefried W. Lifestyle interventions in cancer survivors: designing programs that meet the needs of this vulnerable and growing population. *J Nutrition.* 2007;137:243S–248S.
27. Demark-Wahnefried W, Pinto BM, Gritz ER. Promoting health and physical function among cancer survivors: potential for prevention and questions that remain. *J Clin Oncol.* 2006;32:5125–5131.
28. Jones LW, Demark-Wahnefried W. Diet, exercise, and complementary therapies after primary treatment for cancer. *Lancet Oncol.* 2006;7:1017–1026.
29. Jones LW, Guill B, Keir ST, et al. Exercise interest and preferences among patients diagnosed with primary brain cancer. *Supp Care Cancer.* 2007;15:47–55.

Chapter 23
Integrative Oncology as Part of the Treatment for Brain Tumors

David S. Rosenthal, Christopher D. Turner, Anne M. Doherty-Gilman, and Elizabeth Dean-Clower

Introduction

In his recent book, neurosurgeon Dr. Peter Black relates about the tension that exists in brain tumor patients, the tension between wanting "to go back to their normal lives and the feeling that they've been changed in some significant way because of their brain tumor".[1] He reports that for about 40% of his patients the brain tumor is just a "bump in the road" and they return to their full and active lives after surgery. About 20% continue to have lingering problems after the treatment of their tumor that could go on for months to years. A third group he refers to as "combatants," those who fight daily to manage the complications caused by both the tumor and its treatment during their rehabilitation back to "normal" life.

A large number of brain tumor patients and survivors continue to turn to complementary and alternative medicine (CAM), using these modalities as an adjunct therapy along with their conventional treatment. Patients with brain tumors may feel additional pressure to seek out such treatments in some cases, in part because there may be fewer effective conventional therapies. Recent studies have reported up to 34% of patients with primary brain tumors use CAM.[2] Utilizing CAM therapies will often give patients a sense of empowerment and a feeling of control.

This chapter discusses various CAM therapies that may be helpful to these patients, why so many use them, the expectation derived from using CAM and the importance of discussing the use of CAM with patients. In addition, the evolving discipline of **Integrative Oncology**, i.e., integrating the best of CAM therapies with conventional medicine, is discussed, and current research on the role of complementary therapies in helping to support the brain cancer patient at all phases of their disease and survivorship phases is described.

D.S. Rosenthal (✉)
Leonard P. Zakim Center for Integrative Therapies, Dana-Farber Cancer Institute, 44 Binney Street, Boston, MA 02115, USA
e-mail: drose@uhs.harvard.edu

S. Goldman, C.D. Turner (eds.), *Late Effects of Treatment for Brain Tumors,*
Cancer Treatment and Research 150, DOI 10.1007/b109924_23,
© Springer Science+Business Media, LLC 2009

Complementary and Alternative Medicine: What Is CAM?

According to the National Center for Complementary and Alternative Medicine (NCCAM), the federal government's lead agency for scientific research on CAM housed within the National Institutes of Health (NIH), "CAM is a group of diverse medical and health care systems, practices, and products that are not presently considered to be part of conventional medicine".[3] While some scientific evidence exists regarding some CAM therapies, for most there are questions whether these therapies are safe and/or effective.

By definition, **complementary medicine** is used **alongside or together with** conventional medicine and **alternative medicine** is used **in place of** conventional medicine.

Domains of CAM

NCCAM divides Complementary and Alternative Medicine into five distinct domains (see Table 23.1). *Whole medical systems* include practices such as homeopathic medicine, naturopathy, Tibetan medicine, traditional Chinese medicine (TCM), and Ayurvedic medicine. *Mind-body medicine* includes methods that focus on the mind, body and spirit connection, such as imagery, hypnosis, meditation, prayer, and therapies that use creative outlets such as humor, art, music, or dance therapy. *Biologically based practices* in CAM use substances found in nature, such as herbs, foods, vitamins, dietary supplements and herbal products. *Manipulative and body-based practices* include modalities such as chiropractic, osteopathic manipulation, and massage. *Energy therapies* involve the use of energy fields, such as biofield therapies and bioelectromagnetic-based therapies. The existence of such fields has not yet been scientifically proven, but examples of biofield therapies include *qi gong*, a component of TCM that combines movement, meditation, and controlled breathing to improve circulation and flow of qi ("life force"), and *Reiki* therapy, which is said to transmit a universal energy to a person, usually by placing hands on a patient in specified positions by trained professionals.

Table 23.1 Domains of CAM recognized by the National Center for Complementary and Alternative Medicine

1. Whole medical systems
2. Mind-body medicine
3. Biologically based practices
4. Manipulative and body-based practices
5. Energy medicine

CAM Utilization by Cancer Survivors

Cancer survivors are high utilizers of CAM therapies, embracing these practices to assist with controlling symptoms, improving quality of life, and boosting the immune system. The major driving forces for cancer patients' use of CAM has been a lack of cure of their disease or symptoms, attempted prevention of recurrence, and difficulty with navigating the health care system[4]. CAM has become a massive industry in the United States, an expected 45 billion dollar industry in 2008. In 1997, there were over 600 million visits to CAM practitioners in the United States, and less than 400 million to primary care practitioners.[5] Thirty-three million visits occurred for advice regarding herbs and high-dose vitamins. While 70% of CAM users saw their physicians concurrently with their CAM provider, fewer than 40% disclosed their use of CAM therapy to their physician. These CAM users were surveyed about their lack of communication with their physician about CAM therapy use; 61% felt it was not important for the doctor to know, 60% said the doctor never asked, 31% said it "was none of the doctor's business" and 34% felt the doctor wouldn't understand or would disapprove and discourage the use.[6]

The use of CAM therapies across a broad spectrum of patients with various cancers is high, with one study reporting an 83% usage rate and the highest use in the category of vitamins/herbs, movement and physical therapies. Patients used CAM for hopefulness, to reduce toxicity of the disease and its treatment, and to gain a sense of control.[4] CAM use occurs across the entire spectrum of the disease from genetic predisposition and early stage disease to locally advanced, palliative care and long-term survivorship.[7–11]

Ethical and Safety Concerns

There are many ethical concerns for the clinician regarding CAM. These include issues of safety and efficacy, the lack of standardization of many products, and the accessibility and affordability of CAM services. The safety concerns include direct toxic effects of a substance[12,13] and the potential for interactions with other medicines. There are known drug/drug, drug/herb,[14,15] and antioxidant/radiation interactions that could cause serious harm and/or reduce effectiveness of conventional therapy. A significant concern of oncologists is that if patients choose CAM for a "cure," they may delay use of a known effective therapy.[16,17]

In order to assure that the patient and the oncologist are working together, it is essential that (1) all patients with brain tumors, whether currently on or off of therapy, be asked specifically about their use of CAM therapies, and (2) that all patients receive guidance about the advantages and limitations of CAM therapies in an open, evidence-based and patient-centered manner by a qualified professional.[18]

In making recommendations to patients about CAM therapies, clinicians must consider at least two factors, efficacy and safety.[19] If a CAM therapy is safe and effective, that intervention can be recommended, e.g., acupuncture for chemotherapy-induced nausea and vomiting[20] or massage for anxiety.[20]

If there is evidence that a CAM therapy is ineffective and that it can cause serious risk, that therapy should be discouraged or be considered unacceptable, e.g., laetrile which has been shown to be ineffective and can cause cyanide toxicity or hydrazine sulfate which can cause hepatorenal failure.[13,21]

Many CAM therapies, however, will fall in the category of being safe, but not proven to be effective. In this very large category of CAM therapies, one must consider possible interactions with conventional therapy. If there are none, then one may recommend that these therapies be accepted for use, but with the provision that there is no known evidence of efficacy.

Integrative Oncology

Integrative oncology as a discipline refers to the unified approach in managing patients with cancer using both allopathic and complementary approaches, thereby attempting to eliminate the "alternative" in the term CAM. This evolving discipline is based on an attention to the patient's quality of life issues, symptom management and lifestyle, and communication about CAM use. Through this new field, a research agenda is developing to determine which CAM interventions may be evidence-based by impacting survival, symptom management, improved well-being and quality of life. Complementary therapies should be part of the armamentarium of our medical, surgical and radiation oncologists alongside pain and palliative care, survivors groups, psychosocial oncology, patient advocacy, etc.

Can CAM and Allopathic Medicine Truly Be Integrated?

Too often, the current practice of conventional allopathic medicine and CAM therapies are separated by different facilities and different practitioners. Historically, there has been very little communication between such different types of practitioners. This artificial separation need not exist. Increasingly, large mainstream medical centers are recognizing the benefit of integrating CAM services into conventional cancer and survivorship care. One example of such an integrated approach exists at Dana-Farber Cancer Institute. The Leonard P. Zakim Center for Integrative Therapies (ZCIT) was established in 2000 to enhance the quality of life for cancer patients by integrating complementary therapies into conventional cancer care at one of this country's prominent cancer centers. The Center provides individual CAM services within the conventional medical setting such as acupuncture, massage therapy, reiki, Integrative Medicine and Integrative Nutrition consultations. In addition there are group programs on Qi Gong, yoga, dance, meditation, expressive arts, and music therapy as well as educational, conventional and CAM programs. The program is truly integrated with highly qualified practitioners with cancer patient experience working with the oncologist. Practitioner notes are available in the electronic medical record and patient eligibility letters are sent to the treating oncologist before any patient is treated, making them aware of the intended complementary service. At DFCI, there is a ZCIT/pediatric brain tumor collaboration in which the ZCIT CAM providers are considered part of the patient's care team and participate in clinical case conferences.

Approximately 8% of ZCIT referrals are from the neuro-oncology service. The primary patient complaints when presenting for a CAM intervention at DFCI are a combination of pain, fatigue and anxiety. In addition to seeking relief of symptoms and improved quality of life, many are seeking nutritional advice and have questions about over-the-counter supplements and herbs.[22] Integrative Medicine Consultations serve to discuss the safety and efficacy of complementary therapies and assist the patient in deciding which product to use and when, and what complementary therapy may be beneficial. Prior to any discussion of herbs and botanicals and over-the-counter antioxidants and other supplements, it is important to talk about what comprises a healthy diet and lifestyle during cancer treatment, recommendations about physical therapy and activity and what complementary therapies may be beneficial to the patient with a brain tumor, depending upon their symptoms and quality of life.

Integrating Complementary Therapies into Cancer Care

As discussed in the previous section, many cancer patients and survivors have questions about nutrition, nutritional supplements, physical activity and a range of complementary therapies. Complementary therapies can be used to supplement good nutrition and physical activity and should be aimed at improving the overall quality of life of a cancer patient, and reduce the symptomatology that may be either related to the disease or the treatment of the disease. Individual complementary therapies such as acupuncture, massage and reiki have been shown to be very helpful in the overall improvement of cancer patients' quality of life.[23] One major goal of the complementary or integrative therapy is to allow the patient to be able to fully tolerate the recommended therapies that have the best chance of treating the disease. This section will provide some basic information about complementary therapies for clinicians that can be integrated into their everyday practice.

Nutrition

Good nutrition is essential in people dealing with chronic illnesses such as cancer and brain tumors. Many herbs and spices have antimicrobial properties.[24]

Natural foods that are rich in phytonutrients can increase the plasma antioxidant level in the blood stream[25] helping one to heal faster, rebound from low blood counts faster, have fewer colds, and improve the quality of life . Additionally, according to a study of early stage breast cancer patients, higher vegetable and fruit consumption possibly contributed to increased survival, in combination with moderate physical activity,[26] and warrants further study for other cancer types. The current recommendation is 5–10 servings of fruits and vegetables per day. In addition, one should consume enough fluids as well as the right fatty acids, omega 3 fatty acids. The fatty acids could be either in the form of fish or fish oil capsules. These are available in one-half gram to one gram EHA/DHA, taken orally once or twice per day. In addition, one should get enough protein to supplement the phytonutrient-rich diet. Many of the over–the-counter herbs and botanicals are antioxidants and, generally, are not necessary with the above diet. In addition, most of the botanicals and herbs purchased over-the-counter are unregulated by the FDA and may not be standardized from one lot to another. Generally when a patient asks to use a botanical and/or an herb the first thing to consider is whether it is safe, has any effectiveness either against the cancer or improving the quality of life. If the drug or herb has significant side effects, such as increased bruising or bleeding or liver or kidney damage, and evidence-based medicine has shown it to be ineffective, the treating physician should strongly recommend against the patient taking that agent.

Physical Activity

It is becoming clear that physical activity also plays a significant role along with nutrition in improving the overall quality of life of cancer patients. Generally, the CDC recommendation for physical activity is 30–60 minutes per day, six days a week. Not all of the activity has to be cardiac in nature, but could consist of simple stretching, walking, swimming, or working with a physical trainer. It has been suggested that physical activity, together with nutrition, does boost one's immune response.[27,28] There are a number of clinical studies underway attempting to show whether or not physical activity can reduce the risk of secondary cancers or primary cancers in people with a high risk for disease.

Acupuncture

Acupuncture can be beneficial in reducing chemotherapy-induced nausea and vomiting and cancer-related pain.[29] Randomized clinical trials have demonstrated the efficacy of acupuncture as well as its safety.[30] In addition, pilot studies suggest that acupuncture does improve the quality of life for most patients with cancer, even those with advanced cancer receiving palliative care.[8] Acupuncture has many potentially beneficial effects for cancer patients.[31] it can decrease anxiety, improve cancer-related fatigue unrelated to anemia, reduce chemotherapy-related neuropathies and radiation-induced xerostomia,[32] and reduce insomnia in some cases. In a recent small randomized clinical trial, acupuncture was shown to reduce chemotherapy-induced neutropenia.[33] Acupuncture remains an underutilized complementary or integrative therapy, despite the fact that it is extremely safe even in patients with low blood counts. The number of randomized clinical trials with acupuncture is increasing, as is the use of acupuncture at mainstream cancer centers. It is hoped that, with acupuncture, patients may be able to reduce their antinausea medication and antianxiety and antidepressants as well.

Massage Therapy and Reiki

Massage therapy and reiki are reported to decrease anxiety, alleviate discomfort and improve quality of life.[20,34,35] Although the necessary "dose" of these integrative therapies is unclear, one usually recommends that once or twice per week treatment for two weeks can be enough to determine whether one is a responder to the intervention. At the present time, most of the individual therapies are fee-for-service as insurers have not yet accepted the evidence that these are favorably affecting cancer patients or survivors. This does create a barrier to access of these therapies for patients, but in many cancer institutions, philanthropy has helped patients have access to these interventions at minimal cost.

Mind-Body Techniques

Mind-body techniques such as yoga, tai chi, Qi gong, modified exercise programs, meditation and relaxation programs can benefit patients by improving their general well-being and inducing a relaxation response.[36] Meditation, imagery, and hypnosis are techniques that can reduce anxiety and stress[37] and assist patients' ability to tolerate conventional cancer therapy and symptoms related to their disease.[38] They may be useful during the diagnostic phase, such as undergoing an MRI, during a stressful or painful invasive procedure, or chemotherapy infusion. Patients with brain tumors experience headaches, pain, anxiety and fatigue; these symptoms can be helped by many of the integrative therapies discussed. Practicing the relaxation response and using hypnosis and guided imagery may not eliminate the cancer-related pain, but it may reduce the level of stress by decreasing pain to a more tolerable level and allow the patient to reduce the amount of pain medication required to a more tolerable dosage.

Hypnosis can also reduce pain, nausea and fatigue after surgery,[5] and anticipatory nausea associated with chemotherapy.[39]

Music Therapy and Expressive Art Therapy

Music therapy and expressive art therapy have long been used in hospital
settings and have now been shown to improve the quality of life by reducing
stress and anxiety.[40–42] Music therapy can also improve fine motor skills.

Clinical and Research Collaborations

In 2003, DFCI joined forces with Memorial Sloan-Kettering Cancer Center and
M.D. Anderson Cancer Center to create the Society for Integrative Oncology
(SIO) as a new and evolving organization for health professionals committed to
the study and application of complementary therapies and botanicals for cancer
patients. "This society provides a convenient forum for presentation, discussion
and peer review of evidence-based research and treatment modalities in the
discipline known as integrative medicine"[43]. Research and education is of major
importance in understanding complementary therapies and integrative oncology. The Society for Integrative Oncology serves as a forum for the presentation
of such research in a peer review fashion. Both physicians and patients need to
have all the evidenced-based, relevant information about the use herbs and
botanicals, in conjunction with radiation therapy and chemotherapy, and need
to understand the current evidence on the effectiveness and safety of other
various complementary therapies described above. The effectiveness of these
therapies should be held to the same standards as chemotherapy, biological
agents, and radiation therapy.

Resources and Additional Information

There are many reliable support resources and educational websites for both
patients and providers dealing with brain tumors. A few of these websites are
listed here.

The Brain Tumor Society: www.tbts.org
American Cancer Society: www.cancer.org
Complementary/Integrative Medicine Education Resources (CIMER):
   http://www.mdanderson.org/departments/CIMER/
National Center for Complementary and Alternative Medicine (NCCAM):
   www.nccam.nih.gov
The Wellness Community: www.thewellnesscommunity.org

References

1. Black P, Hogan SC. *Living with a Brain Tumor: Dr. Black's Guide to Taking Control of Your Treatment.* 1st ed. New York: Owl Books; 2006.
2. Armstrong T, Cohen MZ, Hess KR, et al. Complementary and alternative medicine use and quality of life in patients with primary brain tumors. *J Pain Symptom Manage.* 2006;32:148–154.
3. NCCAM Publication No. D347: CAM Basics: What is CAM?, 2007. (Accessed 2008, at http://nccam.nih.gov/health/whatiscam/.)
4. Richardson MA, Sanders T, Palmer JL, et al. Complementary/alternative medicine use in a comprehensive cancer center and the implications for oncology. *J Clin Oncol.* 2000;18:2505–2514.
5. Eisenberg D, Davis R, Ettner S. Trends in alternative medicine use in the United States. *JAMA.* 1998;280:1569–1575.
6. Eisenberg DM, Kessler RC, Van Rompay MI, et al. Perceptions about complementary therapies relative to conventional therapies among adults who use both: results from a national survey. *Ann Intern Med.* 2001;135:344–351.
7. Burstein HJ, Gelber S, Guadagnoli E, et al. Use of alternative medicine by women with early-stage breast cancer. *N Engl J Med.* 1999;340:1733–1739.
8. Dean-Clower E. Acupuncture for common physical symptoms in cancer patient care. *J Soc Integr Oncol.* 2005;3:130–133.
9. DiGianni LM, Garber JE, Winer EP. Complementary and alternative medicine use among women with breast cancer. *J Clin Oncol.* 2002;20:34S–38S.
10. Hann D, Baker F, Denniston M, et al. Long-term breast cancer survivors' use of complementary therapies: perceived impact on recovery and prevention of recurrence. *Integr Cancer Ther.* 2005;4:14–20.
11. Tagliaferri M, Cohen I, Tripathy D. Complementary and alternative medicine in early-stage breast cancer. *Semin Oncol.* 2001;28:121–134.
12. Ernst E. The risk-benefit profile of commonly used herbal therapies: Ginkgo, St. John's Wort, Ginseng, Echinacea, Saw Palmetto, and Kava. *Ann Intern Med.* 2002;136:42–53.
13. Hainer MI, Tsai N, Komura ST, et al. Fatal hepatorenal failure associated with hydrazine sulfate. *Ann Intern Med.* 2000;133:877–880.
14. Mathijssen RHJ. *Proc AACR.* 2002;43:492.
15. Sparreboom A, Cox MC, Acharya MR, et al. Herbal remedies in the United States: potential adverse interactions with anticancer agents. *J Clin Oncol.* 2004;22:2489–2503.
16. Coppes MJ, Anderson RA, Egeler RM, et al. Alternative therapies for the treatment of childhood cancer. *N Engl J Med.* 1998;339:846–847.
17. Ernst E, White A. Prospective studies of the safety of acupuncture: a systematic review. *Ann J Med.* 2001;110(6):481–485.
18. Deng GE, Cassileth BR, Cohen L, et al. Integrative oncology practice guidelines. *J Soc Integr Oncol.* 2007;5:65–84.
19. Weiger W, Smith M, Boon H, et al. Advising patients who seek complementary and alternative medical therapies for cancer. *Ann Int Med.* 2002;137:889–903.
20. Ahles TA, Tope DM, Pinkson B, et al. Massage therapy for patients undergoing autologous bone marrow transplantation. *J Pain Symptom Manage.* 1999;18:157–163.
21. Moertel CG, Fleming TR, Rubin J, et al. A clinical trial of amygdalin (Laetrile) in the treatment of human cancer. *N Engl J Med.* 1982;306:201–206.
22. Rosenthal DS, Dean-Clower E. Complementary and alternative medicine: current state in oncology care. In: Perry MC, Govindan R, editors. *Proceedings of the 42nd Annual Meeting of the American Society of Clinical Oncology*; 2006 June 2–6; Atlanta, Georgia; 2006. pp. 70–74.
23. Joske DJ, Rao A, Kristjanson L. Critical review of complementary therapies in haemato-oncology. *Intern Med J.* 2006;36:579–586.

24. Lai PK, Roy J. Antimicrobial and chemopreventive properties of herbs and spices. *Curr Med Chem.* 2004;11:1451–1460.
25. Prior RL, Gu L, Wu X, et al. Plasma antioxidant capacity changes following a meal as a measure of the ability of a food to alter in vivo antioxidant status. *J Am Coll Nutr.* 2007;26:170–181.
26. Pierce JP, Stefanick ML, Flatt SW, et al. Greater survival after breast cancer in physically active women with high vegetable-fruit intake regardless of obesity. *J Clin Oncol.* 2007;25:2345–2351.
27. Dimeo FC, Stieglitz RD, Novelli-Fischer U, et al. Effects of physical activity on the fatigue and psychologic status of cancer patients during chemotherapy. *Cancer.* 1999;85:2273–2277.
28. Segal R, Evans W, Johnson D, et al. Structured exercise improves physical functioning in women with stages I and II breast cancer: results of a randomized controlled trial. *J Clin Oncol.* 2001;19:657–665.
29. Alimi D, Rubino C, Pichard-Leandri E, et al. Analgesic effect of auricular acupuncture for cancer pain: a randomized, blinded, controlled trial. *J Clin Oncol.* 2003;21:4120–4126.
30. MacPherson H, Thomas K, Walters S, et al. The York acupuncture safety study: prospective survey of 34,000 treatments by traditional acupuncturists. *BMJ.* 2001;323(7311):486–487.
31. Lu W, Dean-Clower E, Doherty-Gilman A, et al. The value of acupuncture in cancer care. *Hematol Oncol Clin North Am.* 2008;22:631–648, viii.
32. Johnstone PA, Peng YP, May BC, et al. Acupuncture for pilocarpine-resistant xerostomia following radiotherapy for head and neck malignancies. *Int J Radiat Oncol Biol Phys.* 2001;50:353–357.
33. Lu W, Hu D, Dean-Clower E, et al. Acupuncture for chemotherapy-induced leukopenia: exploratory meta-analysis of randomized controlled trials. *J Soc Integr Oncol.* 2007;5:1–10.
34. Spence D, Kayumov L, Chen Aea. Acupuncture increases nocturnal melatonin secretion and reduces insomnia and anxiety: a preliminary report. *J Neuropsychiatry Clin Neurosci.* 2004;16(1):19–28.
35. Wilkie DJ, Kampbell J, Cutshall S, et al. Effects of massage on pain intensity, analgesics and quality of life in patients with cancer pain: a pilot study of a randomized clinical trial conducted within hospice care delivery. *Hosp J.* 2000;15:31–53.
36. Bindemann S, Soukop M, Kaye SB. Randomised controlled study of relaxation training. *Eur J Cancer.* 1991;27:170–174.
37. Speca M, Carlson LE, Goodey E, et al. A randomized, wait-list controlled clinical trial: the effect of a mindfulness meditation-based stress reduction program on mood and symptoms of stress in cancer outpatients. *Psychosom Med.* 2000;62:613–622.
38. Walker L, Walker M, Ogston K, et al. Psychological, clinical and pathological effects of relaxation training and guided imagery during primary chemotherapy. *Br J Cancer.* 1999;80:262–268.
39. Redd WH, Montgomery GH, DuHamel KN. Behavioral intervention for cancer treatment side effects. *J Natl Cancer Inst.* 2001;93:810–823.
40. Barrera ME, Rykov MH, Doyle SL. The effects of interactive music therapy on hospitalized children with cancer: a pilot study. *Psychooncology.* 2002;11:379–388.
41. Igawa-Silva W, Wu S, Harrigan R. Music and cancer pain management. *Hawaii Med J.* 2007;66:292–295.
42. Wikstrom BM. Communicating via expressive arts: the natural medium of self-expression for hospitalized children. *Pediatr Nurs.* 2005;31:480–485.
43. Society of Integrative Oncology Home Page. 2008. (Accessed 2008, at http://www.integrativeonc.org.)

Chapter 24
Legal Issues and Laws Relevant to Brain Tumor Survivors

G.P. Monaco and Gilbert Smith

Introduction

The challenges of cancer – obstacles and opportunities – do not stop at the end of active treatment. For many survivors, the challenges posed by late effects from the treatment for brain tumors require ongoing medical vigilance and surveillance. The brain tumor survivor's world of education, work, and everyday life presents daily obstacles and opportunities. Clinicians should ask themselves, are my patients equipped and ready to handle these challenges? Too often the answer is, "no." Fortunately, there are a number of laws and programs available to brain tumor survivors to assist in these day-to-day challenges.

The purpose of this chapter is to provide an overview of the laws that brain tumor survivors can utilize as they move forward with their lives. The law is constantly changing, if not always in word, then in interpretation by the courts and regulatory agencies. That said, this chapter is not an immutable bible. Rather it is a tool to help clinicians recognize and address the legal issues that may confront the survivors they care for and how to obtain helpful resources and a helpful network of support, should it be needed. This chapter presumes that brain tumor patients have completed most of their treatments, with the exception of some maintenance therapy or appropriate medical follow-up guidance and participation in late effects studies.[1]

Overview of Legislation

Education

With regard to education, there are three resources that provide needed educational services for cancer survivors:

G.P. Monaco (✉)
Medical Care Management Corporation, The Candlelighters Childhood Cancer
Foundation, Washington, DC, USA
e-mail: gpmonaco@hughes.net

S. Goldman, C.D. Turner (eds.), *Late Effects of Treatment for Brain Tumors*,
Cancer Treatment and Research 150, DOI 10.1007/b109924_24,
© Springer Science+Business Media, LLC 2009

- Federal Individuals with Disabilities Education Act (IDEA) (PL 94-142 and PL 99-457 amendments) and the respective state laws that implement this law
- Federal Rehabilitation Act of 1973 (Rehab Act) (PL 93-112, section 504) [2]
- Americans with Disabilities Act of 1990 (PL 101-336)

Generally, these laws protect the rights of cancer survivors who may be left with learning disabilities, attention disorders, high risk of infection, amputations, or other physical limitations that prevent use of the full range of educational programs. These laws, which apply to primary and secondary education, to infant, toddler, and preschool interventions, and to college, university, and vocational education, are premised on education as a right guaranteed to every citizen regardless of physical, mental, or health impairments. Although these laws have the authority of federal mandate, state governments implement them and may interpret provisions differently.

In September 2008 Congress approved an expansion of protections for people with disabilities which overturned several recent Supreme Court decisions which were considered to restrict their rights, and President Bush was expected to sign the bill into law. The court decisions overturned are: *Sutton v. United Air Lines*, 527 U.S. 471 (1999), and *Toyota Motor Mfg. v. Williams*, 534 U.S. 184 (2002).

The legislation expands the definition of disability and makes it easier for workers to prove discrimination. It explicitly rejects the strict standards used by the Supreme Court to determine who is disabled, specifically the rights of those with epilepsy, diabetes, cancer, multiple sclerosis, and other ailments had been improperly denied protection because their conditions could be controlled by medications or other measures. The effect of the legislation is that in deciding whether a person is disabled under the Act, courts shouldn't consider the effects of mitigating measures such as prescription drugs, hearing aids, and artificial limbs. In addition, a disability that is in remission or episodic fits the definitions requiring protection if, when it is active, it would substantially limit a major life activity. The legislation makes it clear that Congress originally intended and continues to intend that the ADA have broad and generous coverage.

Employment

There are various laws that potentially apply to cancer survivors with regard to employment, insurance and benefits. Some of these laws are listed below:

- The Americans with Disabilities Act [ADA]
- Health Insurance Portability and Accountability Acts (HIPPA)
- Consolidated Omnibus Budget Reconciliation Act (COBRA)
- Employee Retirement and Income Security Act (ERISA)

Viewed in toto, these laws represent a concerted approach on the federal level to provide a level and equal playing field for cancer patients and survivors regarding access to employment and insurance. Listed below are some of the protections survivors are afforded under these laws.

- Generally, no associational discrimination is allowed. For example, denial of benefits or job to a spouse solely on his or her relationship to a person with a disability is prohibited.
- Prevention of discrimination on the basis of genetic information relating to illness, disease or other disorders.
- Ensure equal insurance to all workers and no diminution in benefits unless there is either legitimate actuarial data or reasonably anticipated experience [current statistics] that shows the person is still at risk. Whether, in the rare instance a person has to put up with diminished benefits (a "rated" policy) depends on when they will be a normal risk, and that also depends on legitimate actuarial data.
- If a person is fired or laid off they have a right to continue group health coverage at their own expense and, if they are disabled, obtain coverage up to 29 months to bridge the gap to other insured employment or, depending on the nature of the disability, to bridge the gap to Medicare coverage.
- The law also provides assistance in combating discrimination in the collection of employee benefits by parents, spouse or survivor forced into retirement or fired, or assigned part-time status which would remove their insurance benefits.

Education

IDEA, the ADA, and the Rehab Act all apply to public schools. Specifically, Title II of the ADA applies to state and local government, and that includes public schools. Children with cancer and other eligible disabilities are entitled to and guaranteed a free and appropriate public education. They are entitled to specially designed instruction and related services such as OT/PT and transportation for example, as well as accommodations such as a modification in policies that they may need in order to have the equal opportunity to participate in academic and athletic instruction and extracurricular activities at school. The ADA further states the disabled cannot be forced to accept an accommodation. In other words, childhood cancer survivors cannot be forced to accept educational plans, such as separate classes, that they do not wish to take. If an appropriate public placement is unavailable, the school system must provide an appropriate private placement to substitute for, or supplement, the public school's package. The ADA also applies to institutions of higher education.

Children covered by IDEA are entitled to a *free and appropriate public education*. Special education means specially designed instruction based on the needs of the individual survivor, and includes related services such as transportation, counseling, and physical therapy. Related services may be provided by public schools to students who are enrolled in private schools. Again the Rehabilitation

Act and the ADA require schools to make accommodations so that the survivor is afforded equal opportunity to participate and benefit from his education.

While not all children who go off treatment will qualify under the IDEA, it is important to understand that they will all qualify under the ADA and the Rehabilitation Act because they all have a record of having survived cancer or other tumors. This usually takes the form of what are known as Student-Study Teams (or Child-Study Teams) that help institute various accommodations such as providing two sets of books, one for school and one for home.

It is a good idea to check with the local state vocational and rehabilitation agency. Assistance may be available for state college tuition or vocational training, so the survivor could get paid to go to school and fill any educational gaps.

In working with families facing education and placement issues, the Supreme Court recently ruled in *Winkelman v. Parma City School District* that parents of disabled children do not have to hire lawyers to sue school districts when they attempt to ensure that their children's special needs are adequately met. The court held that the federal Individuals With Disabilities Education Act (IDEA), which guarantees children a "free appropriate public education," gives rights to parents as well. Parents may represent themselves in federal court when disputes arise between them and a school district over what is best for the child.

Employment and the Americans with Disabilities Act (ADA)

Most employment rights cases will involve the ADA, which is a federal civil rights law. It prohibits discrimination by requiring that disabled people be given the same chances and opportunities as able-bodied people. The key word here is **SAME**; not special or more, just the SAME opportunities that people who aren't disabled have always received. If another federal or state law grants greater protection to the disabled than the ADA would in certain circumstances, than that law controls. The ADA is a **floor**, not a **ceiling.** It is important to know your state's provisions. Often a survivor's original cancer diagnosis is considered to have substantially limited that person. So, while the survivor may not currently consider himself or herself to be disabled, they may be legally, as disability is a term of art in the legal profession. In other words, it does not describe the person's actual status, but their assumed status for the purposes of the rights to which they may be entitled. ADA coverage is determined on a case-by-case basis.

The ADA is **NOT** an affirmative action statute; there are no quotas, goals or "bonus points" for hiring the disabled. The disabled don't receive special job **protection** once they are hired. An employer can still decline to hire the disabled, but the decision must be based on the essential functions of the job and the applicant's qualifications, not because of their disability.

The ADA applies to any **qualified** individual with a disability who can perform the essential functions of the job, regardless of whether the job applicant will need a reasonable accommodation from the employer. Reasonable accommodations are defined later in this chapter.

Defining Disability Under the ADA

Generally, a qualified individual with a disability is defined as someone who is substantially impaired in a major life activity. That means they cannot perform an activity that a non-disabled person can. Major life activities include walking, talking, eating, breathing, seeing, and hearing. For example, if disabled people use drugs or devices such as insulin, prosthetic devices, or antidepressants to perform major life activities, and mitigate the disability, they are not automatically considered disabled. As discussed above, the court interpretations that mitigating measures have a bearing on disability status were removed in the expansion and reinforcement of the ADA in September 2008. Cancer patients and survivors are covered under other definitions of disability[3] discussed in more detail below. Briefly, these provisions relate to a record of disability (substantially limited in the past) or being **regarded** in the workplace as "having a disability" (the employer perceives the person as being substantially limited in performing a major life activity).

Most important for cancer survivors, the ADA protects someone with **a record of impairment**. Every cancer survivor has a record of substantial impairment. Consequently, the ADA will apply to them for the rest of their lives. The ADA protects cancer survivors, whether the cancer is cured, controlled or in remission. However, depending upon how successful a survivor is through the use, for example, of medicines or devices to counter or moderate an effect of the cancer or the treatment, that survivor may not be considered to have a disability under the ADA **that requires intervention or accommodation**.

Employers can no longer discriminate against the disabled in any phase of employment: hiring, training, job assignment, classification, promotion, transfer, benefits, leave of absence, layoff or termination. While employers can't ask about a disability, they can ask an applicant to show they could perform the essential functions of a job. An applicant might want to have a scrapbook of photographs showing him performing these or similar tasks. An applicant has a right to request a reasonable accommodation in testing, and can return to take an employment test after the accommodation has been provided.

Employers will be held to their job descriptions and advertising; a person cannot be hired and then fired because they could not perform assumed or secondary job functions. Employees cannot be asked, nor do they have to disclose, whether they have any disability that would affect their job performance. If a person can do the job – that is all that matters. This applies both to oral interviews and written applications. Employees do not have to explain why there are gaps in their employment history. On the job, employees are entitled to a non-hostile work environment free from severe and pervasive workplace harassment. However, legitimate questions concerning performance or whether health problems are adversely affecting performance are not tantamount to regarding an employee as disabled.

Additional ADA Protections

Associational Discrimination

Unlike the other civil rights laws, the ADA also protects those who associate with a disabled person. The parent or spouse of a cancer survivor cannot be denied employment or fired because the employer assumes the parent or spouse will need time off to deal with treatment-related issues. The employer cannot refuse to hire the associated individual because of a belief that it may increase health care/insurance premium costs. And the employer cannot refuse to insure an individual because he has a disabled spouse or dependent. However, an employer does not have to provide a reasonable accommodation, such as a modified work schedule, to the associated individual.

Reasonable Accommodation

In the workplace, the ADA requires employers to make reasonable accommodations for the disabled. This means an accommodation that would not cause undue hardship for the business. If a disabled employee requests a reasonable accommodation, the employer must analyze the possible accommodations and seek technical assistance. Failure to seek this assistance is not a defense under the law. The burden is on the employer, not on the employee, regarding issues relating to reasonable accommodation.

If the employee can no longer do his current job and there is a vacant job he or she can do with or without reasonable accommodation, reassignment may be a necessary reasonable accommodation. If the survivor is no longer able to provide his or her job function, even with a reasonable accommodation, and no other jobs for which that person is qualified are available, the employer is not required to retain the employee. For example, if the job description legitimately calls for a 55-hour week and the survivor can only provide 40, accommodating that person would destroy the nature of the position, which is not required under the ADA.

Employers are not required to provide personal aids, such as wheelchairs or hearing aids, or personal assistance. This includes assistance a disabled person might need in eating, dressing or toileting. If the survivor requires some accommodation to deal with medical management of a side effect of treatment, provided the survivor can still do the essential functions of the job, the ADA provides flextime as a reasonable accommodation. Additionally, the Family and Medical Leave Act (FMLA)[4] entitles eligible employees to take up to 12 weeks of unpaid, job-protected leave and continued benefits in a 12-month period for specified family and medical reasons, including childbirth, adoption, or a family medical emergency, and also covers intermittent leave time. Either law can be used to achieve this desired result. If pending federal executive orders and legislative efforts prevail, they will permit unemployment benefits to be collected under the FMLA to reduce financial hardship. Additionally, state medical leave laws should be checked as some may provide more coverage than the federal law. A good source of this information is the agency that enforces the state civil rights laws.

It is important to stress that employment rights are always dependent upon whether the employee can do the job satisfactorily. If the employee would have been terminated, but for FMLA,[5] upon return the employee would not be entitled to the same job. An employee who is unable to perform the essential functions of a job, apart from an inability to work a full-time schedule, is not entitled to an intermittent or reduced schedule leave under the FMLA. If the employee has available paid sick leave and FMLA leave, it is the employee's choice, not the employer's, which one he wishes to use.

Health Care, Insurance and Other Benefits

In this section we provide an overview of the various legislation most significantly impacting the cancer survivor regarding health care, insurance, and other benefits. Again, as previously mentioned, it is also important to check local and state law for provisions that may expand a person's federal rights.

ADA Protections

The ADA, as it pertains to insurance, is discussed below under the employment section of this chapter. In general, on access to insurance by cancer survivors, apart from the employment protections, the ADA also requires that denials must be based on either legitimate actuarial data or the reasonably anticipated experience of the persons at risk. This means that the insurance company must have current statistics that show that this person is still at risk.

The Health Insurance Portability and Accountability Act (HIPAA) (Public Law. 104-191)

HIPAA was passed into law in 1996, and allows millions of Americans with preexisting conditions to secure comprehensive health insurance. HIPAA also helps people maintain their coverage if they need to change insurance or jobs. It makes insurance more accessible for those that work for small businesses, and expands the rights of cancer survivors. In brief, HIPAA offers the following rights, some of which overlap with the ADA:

(a) Prevents denial of enrollment based on health status, health factors, medical condition, claims history, medical history, or genetic information;[6]

(b) Prevents higher premiums among workers on group plans (see previous footnote; the insurer can charge higher premiums under the individual coverage plan);
(c) Provides uniform benefits to all workers;
(d) Provides individual coverage to a person who leaves a group health plan due to loss of employment or because the new employer does not offer insurance coverage;
(e) Prevents waiting periods or preexisting condition exclusions, as long as the individual opted for and exhausted COBRA continuation coverage, has had at least 18 months of prior health insurance coverage, and there has been no gap in insurance coverage of more than 63 days, excluding employer waiting periods;
(f) Provides a credit for the time an individual was insured against the preexisting waiting period if an individual had prior insurance, but it was not in effect at the time of job switch;
(g) Provides for renewal of group and individual plans, and
(h) Provides genetic information from being used to establish a preexisting condition unless there is a diagnosis of a related condition.

The Center for Medicare and Medicaid Services (CMS) recently released a program memorandum in which it addressed the situation where an employer with a disabled employee switches its group health insurance plan from one carrier to a new succeeding carrier. According to Program Memorandum 00-04, the new succeeding carrier cannot preclude coverage for disabled employees or dependents by using "actively-at-work clauses." CMS emphasized that, under HIPAA, state-sponsored succeeding carrier laws cannot eliminate a succeeding carrier's obligation to enroll individuals who were disabled at the time that the original plan is terminated.

State Mandated External Review

For those survivors with health insurance coverage, state-mandated external review offers them a important tool when it comes to insurance reimbursement and coverage denials. Forty-four states and the District of Columbia offer an independent external review option. If the survivor is not satisfied with the health plan's decision regarding a treatment/drug/service decision and the survivor has exhausted the plan's internal appeal process, they may be able to appeal the plan's denial to their state's external review program.

These reviews are performed by Independent Review Organizations (IRO) that have no affiliation with the health plan. These IRO programs are designed to ensure that health plans make the correct coverage decisions and hold the health plans accountable for their decisions. Please note that these IRO programs are free to plan enrollees and are also overseen by State Departments of Insurance.

External review programs differ from state to state in the types of disputes that are eligible for appeal, the process used to resolve the appeal, and the time limits imposed at each step of the process. For more information about the states that offer external review and their appeal processes, please visit the Kaiser Family Foundation at www.kffkorg. This Website describes the variations found in states' external review programs and provides a guide that outlines the specific requirements for a particular state and who to contact in that state for further information.

The Consolidated Omnibus Budget Reconciliation Act (COBRA)

COBRA mandates that both public and private employers with 20 or more employees for half of the working days in the previous calendar year must make insurance coverage available for a limited period of time to employees and their dependents. Under COBRA, employees who have been fired or laid off have a right to continue their group health coverage at their own expense and at a rate no higher than 102% of the employer's group insurance premium for 18 months. Beginning in 1989, it provided the same benefits for the disabled for up to 29 months to bridge the gap to Medicare. The premium for the disabled from the 18th to the 29th month can be up to 150% of the premium charged. Listed below are some important facts about COBRA:

- An employer has a duty to inform employees of their COBRA rights and to notify the group health plan of an employee death, termination, or reduction in hours. Coverage may extend to a spouse, for example, after the death of an eligible employee or after divorce or legal separation, and to a dependent under the same conditions or if the child leaves dependent status during the COBRA period.
- The employee or family member has the responsibility of informing the group health plan administrator of a legal separation, divorce or of a child losing dependent status. The employee or beneficiary has 60 days from the date he or she would lose coverage to make a decision about the continuation of coverage.
- COBRA coverage is not available if the terminated employee is already covered by the spouse's plan unless the spouse's plan contains any exclusions or limitations with respect to any preexisting condition of the terminated beneficiary.
- COBRA coverage may be terminated if the employer stops providing employee group health insurance or if the employee becomes covered under another plan, including Medicare, or ceases payment of COBRA continuation premiums.

For further information about COBRA contact the Pension and Welfare Benefits Administration at the United States Department of Labor (DOL). DOL will notify eligible employees utilizing COBRA by mid-March 2009 about a subsidy to drfray some COBRA costs.

Employee Retirement and Income Security Act (ERISA)[7]

ERISA prohibits an employer from discriminating against an employee for the purpose of preventing collection of health benefits under an employee benefit plan; that is, a plan providing benefits in the event of sickness, accident, disability, death, or unemployment. This protection does not apply to persons denied a "new" job due to a history of cancer; the ADA covers this (see the discussion above).

ERISA is an additional tool to be considered by employees facing forced retirement, firing, or placement in part-time status with removal of insurance benefits. For example, in a case involving an employee who enrolled in a plan with out-of-network benefits in order to continue treatment with her original cancer care provider, the plan refused coverage and the case went to court. The court held that unless charges exceeded the usual and customary rates of other local comprehensive cancer centers, the insurer was required to reimburse for all charges.

Note: In all insurance cases, unless the health benefit plan waives the requirement, the employee survivor is required to exhaust administrative remedies under the plan before suit is brought. Further, arbitration cannot be compelled if it is not in a person's insurance contract and if they have not been notified of its inclusion in a change of benefits.

Access of Benefits Through Employment

The ADA mandates that employers provide equal access to health care benefits for the disabled and those who associate with them. This includes disability benefits. An employer cannot consider what effect hiring a disabled person would have on their insurance premium. That also applies to considering whether to hire the parent or spouse of a cancer survivor.

The ADA permits insurers to discriminate provided that those risks that are the basis for discrimination are not inconsistent with state law and are not a means to evade the ADA's purposes. It is still unclear when and whether insurance discrimination violations will be subject to state or federal remedies.

For example, although infertility is considered a disability, an employer may offer insurance that precludes fertility coverage, or some aspects thereof, for all employees providing it is done on an equal basis. However, this applies in general to fertility and, **in the opinion of these authors**, does not apply to infertility that is the result/side effect of the treatment of a disease. Although there is no reported case law related to cancer treatment vis a vis infertility and its remediation, insurers and employers have permitted fertility treatment under the same scenario as they would permit breast reconstruction or hearing aids for cisplatin-related deafness.

The ADA also regulates how health care providers treat the disabled. Health care providers cannot deny medical treatment to a person with a disability if they are qualified to provide it. For example, a dermatologist can refer an HIV-positive person with a broken arm to an orthopedic surgeon, but cannot refuse to treat that person for a skin disorder.

Additional Programs

In 2000, the Department of Health and Human Services announced[8] two new initiatives to enable people with disabilities to become and stay competitively employed. The first, the Demonstration Project to Maintain Independence and Employment, will fund cutting-edge program demonstrations that enable people with chronic, disabling conditions to get medical benefits without having to quit their jobs to obtain needed care. The second, Medicaid Infrastructure Grants, will help states build the systems they need to allow individuals with a disability to purchase health coverage through Medicaid. Both the grants and the demonstrations help advance the goals of the Ticket to Work and Work Incentives Improvement Act of 1999, a law passed by Congress to encourage people with disabilities to work without fear of losing their Medicare, Medicaid or similar health benefits.[9] If a survivor receives a denial, they should request a "Notice of Action" in writing, which states the denial and provides appeal information, and apply for a "Fair Hearing" review of the denial.

There is pending federal legislationand a growing trend in state policy to require parity between medical and mental health benefits (Mental Health Parity and Addiction Equity Act of 2008, Public Law 110–343 Section 512, effective date 10/3/2009). This could benefit the cancer survivor because it may enhance the ability of survivors to obtain assistance in dealing with any post-traumatic stress problems relating to cancer and its treatment.

If the survivor is in the military or a military dependent, the Interagency Agreement Between the Department of Defense and National Cancer Institute for Partnership In Clinical Trials For Cancer Prevention And Treatment dated 10/18/99 was expanded and made permanentunder a final rule effective 3/2/01 and codified in 32 CFR 1999. This agreement provides the opportunity to participate in Phase II and Phase III NCI-sponsored cancer treatment clinical trials for cancer, either in the direct care system or through civilian providers who are reimbursed through TRICARE/CHAMPUS. At this point, we are unaware of any effort to invoke this agreement to participate in late effects trials, but it certainly provides food for thought. In general, it may be argued that failure to cover general specialized monitoring and surveillance post-cancer treatment places the survivor's life at risk, much along the arguments made for coverage of mammography.

Conclusion

The legal issues that affect survivors are not unique. They cross many different diseases, thereby providing a common bond with others that experience chronic illnesses or disabilities to help form focused coalitions. Collectively, survivors and those that care for them need to advocate for the medical, social, political, and the legal infrastructure changes necessary to improve access to care, cure the primary disease, control late effects, and provide enhancement of life expectations for our cancer survivors.

References

1. For general legal issues resources focused on patient issues, see: Childhood Cancer Ombudsman Program (CCOP) gpmonaco@ hughes.nett; The National Coalition for Cancer Survivorship (NCCS) (301) 650-8868; the Childhood Brain Tumor Foundation [CBTF] [add contact info] and Candlelighters Childhood Cancer Foundation (CCCF) info@candlelighters.org . **CBTF has family/patient specific materials on its web side: [insert website].**
2. This Act bans both public and private employers receiving public funds from discriminating on the basis of disability. Information and assistance available from the Access Unit of the Civil Rights Division, Department of Justice, Washington, DC.
3. The definition of disability under Section 501 of the Rehabilitation Act is identical to the definition under the ADA.
4. The Family and Medical Leave Act (29 U.S.C. Section 2612(a)(1); 5 U.S. C. Section 6282 (a)(1)). Excellent source of information: National Partnership for Women & Families, 202-986-2600.
5. 29 U.S.C.A. § 2614(a)(1).
6. interim final rule, 66 Fed. Reg. 1378, at http://www.access.gpo.gov/su_docs/fedreg/a010112c.html.
7. ERISA, Employee Retirement Income Security Act of 1974 as amended, 29 U.S. Section 1001 et seq.
8. Insert citation to announcement from DHHS' press release, go to http://www.hhs.gov/news/press/2000pres/20001025.html.
9. Helpful resource: www.disability.gov; and www.business-disability.com

Chapter 25
Pathways to Brain Tumor Advocacy

Susan L. Weiner and Craig Lustig

Brain tumors represent a unique challenge in that they affect the organ that is the essence of the 'self'[1].

Introduction

Advocacy by and for brain tumor survivors, their families and friends is driven by the fundamental and dramatic nature of the disease and its consequences. For adult patients and for parents of affected children, the trauma of diagnosis, the potential life-threatening nature of the disease, and the anguish of deciding amongst intensive treatment alternatives are life altering events. The current chapter describes how brain tumor advocacy has evolved from these experiences into local and national action intended to improve the pace of research and the quality of care for survivors and families. It is based upon the experiences of a parent who lost a child to a brain tumor and from a long-term survivor, both of whom, like hundreds of others across the country, have served this community.

Brain tumors differ from other cancers in how they affect patients, families and survivors.[2] Brain tumors are not just rare, they are heterogeneous relative to other cancers. Over 44,500 people in the United States and 10,000 people in Canada are diagnosed annually with primary brain tumors.[3] There are more than 126 different histological types of brain tumors, according the World Health Organization classification, and many more subtypes of disease are being discovered with newer genomic and proteomic classifications.

Mortality for brain tumor patients, which has somewhat improved for children, remains unacceptably high. Five-year survival rates for adults have remained the same for over a decade[4] at about 33%.[5] Five-year survival rates

S.L. Weiner (✉)
Children's Brain Tumor Foundation, 274 Madison Avenue, New York, NY 10016, USA
e-mail: slweiner@childrenscause.org

S. Goldman, C.D. Turner (eds.), *Late Effects of Treatment for Brain Tumors*, Cancer Treatment and Research 150, DOI 10.1007/b109924_25, © Springer Science+Business Media, LLC 2009

for children have risen to about 65%,[6] but many survivors struggle with significantly compromised growth and development, impeding their independence as adults.

A major consequence of the significant mortality and morbidity in the brain tumor population is that there are relatively few brain tumor survivors available to become advocates, and those that can participate do not manifest the more severely disabling conditions. Accordingly, it is the families and friends of brain tumor patients who have tended to be the most active brain tumor advocates.

Advocacy is conceptualized here as the public and private activities that individuals and families conduct to ensure their access to services. The challenges that survivors and families experience trying to access treatment, care and follow-up services make evident the need for improvements in the local, state and national policies that govern such access. Brain tumor advocacy is the application of pressure to organizational and governmental systems responsible for these policies.

Brain tumor advocacy is part of the larger cancer advocacy movement, which has evolved rapidly over the past 20 years. Building on the mental health and disability self-help movements of the 1970s, breast cancer advocacy followed the approach and tactics of AIDS activists adopted in the 1990s.[7,8] Brain tumor advocates derived relevant lessons from these models and, as individual groups came together as a coalition in 1993, dreamt of heightened public awareness and increased resources for brain tumor survivors and families. Brain tumor advocates' journey from individual to community to national advocacy in these years has brought both awareness and increased resources to brain tumor concerns.

Individual Advocacy: The Source

Individuals' efforts to optimize care and treatment for themselves or for their loved ones are the roots of subsequent patient advocacy.[9-11] Heretofore medically naïve individuals become schooled in the rituals and procedures associated with diagnosis, surgery, hospitalization, radiation treatment and chemotherapy. Advocacy by and for individuals takes place when survivors and families have an immediate need to decide on a treatment or obtain a needed service. Because brain tumors affect not just the seat of thinking and feeling, but other physiological systems necessary for normal living, e.g., mobility, eating, sleeping, and endocrine function, individual advocacy can involve coordination of multiple providers of specialty care.

When survivors are adults with impaired cognition, individual advocacy for their care typically requires family members to assume considerable responsibility for decision making and case management. For children, parents' responsibilities for rearing an affected child become considerably more complex than is typically required for normal child rearing. Information gathering and engaging professional support services become vital tools for effective individual advocacy. Chapter 24 describes strategies for successfully advocating for individual survivors' quality health care, insurance coverage, educational and employment rights.

Many families and survivors feel powerless when there is so little they can do, given the complexities of the brain tumor experience. Families often feel that they must act to do "something." "Fighting" is often the metaphor used for the struggle with and sometimes against the hospitals, physicians, educational and other systems that offer interventions. As survivors' treatments end and remission ensues, many families "act" by focusing on caring for others, carrying on the fight from what is now a more informed position.

Community Advocacy: Realizing the Need to Help

The desire to transform personal suffering into positive action underlies the founding of hundreds of nonprofit organizations and foundations that serve brain tumor survivors and their families in the United States. These new entities often bear the name of a loved one lost to a brain tumor. Their founders are also making a statement about their desire to bring public attention to them and their loved ones. Over 130 nonprofit groups and foundations provide substantial brain tumor research funding and/or support service programs, and many smaller, unincorporated groups engage in local fund-raising (see Table 25.1). The older established organizations often mentor and advise new support group leaders and young nonprofit organizations all over the country, bringing advocacy lessons to local communities.

Brain tumor organizations offer a rich array of free support and information services that are built upon families' and survivors' knowledge and experience. "Veteran" families and survivors find themselves contacted by others for referrals to physicians and other specialists and for information and advice about treatment decisions. These activities have grown into comprehensive educational and outreach programs in many of the older brain tumor organizations.

Of particular note are the outstanding printed and website materials directed to lay audiences. Brain tumor information is technical and complex, and survivors, parents and families have gone to great lengths to publish professionally reviewed, accurate and interpretable information.[12] These materials have helped thousands of patients and families over the past 25 years.

Other services that started as community activities include face-to-face support and telephone support groups, bereavement support, parent-to-parent networks, teleconference seminars, lay brain tumor conferences and information meetings, caregiver trainings, camps and recreation experiences, financial help and free access to professional social worker case advocacy.

A few local tumor groups have grown to become advocates for change in their home states, e.g., in California and Oklahoma. Groups have lobbied for

Table 25.1 Nonprofit brain tumor funding and/or support organizations

Accelerate Brain Cancer Cure, Inc.
Acoustic Neuroma Association USA
Acoustic Neuroma Association of New Jersey, Inc.
Allison's Hope Pediatric Brain Tumor Foundation
American Brain Tumor Association
Ben & Catherine Ivy Foundation
Brad Kaminsky Foundation
Brain Science Foundation
Brain Tumor and Air Pollution Foundation
Brain Tumor and Cancer Research Foundation
Brain Tumor Awareness Organization
Brain Tumor Foundation (NY)
Brain Tumor Foundation (FL)
Brain Tumor Foundation for Children, Inc.
Brain Tumor Foundation of Michigan
Brain Tumor Fund for the Carolinas
Brain Tumor Network
Brain Tumor Support Network of St. Louis
Brain Tumor Research & Education Funds, Inc.
Brain Tumor Research Foundation
Brain Tumor Research Trust, Inc.
Brain Tumor Resource and Information Network
Brave Kids
The Brea Education Foundation
Brent Eley Foundation
Brian Bedell 2-Young Foundation, Inc.
The Bruce Kaye Brain Tumor Foundation, Inc.
Burnham Institute
Cancer Research Foundation of North Texas
Cancer Research Institute, Inc.
Carol Jean Cancer Foundation, Inc.
Central Brain Tumor Registry of the United States
Central New Jersey Brain Tumor Support Group & Resource Center
The Charlie Sears Police & Fire Brain Tumor Foundation, Inc.
The Charles Warren Brain Tumor Awareness Foundation, Inc.
Chelis Children's Foundation
Childhood Brain Tumor Foundation
Children's Brain Tumor Foundation, Inc.
Children's Brain Tumor Foundation of the Southwest
Children's Brain Tumor Research & Family Relief Foundation
Children's Tumor Foundation
Chordoma Foundation
Collaborative Ependymoma Research Network
Connecting for the Cure Foundation Corp.
Conner's Cause for Children
David Tubbs Hole in the Head Foundation
Debbie Romano Memorial Foundation

Table 25.1 (continued)

Doreen Grace Fund Inc
Emily's Foundation
Endurance Trust, Incorporated
Fox Valley Brain Tumor Coalition, Inc.
George Bartol Memorial Scholarship Fund, LLC
Goldhirsh Foundation
Golf Fights Cancer, Inc.
Grey Matters Brain Tumor Support Group
Gruson Fund for Brain Tumor Support Group
Guardian Brain Foundation, Inc.
The Gus Foundation
IronMatt-The Matthew Larson Foundation
Jerry Cantwell Brain Tumor Foundation, Inc.
Joel A Gingras Jr. Memorial Foundation, Inc.
James S. McDonnell Foundation
Katie's Kids
Kelly Heinz-Grundner Foundation, Inc.
Kelly Swim Fund for Pediatric Brain Tumor Research
Kevin J. Mullin Memorial Fund for Brain Tumor Research
Kimberly Jaye Brain Tumor Foundation, Inc.
Kiona Foundation
The Krempels Foundation
Kristin's Friends, Inc.
Kyle O'Connell Foundation
Liat Chanina Foundation
Lin Fam Supporting Organization
Logan P. Graves Foundation
Making Headway Foundation, Inc.
Mark R Harris Foundation, Inc.
The Matthew Larson Pediatric Brain Tumor Research Foundation
MDTW Memorial, Inc.
Meningioma Mommas, Inc.
Michael Quinlan Brain Cancer Foundation
Mid Atlantic Brain Tumor Foundation LTD
Mississippi Brain Tumor Foundation, Inc.
Molly's Angels
Monmouth and Ocean County Brain Tumor Support Group, Inc.
Morgan Adams Foundation
Musella Foundation for Brain Tumor Research & Information, Inc.
Nancy A Herrin Foundation, Inc.
National Brain Tumor Society
National Cancer Coalition, Inc.
National Disease Research Interchange
Neurofibromatosis, Inc. Massachusetts Bay Area
The Nick Gonzales Foundation for Brain Tumor Research TX
The North American Brain Tumor Coalition
Noyes Brain Tumor Foundation
Oklahoma Brain Tumor Foundation
Owen T. Wheeler Foundation
Ozer Foundation
Pediatric Brain Tumor Consortium Foundation
Pediatric Brain Tumor Foundation

Table 25.1 (continued)

Pediatric Brain Tumor Foundation of the United States
Pediatric Brain Tumor Research Foundation
Pediatric Cancer Foundation
Pediatric Cancer Foundation of Lehigh Valley
Pediatric Low-Grade Astrocytoma Foundation
Pediatric Oncology Treasure Chest Foundation
Peter A. Bednarski Fund for Brain Tumor Research, Inc.
The Preuss Foundation
Tara Bean Foundation, Inc.
The Rainbow Foundation for Brain Tumor Research, Inc.
Raleigh Area Brain Tumor Support Group
Richmond Brain Tumor Support Group
Rory David Deutsch Foundation
St. Louis Brain Tumor Research Foundation
Sami Disharoon Brain Tumor Research Foundation
Samuel J. Foundation
San Diego Brain Tumor Foundation
Sean McCauley Hope Foundation, Inc.
Sidney Kimmel Cancer Center Foundation
Smyth Brain Tumor Foundation Ltd.
Sontag Foundation, Inc.
Southeastern Brain Tumor Foundation, Inc.
Students Supporting Brain Tumor Research
Tanner Seebaum Foundation
Team Ryan
Teresa Reese Brain Tumor Research Fund
Tim & Tom Gullikson Foundation
Tug McGraw Foundation
Tumble Weed Foundation
Turn the Corner Foundation
Under His Wings The Gunnar Sterk Pediatric Brain Tumor Foundation
Unlocking Brain Tumors, Inc.
Voices Against Brain Cancer
We Can Pediatric Brain Tumor Network
Wellness Community – West Los Angeles
Wylie's Day Foundation

This list is derived from http://www.guidestar.org, among other internet sources. It excludes medical centers, United Ways, business corporations, religious and professional societies and foundations whose sole purpose is to support a specific medical center. It is not intended as a complete listing.

state legislation that would require insurance companies to cover the routine health care costs for patients who participate in cancer clinical trials. The research costs of cancer clinical trials are typically covered by their sponsors, either a pharmaceutical or the National Cancer Institute. However, in the past, insurers would deny reimbursement for the non-research health care costs if a patient was in a clinical trial. The North American Brain Tumor Coalition (see below), partnering with other cancer advocacy groups, worked nationally to change reimbursement policy on this issue. The cancer advocacy community's collective efforts secured federal coverage of these non-research health care costs through Medicare, thereby setting a precedent for private payers to cover them as well. Some brain tumor groups have taken this battle to their state legislatures.

Another approach that families and survivors adopt to remedy feelings of helplessness at seeing a loved one ill or die of a brain tumor is fund-raising for brain tumor research. Raising money is a means of taking action that yields rapid, measurable outcomes and rewards. Families often donate funds first to a research project of a treating physician or to the brain tumor program of local medical center. Families' and survivors' local fund-raising efforts have supplemented government funds and markedly enhanced many brain tumor centers, helping to defray costs for laboratory equipment and staff, to fund post-doctoral and clinical training fellowships, and to support teachers to create school transition programs for children. The desire of families and friends to raise money for brain tumor research and services has been the engine for the formation of many now nationally prominent brain tumor grants programs and foundations.

National Brain Tumor Advocacy: Efforts to Influence the Bigger Policy Picture

As the number of brain tumor foundations and voluntary organizations has grown in the past 25 years, many grant and service delivery programs sponsored by these organizations support centers and communities throughout the United States and Canada. Most brain tumor research funding programs have come from labor intensive, grassroots fundraising activities, while others derive from individual families whose fortunes allow them to create foundations. While organizations are united in their commitment to eradicate brain tumors, each group has its signature operating style and its own donors.

Brain Tumor Research Funders

Private research funding is an opportunity for advocates to claim responsibility for increasing the total funds available for investigating brain tumors. Although public support for brain tumors through NIH vastly exceeds that awarded by private groups, private brain tumor research awards are substantial and often support high-risk projects that do not receive government funding. In 2006, NIH funding for brain and central nervous system tumors was $130.3 million.[13] Private research funding for the same year was approximately $15 million.[14] The NIH number, however, includes all types of brain tumor research, including clinical research. Private research programs fund basic and translational work almost exclusively.

Grants from Foundations and Voluntary Nonprofit Organizations

Private research awards are an advocacy opportunity. They give organizations of survivors, friends and families a way of helping to shape the brain tumor research agenda. Although brain tumor funding organizations maintain peer review for evaluating and selecting their grant applications, each may have its own funding priorities, which may also be subject to influence from its own scientific advisors.

Brain tumor foundations and voluntary organizations support both biomedical research and its infrastructure. Groups favor individual investigator-initiated research awards and can range from $15,000 to $450,000 per year for basic and translational brain tumor science. Private funding is an important opportunity for funders and for researchers to pursue somewhat riskier scientific leads than typically allowed through more traditional NIH funding mechanisms. Family foundations may be more willing to take on research projects where outcomes may be less predictable.[15] Voluntary organizations, whose funds are raised by a community of volunteers, may tend to be less willing to take major risks with their grants.

Private funders are also committed to broadly supporting the brain tumor research enterprise. In Canada, for example, the national Brain Tumor Tissue Bank is made possible through funding from the Brain Tumor Foundation of Canada.[16] Private groups founded and support the Central Brain Tumor Registry of the United States, a nonprofit organization that is a data resource that augments epidemiological resources on all primary brain tumors.[17] Funders support the recruitment and retention of young brain tumor investigators through fellowships and major awards. Examples include the American Brain Tumor Association, the National Brain Tumor Foundation and the Sontag Foundation.[18] Professional associations and NCI-supported research networks have also been the recipients of generous private support, including the Society for Neuro-oncology, the American Association for Cancer Research, the International Symposium on Pediatric Neuro-oncology, the Brain Tumor Specialized Programs of Research Excellence (SPORES),[19] and the Pediatric Brain Tumor Consortium.[20]

Survivors, parents, friends and families of children with brain tumors have been especially effective in fund-raising for pediatric initiatives. Some groups have primarily supported investigator initiated pediatric brain tumor research, such as the Children's Brain Tumor Foundation and the Childhood Brain Tumor Foundation. Others, such as the Pediatric Brain Tumor Foundation and Fight Pediatric Low Grade Glioma, have created major research programs, such as the Pediatric Brain Tumor Institutes at Duke University Medical

Center, University of California at San Francisco (UCSF) Medical Center, Children's Hospital Los Angeles and Hospital for Sick Children in Toronto,[21] and the low-grade glioma programs at UCSF and the Dana-Farber Cancer Institute.[22]

Some groups dedicate most of their research funding and awards to improving the quality of life of brain tumor patients and those that care for them. The Tug McGraw Foundation and the Gullikson Foundation give college scholarships to brain tumor survivors and awards for service to those working to improve the lives of brain tumor patients.[23] Quality of life research awards have gone, for example, to improve survivors' neurocognitive functioning, to investigate the effect of diet on cell growth in tumors, and to examine models for improving caregiver training and support.

Brain Tumor Funders' Collaborative (BTFC)

BTFC is a partnership among foundations and voluntary nonprofits which came together out of a concern for the slow progress in brain tumor treatments.[24] While each organization has its own established investigator-initiated grants program, they were drawn together by the possibility of pooling research funds into a larger, coordinated national grants program. The underlying notion was to use the flexibility of private philanthropy to challenge the brain tumor research community to improve the outlook for people diagnosed with gliomas (see Table 25.2). The groups held several symposia to identify barriers and gaps in progress to successful treatment for brain tumor disease. After considerable deliberation and planning, eight groups, contributing various amounts to the funding pool, chose to collaborate in a first round of grants.

BTFC members agreed to focus on the "translational gap" preventing promising laboratory science from yielding more effective brain tumor therapies. A Request for Application was intended to stimulate less traditional research approaches. It called for new collaborative, interdisciplinary teams of investigators to form novel strategies to improve the interaction of preclinical and clinical data. Grants were awarded to three teams of investigators.

Table 25.2 Members of the brain tumor funders' collaborative

American Brain Tumor Association
Ben & Catherine Ivy Foundation*
Brain Tumour Foundation of Canada
Children's Brain Tumor Foundation
Goldhirsh Foundation
James S. McDonnell Foundation
National Brain Tumor Society
Sontag Foundation

*Membership occurred after the first grants cycle

One interesting feature of BTFC is the collaboration between funders and grantees. The professional and volunteer leadership of BTFC members act as research advocates in that the intent and implementation of the BTFC is to apply pressure to alter both the conduct and pace of brain tumor research. These leaders, who are not researchers, are nonetheless experienced and knowledgeable about brain tumor research and how to fund it. Meetings and decisions between grantees and funders are treated as collaborative activities, in which accommodations are offered and negotiated from both sides.

A second novel feature of the BTFC is that, regardless of how much a member contributes to the funding pool, each group has an equal voice in decision making. BTFC is established on a basis of mutual trust among its participants, committed to a common goal while respecting and maintaining organizations' differences. This is the case despite the fact that brain tumor voluntary organizations, like other cancer advocacy nonprofits, compete for fund-raising and public attention. It is also worth noting that BTFC is not independently incorporated from its members, therefore markedly reducing the administrative and overhead burden.

Other Funding Partnerships

Different types of partnerships are emerging in the brain tumor community with the same motivations – a desire to accelerate the pace of research and treatment. For example, Accelerate Brain Cancer Cure formed a funding partnership with a pharmaceutical company in an attempt to hasten the testing of a new cancer agent in brain tumor patients. Other groups co-fund investigator-initiated grants because of common interests, or in an effort to reduce the cost and burden of administering a small grants program, e.g., the Children's Brain Tumor Foundation and the Childhood Brain Tumor Foundation. Some of the larger groups have recently merged their research and service programs, e.g., the National Brain Tumor Foundation and the Brain Tumor Society has become the National Brain Tumor Society.

National Opportunities for Individuals to Advocate

Pressure from survivors and families, advocates, members of Congress and the research community urged the NIH in the 1990s to adopt direct public participation in the design and conduct of research.[25] The Institute of Medicine (IOM) also formally advised greater public input in NIH priority setting, and in the conduct and application of biomedical science.[26] IOM recommended that NIH formally solicit public input by establishing public liaison offices in the NIH Director's office and in each NIH institute.

Subsequently, opportunities arose for advocates to become involved in many levels of research, scientific review, planning and oversight. Brain tumor advocates have been vigorous in ensuring that the perspectives of the brain tumor community were integrated into as many cancer research, drug review and reimbursement debates and forums as possible. They have also been committed to bringing back to the North American Brain Tumor Coalition and individual groups news of these deliberations. The many settings in which survivors and families have represented the brain tumor community include the NIH Council on Public Representatives, FDA Oncologic Drugs Advisory Committee, NCI's Pediatric Brain Tumor Consortium, the Brain Tumor SPORES, the NCI-supported adult and pediatric consortia,[27] and the Secretary's Advisory Committee on Human Research Protections.

Public Policy and Advocacy

North American Brain Tumor Coalition (NABTC)

Founded in 1993, NABTC is the first attempt to coordinate voices across the United States and Canada on matters of public policy that affect individuals diagnosed and living with brain tumors.[28] Member organizations believed that together they could change national policies more effectively than they could do so acting alone. NABTC's policy agenda is shaped by the priorities of survivors and families through its member organizations. In addition to its agenda, NABTC responds to the current political opportunities and realities in both the United States and Canada.

Brain tumor research has been NABTC's top policy priority since its inception. Each year, NABTC has lobbied for more generous public funding of brain tumor research in the United States and Canada. NABTC collaborated with other research advocates to double NIH funding in the five-year period between 1998 and 2003. As NIH funding levels froze after 2003, NABTC worked with other disease advocacy groups to reverse the reduction in biomedical research funding. NABTC also pressed members of Congress to protect the academic brain tumor research networks, including the brain tumor consortia and the Brain Tumor SPORES.

Early in its history, NABTC advocates entered into extensive discussions with the leaders of the NCI and the NINDS to urge them to engage in more coordination and planning of their national brain tumor research programs. The institutes responded by forming the Neuro-Oncology Branch, that is a jointly sponsored initiative of NCI and NINDS. NABTC was instrumental in securing both institutes' sponsorship of the Brain Tumor Progress Review Group, a meeting of researchers and patient advocates, to develop a national plan for brain tumor research. This report is still a benchmark against which private brain tumor research programs are compared.

NABTC attacked another problem facing brain tumor researchers. Research was hampered by a lack of complete data about all forms of brain tumors, both benign and malignant. NABTC secured the introduction, enactment, funding and implementation of federal legislation in 2002, the Benign Brain Tumor Cancer Registries Amendment Act, to require the state cancer registry program to collect benign as well as malignant brain tumor data.

NABTC has actively sought reforms of the health care system to guarantee that brain tumor patients have access to care of the highest quality. Activities to ensure high quality care include advocating appropriate payment for brain tumor treatments, seeking proper regulatory review of new therapies and removing financial or other barriers to health care. NABTC participated in legislative efforts that require Medicare to cover the routine care costs incurred by patients who participate in clinical trials. It also led advocacy to eliminate the two-year lag between eligibility for Social Security Disability benefits and eligibility for Medicare for those with life-threatening illnesses. This is a period when brain tumor patients are in most urgent need of good health care, yet find themselves without insurance.

NABTC actively collaborates with other national cancer organizations through the Cancer Leadership Council (CLC).[29] The CLC is an alliance of 33 patient organizations, professional societies, and research organizations which advocates for a wide range of research policy, funding and health care access matters that relate to all cancers. NABTC's participation in the CLC ensures that, whenever possible, brain tumor survivors' and families' needs are factored in during national cancer research and health care advocacy efforts.

Canadian Alliance of Brain Tumour Organizations (CABTO)

CABTO, founded in 1991, is an alliance of voluntary organizations, dedicated to enhancing the quality of life of brain tumor patients and families in Canada.[30] CABTO advocates politically and publicly for better patient care, for increased government funding for brain tumor research, and for increased awareness of both the public-at-large and elected officials of the devastating toll brain tumors take on patients and their loved ones. CABTO is a division of the larger Canadian Brain Tumour Network (CBTNet), whose membership includes clinicians, specialists, researchers and patient support organizations.

Recognizing researchers' need for more accurate statistics on brain tumors, CABTO, the Brain Tumour Foundation of Canada and individual brain tumor advocates obtained Canadian Parliament approval for a measure that calls on provincial governments to count benign brain tumors in their statistics, a counterpart of the U.S. initiative. Advocates are working to establish a central registry within Canada for the collection of data on brain tumors.

Other CABTO priorities include reducing patients' wait times for radiation treatments and increasing access to equitable drug coverage. Despite differences in health care insurance systems, Canadian and U.S. brain tumor advocates have equal concerns about better access to supportive care services, including home care, rehabilitation and palliative care.

Future of Brain Tumor Advocacy: Opportunities for Collaboration

Survivors of brain tumors and their families have critical challenges that require their vigorous and strategic focus. Flat funding of federal research threatens progress for treating all diseases, and continued lack of progress in treatments for brain tumors continues to be unacceptable. Advocates need to apply pressure on many other critical issues. A clear definition of surrogate endpoints for brain tumor disease is needed to speed the evaluation of new therapeutic agents. Patient-reported outcomes or quality of life measures must be included as new agents may be approved for treating brain tumors. There continues to be a profound need to develop effective neurocognitive rehabilitation strategies for survivors so they can lead successful and productive lives beyond treatment. As a final example, treatments and care must be affordable if brain tumor patients are to have access to new, more targeted therapies.

These challenges need to be met by mobilizing resources, both internal and external, to the brain tumor community. Collaboration among the many brain tumor groups can improve private research programs by trimming administrative costs and increasing their impact through pooled funds. Services can be available to even more survivors and families through joint programs that use increasingly sophisticated web-based approaches. Strategies that concentrate the energy and capabilities of the relatively small brain tumor community are critical to effectively meeting present and imminent challenges.

The brain tumor community is fortunate to have many seasoned advocates among its ranks who have grown with the cancer advocacy movement and worked to improve the lives of survivors and families. Now, for the first time, there is a growing population of young adult brain tumor survivors whose talents and concerns are emerging. These survivors, their families and friends can build on the accomplishments of more than a decade of advocates' groundwork, offering new energy and insights to advance treatment and care for those with brain tumors.

Acknowledgments The authors would like to thank Elizabeth Goss, long-time policy counsel to NABTC, for her substantive contributions and commitment to advocacy for brain tumor patients, survivors and families.

References

1. http://planning.cancer.gov/pdfprgreports/2000braintumor.pdf
2. This chapter uses the definition of survivor on the NCI website: "An individual is considered a cancer survivor from the time of diagnosis, through the balance of his or her life.

Family members, friends, and caregivers are also impacted by the survivorship experience and are therefore included in this definition. Adapted from the National Coalition for Cancer Survivorship. http://cancercontrol.cancer.gov/ocs/definitions.html.

3. CBTRUS. Statistical Report: Primary Brain Tumors in the United States, 1998–2002. Published by the Central Brain Tumor Registry of the United States, 2005.
4. http://planning.cancer.gov/disease/Brain-Snapshot.pdf
5. http://seer.cancer.gov/statfacts/html/brain_print.html
6. CBTRUS (2005). Statistical Report: Primary Brain Tumors in the United States, 1998–2002. Published by the Central Brain Tumor Registry of the United States.
7. While some brain tumors can be benign or slow growing, all are neoplasia and can be disabling. "Cancer" is used here to apply to all types of brain tumors.
8. Epstein S. *Impure Science: AIDS,Activism,and the Politics of Knowledge*. Berkeley, CA: University of California Press, 1996.
9. Effective Lobbying Increases U.S. Funds for Breast Cancer Research. New York Times, October 19, 1992.
10. Clark E, Stovall E. Advocacy: the cornerstone of cancer survivorship. *Cancer Pract.* 1996;4(5):239–244.
11. Weiner SL, McCabe MS, Smith G, Monaco GP, Fiduccia D. Pediatric cancer: Advocacy, legal, insurance and employment Issues. In: Pizzo P, and Poplack D, eds. *Principles and Practice of Pediatric Oncology*, 4th ed. Philadelphia: Lippincott Raven Publishers, 2001.
12. Hoffman B, Stovall E. Survivorship perspectives and advocacy. *J Clin Oncol.* 2006;24:5154–5159.
13. For example, the American Brain Tumor Association, http://www.abta.org, the National Brain Tumor Foundation, http://www.braintumor.org, and the Children's Brain Tumor Foundation, http://www.cbtf.org.
14. National Cancer Institute 2006 Fact Book, http://obf.cancer.gov/financial/attachments/06Factbk.pdf.
15. Personal communication, Brain Tumor Funders' Collaborative.
16. See for example, the Sontag Foundation at http://www.sontagfoundation.org
17. http://www.braintumour.ca/braintumour.nsf/eng/research
18. American Brain Tumor Association and Pediatric Brain Tumor Foundation of the US.
19. http://abta.org/index.cfm?contentid = 38   http://www.braintumor.org.http://www.sontagfoundation.org.
20. http://spores.nci.nih.gov/current/brain/brain.html
21. http://www.pbtc.org
22. http://www.pbtfus.org
23. http://www.fightplga.org
24. http://www.tugmcgraw.org http://www.gullikson.org
25. http://www.braintumorfunders.org
26. http://getinvolved.nih.gov/
27. Institute of Medicine, Committee on the NIH Research Priority-Setting Process, Scientific Opportunities and Public Needs: Improving Priority Setting and Public Input at the National Institutes of Health, 1998.
28. North American Brain Tumor Consortium and New Approached to Brain Tumor Therapy (which at this writing are merging) and Pediatric Brain Tumor Consortium.
29. http://www.nabraintumor.org
30. http://www.cancerleadership.org
31. http://www.cabto.ca

Chapter 26
Screening for Late Effects in Brain Tumor Survivors

Wendy Landier, Karen E. Kinahan, Susan Shaw, and Smita Bhatia

Introduction

Brain tumor survivors frequently receive therapy that places them at risk for long-term or late sequelae involving multiple organs. These late complications, arising as a result of neurosurgery, radiation, chemotherapy, and bone marrow/ stem cell transplant, have been discussed in detail throughout this book. The focus of this chapter is to provide the clinician with guidance regarding how to methodically assess each survivor's risk for late complications, and how to determine appropriate risk-based surveillance, in order to provide targeted, yet comprehensive, long-term follow-up care for brain tumor survivors. Two case studies of brain tumor survivors are included to illustrate the potential and actual late effects experienced by these survivors and the need for ongoing surveillance for late complications.

Common Therapy-Related Late Sequelae in Brain Tumor Survivors

Long-term complications observed in brain tumor survivors are linked to therapeutic exposures and, as such, the risk in individual patients is determined in part by the intensity and nature of therapeutic exposures. We will briefly review late sequelae associated with the more commonly employed therapeutic strategies in patients with brain tumors.

Chemotherapy

Chemotherapeutic regimens used to treat brain tumors commonly incorporate agents such as platinum analogues (e.g., cisplatin, carboplatin), classical

W. Landier (✉)
Department of Population Sciences, Center for Cancer Survivorship, City of Hope
National Medical Center, Duarte, CA, USA
e-mail: wlandier@coh.org

S. Goldman, C.D. Turner (eds.), *Late Effects of Treatment for Brain Tumors*,
Cancer Treatment and Research 150, DOI 10.1007/b109924_26,
© Springer Science+Business Media, LLC 2009

alkylators (e.g., cyclophosphamide, procarbazine), nonclassical alkylators (e.g., temozolomide), nitrosureas (e.g., CCNU), vinca alkaloids (e.g., vincristine, vinblastine), antimetabolites (e.g., 6-thioguanine), epipodophyllotoxins (e.g., etoposide), and/or corticosteroids (e.g., prednisone, dexamethasone).[1] Common agents typically used to treat specific brain tumor types are presented in Table 26.1. Late sequelae of the common chemotherapeutic agents used to treat brain tumors include gonadal dysfunction[2-4] (alkylators, platinum analogues, nitrosureas), acute myeloid leukemia or myelodysplasia[5,6] (alkylators, platinum analogues, epipodophyllotoxins, nitrosureas), urinary tract toxicity[7,8]

Table 26.1 Chemotherapeutic agents commonly used to treat specific brain tumor types

Tumor type	Commonly used agents	Chemotherapy class
Medulloblastoma	Cisplatin	Platinum analogues
	Carboplatin	
	Cyclophosphamide	Alkylators
	CCNU	
	Vincristine	Vinca alkaloids
	Etoposide	Epipodophyllotoxins
Optic pathway tumors	Carboplatin	Platinum analogues
	Cisplatin	
	Procarbazine	Alkylators
	Vincristine	Vinca alkaloids
	6-Thioguanine	Antimetabolites
	Actinomycin-D	
Ependymoma	Cisplatin	Platinum analogues
	Carboplatin	
	Cyclophosphamide	Alkylators
	Vincristine	Vinca alkaloids
	Etoposide	Epipodophyllotoxins
Low-grade gliomas (non-brain stem)	Carboplatin	Platinum analogues
	Procarbazine	Alkylators
	Dibromodulcitol	
	CCNU	
	Vincristine	Vinca alkaloids
	6-Thioguanine	Antimetabolites
High-grade gliomas (non-brain stem)	Procarbazine	Alkylators
	CCNU	
	Cyclophosphamide	
	Temozolomide	
	Vincristine	Vinca alkaloids
	Prednisone	Corticosteroid
Germ cell tumors	Carboplatin	Platinum analogues
	Cisplatin	
	Bleomycin	Anti-tumor antibiotics
	Vincristine	Vinca alkaloids
	Vinblastine	
	Etoposide	Epipodophyllotoxins

Data from Blaney et al.[1]

(cyclophosphamide, ifosfamide, platinum analogues), ototoxicity[9] (platinum analogues), peripheral neuropathy[10] (platinum analogues, vinca alkaloids), dyslipidemia[11] (platinum analogues), pulmonary toxicity[12] (nitrosureas, bleomycin), hepatic dysfunction[13] (thioguanine), osteopenia/osteoporosis,[14] osteonecrosis,[15] and cataracts (corticosteroids).[16] The late sequelae frequently associated with chemotherapeutic agents used to treat brain tumors are summarized in Table 26.2.

Table 26.2 Common sequelae of chemotherapeutic agents used to treat brain tumors

Chemotherapy class	Associated late sequelae
Alkylators	Gonadal dysfunction
	Acute myeloid leukemia/myelodysplasia
	Urinary tract toxicity (cyclophosphamide/ifosfamide)
Platinum analogues	Gonadal dysfunction
	Acute myeloid leukemia/myelodysplasia
	Ototoxicity
	Renal toxicity
	Peripheral neuropathy
	Dyslipidemia
Vinca alkaloids	Peripheral neuropathy
	Raynaud's phenomenon
Epipodophyllotoxins	Acute myeloid leukemia
Nitrosureas	Gonadal dysfunction
	Acute myeloid leukemia/myelodysplasia
	Pulmonary fibrosis
Antimetabolites	Hepatic dysfunction (thioguanine)
Corticosteroids	Osteopenia/osteoporosis
	Osteonecrosis
	Cataracts
Anti-tumor antibiotics	Pulmonary toxicity (bleomycin)

Data from[50]

Radiation

Radiation is commonly employed as primary, adjuvant or neoadjuvant therapy for patients with brain tumors.[1] Radiation-related sequelae depend on multiple factors, including the target, volume, and field irradiated, as well as the patient's age at the time of irradiation. Common sequelae resulting from conventional radiation to the cranium include secondary benign or malignant neoplasms (e.g., skin, brain, thyroid, bone, soft tissue),[17] dermatologic changes including alopecia,[18] neurocognitive deficits,[19] clinical leukoencephalopathy,[20] cerebrovascular complications (e.g., stroke, moyamoya, occlusive cerebral vasculopathy),[21–23] craniofacial abnormalities,[24] chronic sinusitis,[25] cataracts and other ocular toxicities,[26] ototoxicity,[27] xerostomia,[28] dental abnormalities,[29] osteoradionecrosis,[30] carotid/subclavian artery disease,[21] obesity,[31] metabolic syndrome,[32] and endocrinopathies,[33] (including growth hormone deficiency,[34] precocious puberty,[35] hypo- and hyperthyroidism,[36] gonadotropin deficiency,[37] central adrenal insufficiency,[38] hyperprolactinemia,[33] and panhypopituitarism[31]). The late sequelae of newer radiation modalities (e.g., protons, intensity-modulated radiation therapy [IMRT]) are largely unknown at this time; however, there is some concern that the additional fields required for IMRT and the higher doses of radiation delivered by protons administered without a scanning beam may potentially result in an increased incidence of second neoplasms and other radiation-related late sequelae.[39]

Neurosurgery

The late sequelae of neurosurgical procedures depend on tumor location and the surgical approach; however, complications include neurocognitive deficits,[40] motor and/or sensory deficits,[41,42] (including paralysis, movement disorders, ataxia, and ocular sequelae), and seizures.[41]

Bone Marrow/Stem Cell Transplant

High-dose consolidative therapy followed by autologous stem cell rescue for treatment of brain tumors may result in significant late complications, including myelodysplasia/acute myeloid leukemia,[43] solid tumors,[44] lymphoma,[45] hepatotoxicity,[46] osteonecrosis,[47] and osteopenia or osteoporosis.[48]

Long-Term Follow-Up After Treatment for Brain Tumors

Virtually every organ system can be affected by the chemotherapy, radiation, and/or surgery required to treat brain tumors, and potential late complications, as reviewed above and throughout this book, may include organ dysfunction, growth and developmental delay (in children), neurocognitive impairment, and subsequent malignant neoplasms. In addition, psychosocial sequelae of cancer treatment may adversely affect family and peer relationships, vocational and employment opportunities, and insurance and health care access. These long-term problems after cancer treatment have been particularly well documented in survivors of pediatric malignancies. Unfortunately, two out of every three childhood cancer survivors will develop at least one late therapy-related complication, and in one of every four cases, the complication will be severe or life-threatening.[49]

The Children's Oncology Group Long-Term Follow-Up Guidelines

To facilitate and standardize risk-based, exposure-related, long-term, follow-up evaluations of childhood cancer survivors, the Children's Oncology Group's Late Effects Committee and Nursing Discipline developed *Long-Term Follow-Up Guidelines for Survivors of Childhood, Adolescent, and Young Adult Cancers*[50] (COG LTFU Guidelines).[51] The COG LTFU Guidelines are both evidence-based (utilizing established associations between thera- peutic exposures and late effects to identify high-risk categories) and grounded in the collective clinical experience of late effects experts (matching the magnitude of risk with the intensity of the recommended screening), and are designed to optimize the early identification of and intervention for treatment-related complications in childhood cancer survivors. The screening recommendations outlined in the COG LTFU Guidelines are appropriate for asymptomatic survivors presenting for routine exposure-based medical follow-up two or more years after completion of therapy. More extensive evaluations should be provided, as clinically indicated, for survivors presenting with signs and symptoms suggestive of illness or organ dysfunction. Patient education materials, known as "Health Links," complement a variety of survi- vorship topics addressed in the Guidelines.[52] The COG LTFU Guidelines and their associated Health Links can be downloaded from www.survivorship guidelines.org.

Currently, there are no comparable guidelines designed for the adult popula- tion of cancer survivors;[53] however, many of the recommendations within the COG LTFU Guidelines are applicable to adult patients, with the exception of those specifically associated with growth and developmental issues unique to children and adolescents.

Using the LTFU Guidelines in Clinical Practice

In order to effectively utilize the COG LTFU Guidelines in clinical prac- tice, steps must be taken to assure that adequate information is available in order to customize recommendations for individual survivors based on their treatment history. Therefore, the initial step in providing long-term follow-up care for brain tumor survivors involves compilation of a ther- apeutic summary for each patient. Once the treatment summary is pre- pared, the COG LTFU Guidelines can be used as a guide for developing individualized screening recommendations for each survivor. Applicable patient education materials can then be selected in preparation for the long-term follow-up visit. The preparation culminates in a focused yet comprehensive evaluation of each patient's physical and psychosocial health and long-term follow-up needs. The long-term follow-up evaluation is gen- erally carried out on an annual basis in order to provide ongoing surveillance and early intervention for any late therapy-related complications; however, younger survivors may need more frequent evaluations, particularly during periods of rapid growth.[50]

Summarizing Therapeutic Exposures

In order to identify appropriate risk-based screening recommendations for brain tumor survivors, preparing a therapeutic summary is an essential first step. Key information in the therapeutic summary includes diagnosis, treatment protocol, names of all chemotherapeutic agents (with cumulative doses, if available), radiation therapy dates, fields, laterality and doses, surgical procedures (including surgeon, date, site and laterality), and other modalities if indicated (e.g., hematopoietic cell transplant, biotherapy). See Fig. 26.1 for a sample therapeutic summary form.

Individualizing Screening Recommendations

Once the therapeutic summary is complete, the next step in preparing to provide survivorship care for brain tumor survivors is determining the appropriate recommendations for screening by assessing the patient's treatment history and other relevant risk factors (e.g., age, gender, family history, health behaviors, comorbidities, and time since diagnosis/treatment). This can be accomplished by using the COG LTFU Guidelines to identify the potential late effects and associated risk factors for each therapeutic exposure within the treatment summary. For example, if a patient received carboplatin and vincristine for treatment of a low-grade diencepehalic glioma, the clinician should identify the relevant Guideline sections for each individual agent (carboplatin, vincristine), and make note of the potential late effects, associated risk factors, and recommended screening for each agent. In this example, screening would be indicated for the potential renal and gonadal dysfunction, dyslipidemia, and secondary myelodysplasia/acute myeloid leukemia associated with carboplatin, and for the peripheral neuropathy associated with vincristine. In addition, the clinician should incorporate the appropriate general recommendations from the COG LTFU Guidelines into each patient's follow-up plan. Some of these general recommendations are applicable to all patients regardless of therapeutic exposures (e.g., psychosocial sequelae), and others are applicable only to specific subgroups (e.g., patients who received radiation or chemotherapy). An algorithm is available to assist with this process (see Appendix 1 of the COG LTFU Guidelines, available at www.survivorshipguidelines.org). Once a comprehensive list of potential late effects and screening recommendations has been compiled, the follow-up visit can be planned and appropriate screening tests scheduled as indicated.

Use of Patient Education Materials (Health Links)

While reviewing the COG LTFU Guidelines to identify potential late effects and associated screening recommendations, the clinician should also make note

SUMMARY OF CANCER TREATMENT

Demographics

Name:		Sex:		Date of Birth:	
Address:					
Phone:	SS#		Race/Ethnicity:		
Alternate contact:		Relationship:		Phone:	

Cancer Diagnosis

Diagnosis:			
Date of Diagnosis:	Age at Diagnosis:	Date Therapy Completed:	
Sites involved/stage/diagnostic details:			Laterality:
Hereditary/congenital history:			
Pertinent history/Past medical history/Family history:			
Treatment Center:		Medical Record #:	
MD/APN Contact Information:			

Relapse(s)

Date:	Site(s):	Laterality:	Date Therapy Completed:

CANCER TREATMENT SUMMARY

Protocol

Acronym/Number	Title/Description	Initiated	Completed	On-Study

Surgery

Date	Procedure	Site (if applicable)	Laterality	Surgeon/Institution

Chemotherapy

Drug Name	Route	Cumulative Dose
		mg/m^2
		mg/m^2

Bioimmunotherapy

Drug Name	Route	Cumulative Dose

Radiation

Site/Field	Laterality	Start	Stop	Fractions	Dose per Fraction (cGy)	Total Dose (cGy)	Type
Radiation oncologist:		Institution:					

Transplant

Type	Source	Date	Conditioning Regimen	Institution/Treating MD

Blood Products

Complications/Late Effects

Problem	Date onset	Date resolved	Status

Adverse Drug Reactions/Allergies

Drug	Reaction	Date	Status

Additional Information/Comments

Summary prepared by:	Date prepared:
Summary updated by: ---	Date updated: ---

Fig. 26.1 Sample therapeutic summary form (Used with permission from: Children's Oncology Group: Long-Term Follow-Up Guidelines for Survivors of Childhood, Adolescent, and Young Adult Cancers, Version 2.0. March 2006)

of the available patient education materials associated with each applicable Guideline section.[52] These materials, identified as "Health Links," are easily accessible for printing and distribution to patients via the www.survivorship guidelines.org website.

Implementing Risk-Based Care

Once the individualized surveillance recommendations and patient education materials have been compiled, based on the therapeutic summary, the process of long-term follow-up care begins in earnest. Each survivor should undergo a thorough history and physical examination, with emphasis placed on high-risk areas identified through review of the therapeutic summary and COG LTFU Guidelines. The annual long-term follow-up visit should be health-oriented in focus, with strategies for health promotion incorporated throughout, both by the clinician (e.g., by providing anticipatory guidance and health education), and by other members of the multidisciplinary team, as applicable and available (see Chapters 7 and 22).

Case Study 1: Pediatric Brain Tumor Survivor

Diagnosis: S.J. was diagnosed with stage IIIB medulloblastoma at the age of 11 years, seven months. He presented with bitemporal headaches, blurred vision and head tilt. Physical examination was remarkable for mild neck rigidity, mild discomfort with flexion, bilateral blurred discs, lateral nystagmus, and unsteadiness with tandem walking. Diagnostic CT scan revealed a cystic, hyperdense midline cerebellar tumor with moderate hydrocephalus and enlarged temporal horns.

Therapeutic Exposures: Treatment consisted of surgery, radiation therapy and chemotherapy according to the Pediatric Oncology Group (POG) Protocol #9031, Treatment #2. Surgical intervention included a ventriculostomy, sub-occipital craniotomy with C1 bilateral laminectomy and debulking of the tumor. Pathology was confirmatory for medulloblastoma. Craniospinal axis irradiation to a total dose of 3,520 cGy in 22 equal daily fractions of 160 cGy was delivered over 29 days. A posterior fossa boost of 1,800 cGy was then delivered in 10 fractions, for a total dose of 5,320 cGy delivered to the posterior fossa over 43 days. Cumulative doses of chemotherapeutic agents included cisplatin (157.5 mg/m^2), etoposide (600 mg/m^2), vincristine (16 mg/m^2) and cyclophosphamide (16,000 mg/m^2). He also received numerous red cell and platelet transfusions (subsequent studies for Hepatitis C were negative). Therapy was completed at the age of 12 years, seven months. The only significant complication during therapy was acute renal toxicity, which resolved without sequelae. S.J. has remained in continuous remission since completion of therapy without evidence of recurrent disease.

Late Effects: S.J. exhibited decelerating growth velocity within six months after completing radiation therapy (see Fig. 26.2). Workup revealed evidence of

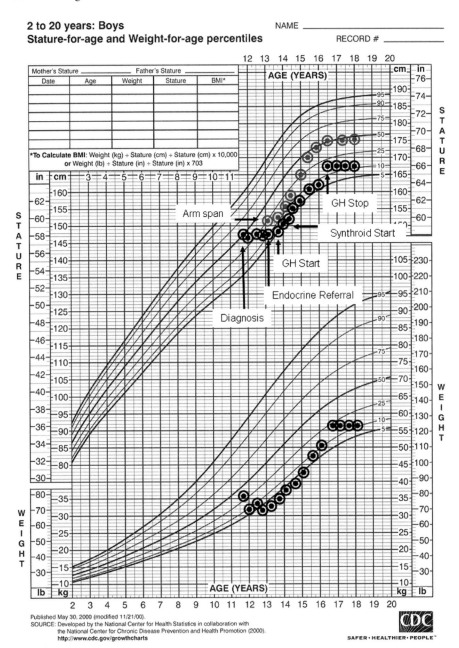

Fig. 26.2 Case study 1: Growth curve with height, weight and arm span

growth hormone deficiency. Growth hormone therapy was initiated at age 13 years, seven months (one year after completion of therapy) and continued through age 16 years, six months. S.J.'s target height was 67.5 inches, with a genetic potential of 65.5 inches to 69.5 inches. His final adult height is 66 inches and his adult arm span is 69 inches, indicative of an approximately three inch loss in final adult height related to spinal irradiation. Growth hormone therapy was reinitiated at the adult replacement dose at the age of 17 years, six months. S.J. developed primary hypothyroidism at age 14 years, three months, and thyroid hormone replacement therapy was initiated. He subsequently developed papillary thyroid carcinoma at age 24 and underwent thyroidectomy. He is maintained on daily thyroid hormone replacement therapy.

S.J. was able to graduate from high school with the assistance of a Section 504 accommodation plan, allowing extended testing time and resource assistance on an as-needed basis. He maintained a low "C" grade point average with extensive time spent studying and completing homework assignments. He subsequently attended a small local college for two semesters, enrolling in an architecture and computer design program. He was unable to complete this program due to poor academic performance despite assistance from a tutor. He subsequently enrolled in night classes for computer programming at a local community college, but this program also proved to be academically challenging and he withdrew from classes after one semester. Problems with processing speed, short-term memory issues, and limited ability to process complex information emerged during this time. S.J. has also sustained additional therapy-related late effects, which are presented in Table 26.3. The potential late effects for which S.J. remains at risk are presented in Table 26.4.

Table 26.3 Case Study 1: S.J.'s actual late effects

Current late effect	Therapeutic agent(s)	Evaluation	Intervention/ counseling
Neurocognitive impairment	Cranial radiation; Neurosurgery	Neurocognitive testing if desired	Appropriate accommodations if returns to school; Referral for vocational testing and job placement if needed; *Educational Issues* Health Link
Possible mild depression	Cancer diagnosis, treatment, and late effects	Yearly psychological assessment	Referral for counseling as indicated; *Emotional Issues* Health Link
Alopecia in radiation field (occiput)	Cranial radiation	Yearly physical exam	Counsel re: hair prosthesis or replacement

Table 26.3 (continued)

Current late effect	Therapeutic agent(s)	Evaluation	Intervention/ counseling
			options; Referral to cosmetologist if desired
Multiple nevi in irradiated fields	Craniospinal radiation	Yearly physical exam	Dermatology referral for suspicious lesions; *Skin Health* Health Link
Cataract (left eye)	Cranial radiation	Follow-up as per ophthalmology	Ophthalmology referral; Sunglasses/sun-protective lenses; *Eye Health* Health Link
Bilateral mild high frequency hearing loss	Cranial radiation, Cisplatin	Follow-up as per otolaryngologist	Otolaryngology referral; Hearing aids (refuses to wear); *Hearing Loss* Health Link
Adult growth hormone deficiency (prior growth hormone deficiency of childhood)	Cranial radiation	Follow-up as per endocrinology	Growth hormone replacement therapy; *Growth Hormone Deficiency* Health Link
Hypothyroidism	Craniospinal radiation; Thyroidectomy	Follow-up as per endocrinology	Thyroid hormone replacement therapy; *Thyroid Problems* Health Link
Papillary thyroid carcinoma (s/p thyroidectomy)	Craniospinal radiation	Follow-up as per surgery and endocrinology	*Thyroid Problems* Health Link
Musculoskeletal hypoplasia (neck)	Spinal radiation	Yearly physical exam	Counsel re: increased fracture risk
Shortened truncal height	Spinal radiation	Yearly physical exam	Counsel re: increased fracture risk; *Bone Health* Health Link
Osteopenia (left hip and spine)	Cranial radiation with resultant hypogonadism and growth hormone deficiency	Follow-up as per endocrinology	Calcium, vitamin D, Bisphosphonates; *Bone Health* Health Link
Infertility	Cyclophosphamide; Craniospinal radiation		Semen analysis and counseling as needed;

Table 26.3 (continued)

Current late effect	Therapeutic agent(s)	Evaluation	Intervention/counseling
Borderline low testosterone level	Craniospinal radiation	Follow-up as per endocrinology	*Male Health Issues* Health Link Testosterone supplementation (refuses at present time); *Male Health Issues* Health Link

Table 26.4 Case Study 1: S.J.'s potential late effects (for which ongoing monitoring is necessary)

Potential late effect	Therapeutic agent	Screening	Intervention/counseling
Psychosocial issues, including employment discrimination and insurance issues	Cancer diagnosis, treatment, late effects	Yearly psychosocial assessment	*Emotional Issues* and *Finding Health Care* Health Links; Legal referral if indicated
Subsequent neoplasm (benign or malignant) in irradiated field	Craniospinal radiation	Yearly history and physical	*Reducing Risk of Cancers* Health Link
Dysplastic nevi/skin cancer; Dermatologic changes in irradiated field	Craniospinal radiation	Yearly history and physical	*Skin Health* and *Reducing Risk of Cancers* Health Links
Cerebrovascular complications, including stroke and occlusive cerebral vasculopathy; Leukoencephalopathy	Craniospinal radiation	Yearly history and physical	Anticipatory guidance
Seizures	Cranial radiation, Neurosurgery	Yearly history and physical	Neurology evaluation as clinically indicated
Motor and/or sensory deficits	Neurosurgery	Yearly evaluation by physiatrist	Neurology evaluation; Speech, physical and occupational therapy evaluations as indicated
Hyperprolactinemia	Cranial radiation	Yearly review of systems, including galactorrhea, decreased libido	*Hyperprolactinemia* Health Link
Chronic sinusitis	Cranial radiation	Yearly history and physical	Anticipatory guidance
Xerostomia; Salivary gland dysfunction; Dental problems;	Craniospinal radiation	Yearly history and physical; Dental visits every 6 months	*Dental Health* Health Link
Osteoradionecrosis	Cranial radiation	Dental evaluation as indicated	*Osteoradionecrosis* Health Link

Table 26.4 (continued)

Potential late effect	Therapeutic agent	Screening	Intervention/ counseling
Carotid artery disease	Cranial radiation	Yearly history (include evaluation of memory) and physical exam	Anticipatory guidance
Esophageal stricture; Bowel obstruction;	Spinal radiation	Yearly history and physical	*GI Health* Health Link
Colorectal cancer	Spinal radiation	Colonoscopy every 5 years starting at age 35	*Colorectal Cancer* Health Link
Cardiac toxicity (e.g., congestive heart failure, cardiomyopathy, pericarditis, pericardial fibrosis, valvular disease, myocardial infarction, arrhythmia, atherosclerotic heart disease)	Spinal radiation	Yearly history and physical; Fasting glucose and lipid profile every 3–5 years; Baseline EKG; Echocardiogram every 2 years	*Heart Health* Health Link
Metabolic syndrome; Overweight/obesity; Dyslipidemia	Cranial radiation; Cisplatin	Yearly history and physical; Fasting glucose, insulin, lipids every 2 - 5 years	*Diet and Physical Activity* Health Link
Hemorrhagic cystitis; Bladder cancer	Cyclophosphamide, Spinal radiation	Yearly urinalysis	*Bladder Health* Health Link
Renal toxicity	Cisplatin	Yearly blood pressure; Baseline renal function panel	*Kidney Health* Health Link
Peripheral neuropathy	Cisplatin, Vincristine	Neurological exam as indicated	*Peripheral Neuropathy* and *Raynaud's Phenomenon* Health Links

Current status: Currently 27-years-old, S.J. is employed in the warehouse of a local department store where he is paid slightly more than minimum wage. He has medical insurance and a small life insurance policy through his employer. He continues to live with his parents in a small rural community. He has a driver's license and has been involved in two minor traffic accidents due to slow reaction time and misjudgment of a turn. His car insurance premium was increased after these accidents. As he has become older, the social gap between S.J. and his peers has widened. Although mild depression has been identified, he has refused psychological intervention. His current medications include daily Levoxyl (synthroid), calcium, and vitamin D, nightly growth hormone injections, and weekly oral bisphosphonate. He is evaluated in the long-term follow-up clinic and the neuro-oncology clinic at his treating institution annually, and is also followed by endocrinology and ophthalmology on a regular basis.

Case Study 2: Adult Brain Tumor Survivor

Diagnosis: R.M. is a Hispanic female who was diagnosed with an intracranial germinoma at 30 years of age after she presented with amenorrhea, galactorrhea and headaches. MRI revealed a large, predominantly suprasellar mass, with extension and invasion into the clivus, suprasellar cistern, and cavernous sinus. She underwent transsphenoidal tumor resection, and pathology was confirmatory for dysgerminoma. She was treated with cranial radiation followed by three cycles of chemotherapy (cisplatin, etoposide, and bleomycin). A complete response was achieved. Unfortunately, nine years following her initial diagnosis, a follow-up MRI revealed a large mass centered in the genu of the corpus callosum involving the septum pellucidum and fornices bilaterally; this proved to be recurrent dysgerminoma. It was felt that this patient's recurrent disease could not be cured with conventional treatment. She, therefore, received two cycles of re-induction chemotherapy with etoposide and carboplatin, followed by autologous stem cell harvest. She subsequently received high-dose consolidative therapy with etoposide, carboplatin, and thiotepa, followed by autologous peripheral stem cell transplant.

Therapeutic exposures: R.M. received cranial radiation to a dose of 4,500 cGy. Her cumulative chemotherapy doses are as follows: cisplatin (300 mg/m^2), carboplatin (2,300 mg/m^2), bleomycin (270 mg/m^2), etoposide (3,050 mg/m^2) and thiotepa (900 mg/m^2). She also underwent autologous hematopoietic stem cell transplant and received numerous transfusions of packed red blood cells and platelets.

Course: R.M.'s initial course was uncomplicated and she was able to work as a cashier for several years prior to her recurrence. At the time of recurrence, there was significant deterioration in her mental function over a period of several months, including labile emotional outbursts. Additionally, she sustained a 50 to 60% increase in body weight over the six-month period prior to her recurrence. She experienced multiple serious complications during her transplant course, including severe epistaxis with subsequent aspiration and respiratory arrest on Day +6, requiring prolonged intubation and mechanical ventilation. She developed ARDS and required ICU care for 38 days. White cell engraftment was achieved on Day +12. She suffered hemorrhagic complications during a tracheostomy on Day +48 due to persistent thrombocytopenia and subsequently received a second stem cell reinfusion on Day +53; her thrombocytopenia resolved three weeks later. A Day +63 MRI for staging of R.M.'s intracranial germinoma revealed marked regression of the corpus callosum tumor. She was transferred to a rehabilitation hospital on Day +65. At the time of transfer, she was alert and oriented x 4. She was speaking, obeying commands and tolerating oral intake. R.M. chose not to stay in the rehabilitation hospital for the recommended length of stay. Once home, she was able to ambulate with a walker around her home, but suffered from mental changes that impacted her ability to communicate effectively.

Late Effects: R.M. developed panhypopituitarism, requiring management with DDAVP (for diabetes insipidus), prednisone (for cortisol deficiency), thyroxine (for hypothyroidism), growth hormone (for adult growth hormone deficiency) and estrogen (for gonadotrophin deficiency). She has also developed type II diabetes requiring management with insulin, osteopenia requiring weekly oral bisphosphonate therapy and daily calcium/vitamin D supplementation, and hearing loss requiring hearing aids (Table 26.5). The potential late effects for which R.M. remains at risk are presented in Table 26.6.

Table 26.5 Case Study 2: R.M.'s actual late effects

Current late effect	Therapeutic agent(s)	Evaluation	Intervention/counseling
Neurocognitive impairment	Cranial radiation; Neurosurgery	Neuropsychological evaluation	Referral for vocational testing and job placement if indicated; Referral for psychotherapy as indicated
Psychosocial difficulties; Psychological maladjustment; Depression	Cancer diagnosis, treatment and late effects	Yearly psychosocial assessment	Referral for counseling and antidepressant medications as indicated; *Emotional Issues* Health Link
Diabetes insipidus	Cranial radiation	Follow-up per endocrinology	DDAVP; *Hypopituitarism* Health Link
Central adrenal insufficiency	Cranial radiation	Follow-up per endocrinology	Cortisol, prednisone; *Hypopituitarism* Health Link
Hypothyroidism	Cranial radiation	Follow-up per endocrinology	Thyroid hormone replacement therapy; *Thyroid Problems* Health Link
Adult growth hormone deficiency	Cranial radiation	Follow-up per endocrinology	Growth hormone replacement therapy; *Growth Hormone* Health Link
Gonadotropin deficiency	Cranial radiation	Follow-up per endocrinology	Hormone replacement therapy; *Female Health Issues* Health Link

Table 26.5 (continued)

Current late effect	Therapeutic agent(s)	Evaluation	Intervention/counseling
Ototoxicity/sensorineural hearing loss	Cranial radiation, Cisplatin, Carboplatin	Follow-up as per otolaryngologist	Audiology referral for hearing aids as indicated; *Hearing Loss* Health Link
Obesity (with associated Type II diabetes)	Cranial radiation	Follow-up per endocrinology	Diet/exercise, insulin; *Diet and Physical Activity* Health Link
Osteopenia	Cranial radiation with resultant hypogonadism and growth hormone deficiency; autologous stem cell transplant	Follow-up per endocrinology	Calcium, vitamin D, bisphosphonates; *Bone Health* Health Link

Table 26.6 Case Study 2: R.M.'s potential late effects (for which ongoing monitoring is necessary)

Potential late effect	Therapeutic agent	Screening	Intervention/counseling
Psychosocial issues, including employment discrimination and insurance issues	Cancer diagnosis, treatment, late effects	Yearly psychosocial assessment	*Emotional Issues* and *Finding Healthcare* Health Links; Legal referral if indicated
Subsequent neoplasm (benign or malignant)	Cranial radiation; Autologous stem cell transplant	Yearly history and physical	*Reducing Risk of Cancers* Health Link
Acute myeloid leukemia or myelodysplasia	Cisplatin, Carboplatin, Etoposide, Thiotepa; Autologous stem cell transplant	Yearly CBC with differential x 10 years	*Reducing Risk of Cancers* Health Link
Dysplastic nevi/skin cancer; Dermatologic changes;	Cranial radiation	Yearly history and physical	*Skin Health* and *Reducing Risk of Cancers* Health Link
Cataracts and other ocular toxicities	Cranial radiation, Corticosteroids	Yearly ophthalmology evaluation	Sunglasses/sun-protective lenses; *Eye Health* Health Link

Table 26.6 (continued)

Potential late effect	Therapeutic agent	Screening	Intervention/ counseling
Cerebrovascular complications, including stroke and occlusive cerebral vasculopathy; Leukoencephalopathy	Cranial radiation	Yearly history and physical	Anticipatory guidance
Seizures	Cranial radiation, Neurosurgery	Yearly history and physical	Neurology evaluation as clinically indicated
Motor and/or sensory deficits	Neurosurgery	Yearly evaluation by physiatrist	Neurology evaluation; Speech, physical and occupational therapy evaluations as indicated
Hyperprolactinemia	Cranial radiation	Yearly review of systems, including galactorrhea and menstrual history	*Hyperprolactinemia* Health Link
Chronic sinusitis	Cranial radiation	Yearly history and physical	Anticipatory guidance
Xerostomia; Salivary gland dysfunction; Dental problems;	Cranial radiation	Yearly history and physical; Dental visits every 6 months	*Dental Health* Health Link
Osteoradionecrosis	Cranial radiation	Dental evaluation as indicated	*Osteoradionecrosis* Health Link
Thyroid nodules; Thyroid cancer	Cranial radiation	Yearly physical exam	*Thyroid Problems* Health Link
Carotid artery disease	Cranial radiation	Yearly history (include evaluation of memory) and physical exam	Anticipatory guidance
Pulmonary toxicity	Bleomycin	Yearly history and physical; Baseline chest X-ray and pulmonary function testing	*Pulmonary Health* and *Bleomycin Alert* Health Links

Table 26.6 (continued)

Potential late effect	Therapeutic agent	Screening	Intervention/counseling
Dyslipidemia	Cisplatin	Fasting lipid profile baseline and as clinically indicated	*Diet and Physical Activity* Health Link
Hepatotoxicity; Iron overload; Renal toxicity	Autologous stem cell transplant Cisplatin, Carboplatin	Serum ferritin at baseline and PRN Yearly BP; baseline renal function panel	Anticipatory guidance *Kidney Health* Health Link
Peripheral neuropathy	Cisplatin, Carboplatin	Neurological exam as indicated	*Peripheral Neuropathy* and *Raynaud's Phenomenon* Health Links
Osteonecrosis	Autologous stem cell transplant, Corticosteroids	Musculoskeletal exam yearly and as clinically indicated	*Osteonecrosis* Health Link

Current status: R.M. continued to gain strength following her transplant, but over the subsequent two years she suffered incapacitating cognitive adverse effects requiring assignment of power of attorney to her mother (her primary caregiver), who also handles all of her financial and medical issues. She has never been able to return to work following her recurrence.

Summary

As one can appreciate from the case studies above, survivors of brain tumors are unfortunately left with serious chronic health conditions. These late effects and other potential complications endured by brain tumor survivors require lifelong follow-up care by an experienced medical team. As adult survivors of brain tumors are typically followed by neuro-oncologists, it is critical that these specialists and their team of nurse practitioners, physician assistants and social support staff monitor not only for recurrence of the brain tumor, but also the deleterious effects on the survivor's quality of life. By utilizing the COG Long-Term Follow-Up Guidelines, practitioners can provide state–of-the-art comprehensive medical care to this complicated population of survivors.

Acknowledgments A special thank you to Jeffrey Raizer, M.D. for his assistance in writing Case Study 2.

References

1. Blaney SM, Kun LE, Hunter J, et al. Tumors of the central nervous system. In: Pizzo PA, Poplack DA, eds. *Principles and Practice of Pediatric Oncology*. 5th ed. Philadelphia: Lippincott Williams & Wilkins; 2006:786–864.
2. Sklar CA, Mertens AC, Mitby P, et al. Premature menopause in survivors of childhood cancer: a report from the childhood cancer survivor study. *J Natl Cancer Inst*. 2006;98: 890–896.
3. Howell SJ, Shalet SM. Spermatogenesis after cancer treatment: damage and recovery. *J Natl Cancer Inst Monogr*. 2005:12–17.
4. Gurney JG, Kadan-Lottick NS, Packer RJ, et al. Endocrine and cardiovascular late effects among adult survivors of childhood brain tumors: Childhood Cancer Survivor Study. *Cancer*.2003;97:663–673.
5. Cheruku R, Hussain M, Tyrkus M, et al. Myelodysplastic syndrome after cisplatin therapy. *Cancer*.1993;72:213–218.
6. Pui CH. Epipodophyllotoxin-related acute myeloid leukaemia. *Lancet*.1991;338:1468.
7. Stillwell TJ, Benson RC, Jr. Cyclophosphamide-induced hemorrhagic cystitis. A review of 100 patients. *Cancer*.1988;61:451–457.
8. Bianchetti MG, Kanaka C, Ridolfi-Luthy A, et al. Persisting renotubular sequelae after cisplatin in children and adolescents. *Am J Nephrol*.1991;11:127–130.
9. Schell MJ, McHaney VA, Green AA, et al. Hearing loss in children and young adults receiving cisplatin with or without prior cranial irradiation. *J Clin Oncol*.1989;7: 754–760.
10. Hilkens PH, ven den Bent MJ. Chemotherapy-induced peripheral neuropathy. *J Peripher Nerv Syst*.1997;2:350–361.
11. Ellis PA, Fitzharris BM, George PM, et al. Fasting plasma lipid measurements following cisplatin chemotherapy in patients with germ cell tumors. *J Clin Oncol*.1992;10: 1609–1614.
12. Mertens AC, Yasui Y, Liu Y, et al. Pulmonary complications in survivors of childhood and adolescent cancer. A report from the Childhood Cancer Survivor Study. *Cancer*. 2002;95:2431–2441.
13. Piel B, Vaidya S, Lancaster D, et al. Chronic hepatotoxicity following 6-thioguanine therapy for childhood acute lymphoblastic leukaemia. *Br J Haematol*.2004;125:410–411; author reply 2.
14. Aisenberg J, Hsieh K, Kalaitzoglou G, et al. Bone mineral density in young adult survivors of childhood cancer. *J Pediatr Hematol Oncol*.1998;20:241–245.
15. Hurel SJ, Kendall-Taylor P. Avascular necrosis secondary to postoperative steroid therapy. *Br J Neurosurg*.1997;11:356–358.
16. Kaye LD, Kalenak JW, Price RL, et al. Ocular implications of long-term prednisone therapy in children. *J Pediatr Ophthalmol Strabismus*. 1993;30:142–144.
17. Neglia JP, Friedman DL, Yutaka Y, et al. Second malignant neoplasms in five-year survivors of childhood cancer: childhood cancer survivor study. *J Natl Cancer Inst*. 2001;93:618–629.
18. Lawenda BD, Gagne HM, Gierga DP, et al. Permanent alopecia after cranial irradiation: dose-response relationship. *Int J Radiat Oncol Biol Phys*. 2004;60:879–887.
19. Reimers TS, Ehrenfels S, Mortensen EL, et al. Cognitive deficits in long-term survivors of childhood brain tumors: Identification of predictive factors. *Medical and pediatric oncology*.2003;40:26–34.
20. Matsumoto K, Takahashi S, Sato A, et al. Leukoencephalopathy in childhood hematopoietic neoplasm caused by moderate-dose methotrexate and prophylactic cranial radiotherapy – an MR analysis. *Int J Radiat Oncol Biol Phys*. 1995;32:913–918.
21. Grenier Y, Tomita T, Marymont MH, et al. Late postirradiation occlusive vasculopathy in childhood medulloblastoma. *J Neurosurg*.1998;89:460–464.

22. Kestle JR, Hoffman HJ, Mock AR. Moyamoya phenomenon after radiation for optic glioma. *J Neurosurg*.1993;79:32–35.
23. Bowers DC, Liu Y, Leisenring W, et al. Late-occurring stroke among long-term survivors of childhood leukemia and brain tumors: a report from the Childhood Cancer Survivor Study. *J Clin Oncol*.2006;24:5277–5282.
24. Kaste SC, Chen G, Fontanesi J, et al. Orbital development in long-term survivors of retinoblastoma. *J Clin Oncol*.1997;15:1183–1189.
25. Ellingwood KE, Million RR. Cancer of the nasal cavity and ethmoid/sphenoid sinuses. *Cancer*.1979;43:1517–1526.
26. Parsons JT, Bova FJ, Mendenhall WM, et al. Response of the normal eye to high dose radiotherapy. *Oncology*(Williston Park, NY). 1996;10:837–847; discussion 47–48, 51–52.
27. Johannesen TB, Rasmussen K, Winther FO, et al. Late radiation effects on hearing, vestibular function, and taste in brain tumor patients. *Int J Radiat Oncol Biol Phys*. 2002;53:86–90.
28. Guchelaar HJ, Vermes A, Meerwaldt JH. Radiation-induced xerostomia: pathophysiology, clinical course and supportive treatment. *Support Care Cancer*.1997;5:281–288.
29. Sonis AL, Tarbell N, Valachovic RW, et al. Dentofacial development in long-term survivors of acute lymphoblastic leukemia. A comparison of three treatment modalities. *Cancer*.1990;66:2645–2652.
30. Nasman M, Forsberg CM, Dahllof G. Long-term dental development in children after treatment for malignant disease. *Eur J Orthod*.1997;19:151–159.
31. Constine LS, Woolf PD, Cann D, et al. Hypothalamic-pituitary dysfunction after radiation for brain tumors. *N Engl J Med*. 1993;328:87–94.
32. Nuver J, Smit AJ, Postma A, et al. The metabolic syndrome in long-term cancer survivors, an important target for secondary preventive measures. *Cancer Treatment Rev*. 2002;28:195–214.
33. Sklar CA, Constine LS. Chronic neuroendocrinological sequelae of radiation therapy. *Int J Radiat Oncol Biol Phys*. 1995;31:1113–1121.
34. Packer RJ, Boyett JM, Janss AJ, et al. Growth hormone replacement therapy in children with medulloblastoma: use and effect on tumor control. *J Clin Oncol*.2001;19:480–487.
35. Oberfield SE, Soranno D, Nirenberg A, et al. Age at onset of puberty following high-dose central nervous system radiation therapy. *Arch Pediatr Adolescent Med*. 1996;150:589–592.
36. Livesey EA, Brook CG. Thyroid dysfunction after radiotherapy and chemotherapy of brain tumours. *Arch Dis Child*.1989;64:593–595.
37. Gleeson HK, Shalet SM. The impact of cancer therapy on the endocrine system in survivors of childhood brain tumours. *Endocrine-related Cancer*. 2004;11:589–602.
38. Schmiegelow M, Feldt-Rasmussen U, Rasmussen AK, et al. Assessment of the hypothalamo-pituitary-adrenal axis in patients treated with radiotherapy and chemotherapy for childhood brain tumor. *J Clin Endocrinol Metabolism*. 2003;88:3149–3154.
39. Hall EJ. Intensity-modulated radiation therapy, protons, and the risk of second cancers. *Int J Radiat Oncol Biol Phys*. 2006;65:1–7.
40. Carpentieri SC, Waber DP, Pomeroy SL, et al. Neuropsychological functioning after surgery in children treated for brain tumor. *Neurosurgery*.2003;52:1348–1356; discussion 56–57.
41. Sonderkaer S, Schmiegelow M, Carstensen H, et al. Long-term neurological outcome of childhood brain tumors treated by surgery only. *J Clin Oncol*.2003;21:1347–1351.
42. Cassidy L, Stirling R, May K, et al. Ophthalmic complications of childhood medulloblastoma. *Med Pediatr Oncol*.2000;34:43–47.
43. Miller JS, Arthur DC, Litz CE, et al. Myelodysplastic syndrome after autologous bone marrow transplantation: an additional late complication of curative cancer therapy. *Blood*.1994;83:3780–3786.
44. Bhatia S, Louie AD, Bhatia R, et al. Solid cancers after bone marrow transplantation. *J Clin Oncol*.2001;19:464–471.

45. Baker KS, DeFor TE, Burns LJ, et al. New malignancies after blood or marrow stem-cell transplantation in children and adults: incidence and risk factors. *J Clin Oncol.*2003;21: 1352–1358.
46. McKay PJ, Murphy JA, Cameron S, et al. Iron overload and liver dysfunction after allogeneic or autologous bone marrow transplantation. *Bone Marrow Transplant.*1996; 17:63–66.
47. Tauchmanova L, De Rosa G, Serio B, et al. Avascular necrosis in long-term survivors after allogeneic or autologous stem cell transplantation: a single center experience and a review. *Cancer.*2003;97:2453–2461.
48. Sklar C, Boulad F, Small T, et al. Endocrine complications of pediatric stem cell transplantation. *Front Biosci.*2001;6:G17–G22.
49. Oeffinger KC, Mertens AC, Sklar CA, et al. Chronic health conditions in adult survivors of childhood cancer. *N Engl J Med.* 2006;355:1572–1582.
50. Children's Oncology Group: Long-Term Follow-Up Guidelines for Survivors of Childhood, Adolescent, and Young Adult Cancers, Version 3.0. September 2008, www.survivor shipguidelines.org
51. Landier W, Bhatia S, Eshelman DA, et al. Development of risk-based guidelines for pediatric cancer survivors: the Children's Oncology Group Long-Term Follow-Up Guidelines from the Children's Oncology Group Late Effects Committee and Nursing Discipline. *J Clin Oncol.*2004;22:4979–4990.
52. Eshelman D, Landier W, Sweeney T, et al. Facilitating care for childhood cancer survivors: integrating children's oncology group long-term follow-up guidelines and health links in clinical practice. *J Pediatr Oncol Nurs.*2004;21:271–280.
53. Hewitt ME, Greenfield S, Stovall E, eds. From cancer patient to cancer survivor: lost in transition: Institute of Medicine. Washington, DC: The National Academies Press; 2006.

Chapter 27
Support Organizations, Resources and Relevent Websites

Dawn Grenier and Sarah Gupta

Introduction

The effects of brain tumors can be complex and often vary widely between individuals. Patients, survivors, caregivers, family members, and other concerned individuals need access to current and relevant information, resources, and support. The following organizations provide a wide range of services relevant to individuals coping with a brain tumor diagnosis.

Brain Tumor Resources – Adults and General

Acoustic Neuroma Association

600 Peachtree Parkway, Suite 108
Cumming, GA 30041-6899
Phone: 770.205.8211
Website: www.anausa.org

Patient-organized mutual aid group offering information and support for people who have experienced an acoustic neuroma or other tumors affecting the cranial nerves. Offers national meetings, local support networks and groups, information booklets, public education, research funding, and a quarterly newsletter.

American Brain Tumor Association

2720 River Road, Suite 146
Des Plains, IL 60018-4110
Phone: 800.886.2282, 847.827.9910
Website: www.abta.org

D. Grenier (✉)
National Brain Tumor Society, 124 Watertown Street, Suite 3H, Watertown, MA 02472-2500, USA
e-mail: grenier@braintumor.org

S. Goldman, C.D. Turner (eds.), *Late Effects of Treatment for Brain Tumors*, Cancer Treatment and Research 150, DOI 10.1007/b109924_27,
© Springer Science+Business Media, LLC 2009

Funds brain tumor research. Provides information on brain tumors, treatments, clinical trials, and quality of life issues. Offers patient conferences, an information and support phone line, and a comprehensive collection of free publications.

Brain Science Foundation

277 Linden Street, Suite 207
Wellesley, MA 02482
Phone: 866.492.2466, 781.239.2903
Website: www.brainsciencefoundation.org

Supports basic and clinical research of promising new treatments, as well as opportunities to improve the quality of patient care relevant to all primary brain tumors. Special focus on nonmalignant, primary brain tumors, especially meningiomas.

Brain Tumor Action Network

5749 Gall Boulevard
Zephyrhills, FL 33542
Website: www.btan.org

Raises public awareness about brain tumors. Educates and empowers brain tumor survivors, their families, and friends to become advocates. Raises funds to support specific research projects.

Brain Tumor Home Page – National Cancer Institute

NCI Public Inquiries Office
6116 Executive Boulevard, Room 3036A
Bethesda, MD 20892-8322
Phone: 800.422.6237, TTY: 800.332.8615
Website: www.cancer.gov/cancertopics/types/brain/

Provides information about brain tumor treatment, clinical trials, research, statistics, and other topics.

Brain Tumour Foundation of Canada

620 Colborne Street, Suite 301
London, ON Canada N6B 3R9
Phone: 519.642.7755
Website: www.braintumour.ca

Funds brain tumor research. Provides patient and family support services. Educates the public. Offers pediatric and adult patient resource guides and a quarterly newsletter.

Central Brain Tumor Registry of the United States

244 East Ogden Avenue, Suite 116
Hinsdale, IL 60521

Phone: 630.655.4786
Website: www.cbtrus.org

Collects data on primary benign and malignant brain tumors in a central database, for the purposes of accurately describing incidence and survival patterns, evaluating diagnosis and treatment, facilitating etiologic studies, establishing awareness of the disease and, ultimately, for the prevention of all brain tumors.

Florida Brain Tumor Association, Inc.

P.O. Box 770182
Coral Springs, FL 33077-0182
Phone: 954.755.4307
Website: www.fbta.info

Raises funds for medical research. Provides educational resources and support services for brain tumor survivors and families. Hosts conferences, seminars, and meetings for survivors, families, and professionals.

Meningioma Mommas

9249 S. Broadway Blvd., Unit 200-PMB#240
Highlands Ranch, CO 80129
Website: www.meningiomamommas.org

Offers an online support group for men and women affected by meningiomas.

Musella Foundation for Brain Tumor Research & Information

Clinical Trials and Noteworthy Treatments for Brain Tumors
1100 Peninsula Boulevard
Hewlett, NY 11557
Phone: 888.295.4740
Website: www.virtualtrials.com

Provides information on brain tumor treatments, with a focus on new and experimental treatments. Uses computer technology to index brain tumor clinical trials, streamline the flow of information, organize the brain tumor community, and raise money for brain tumor research.

National Brain Tumor Society

East Coast Office:
124 Watertown Street, Suite 3H
Watertown, MA 02472
Phone: 800.770.8287, 617.924.9997

West Coast Office:

22 Battery Street, Suite 612
San Francisco, CA 94111-5520
Phone: 800.934.CURE (2873)
Website: www.braintumor.org

Formed from the merger of the National Brain Tumor Foundation and
the Brain Tumor Society, this national organization brings together strong
coast to coast research and patient services in the United States and serves
as a comprehensive resource for patients, families, caregivers, researchers,
and medical professionals. Offers a telephone support line as well as online
support networks for patients and caregivers. Provides information about
treatments, clinical trials, free publications, and local support groups
nationwide. Holds national and regional conferences for patients and
caregivers.

Pituitary Network Association

P.O. Box 1958
Thousand Oaks, CA 91360
Phone: 805.499.9973
Website: www.pituitary.org

Disseminates information to patients, families, and health care providers
regarding early detection, symptoms, treatments, and resources for pituitary
tumors and disorders.

Southeastern Brain Tumor Foundation

P.O. Box 422471
Atlanta, GA 30342
Phone: 404.843.3700
Website: www.sbtf.org
Offers information, education, and support services for brain tumor patients
and their families. Raises funds for research and medical personnel so that a
cure can be found.

The Healing Exchange Brain Trust

186 Hampshire Street
Cambridge, MA 02139-1320
Phone: 617.876.2002, 877.252.8480
Website: www.braintrust.org

Offers over a dozen online support groups, helping people communicate about
brain tumors and related conditions via email to promote a healing exchange of
information and support. Trains people how to use the Internet to get information and support.

The International Brain Tumour Alliance

P.O. Box 244, Tadworth
Surrey KT20 5WQ
United Kingdom
Website: www.theibta.org

Seeks to promote collaboration and coordination between support, advocacy, and information groups for brain tumor patients and caregivers in different countries, as well as the researchers, scientists, clinicians and allied health professionals who work in the area of brain tumors.

Brain Tumor Resources – Children and Adolescents

Brain Tumor Foundation for Children, Inc.

6065 Roswell Road NE #505
Atlanta, GA 30328
Phone: 404.252.4107, 404.252.4108
Website: www.braintumorkids.org

Promotes public awareness and information, activities, family support, and educational programs. Funds research and offers a newsletter.

Childhood Brain Tumor Foundation

20312 Watkins Meadow Drive
Germantown, MD 20876
Phone: 301.515.2900, 877.217.4166
Website: www.childhoodbraintumor.org

Heightens public awareness of childhood brain tumors. Raises funds for clinical as well as basic scientific research. Enhances efforts to develop safer and more effective therapies. Serves as an advocate for children disabled by this disease.

Children's Brain Tumor Foundation

274 Madison Avenue, Suite 1004
New York, NY 10016
Phone: 212.448.9494
Website: www.cbtf.org

Raises funds for research programs and medical personnel training. Hosts monthly parent support meetings in New York City. Provides a free resource guide for parents of children with brain and spinal cord tumors.

Pediatric Brain Tumor Foundation of the United States

302 Ridgefield Court
Asheville, NC 28806
Phone: 800.253.6530, 828.665.6891
Website: www.pbtfus.org

Supports medical research and increases public awareness about the severity
and prevalence of childhood brain tumors. Aids in the early detection and
treatment of childhood brain tumors. Supports a national database on all
primary brain tumors and provides educational and emotional support for
children and families affected by brain tumors.

Pediatric Low-Grade Astrocytoma Foundation (PLGA)

98 Random Farms Drive
Chappaqua, NY 10514
Website: www.fightplga.org

Supports children, parents, and families with pediatric low-grade astrocytomas
(PLGA's). Funds education and innovative research targeted at children's
brain tumors or PLGAs.

Cancer Resources – Adults and General

American Cancer Society

National Headquarters
1559 Clifton Road, N.E.
Atlanta, GA 30329
Phone: 404.320.3333
Website: www.cancer.org

Focuses on preventing cancer, saving lives, and diminishing suffering from
cancer through the support of research, up-to-date cancer diagnosis and treatment information, advocacy and public policy, and community programs and
services.

Association of Cancer Online Resources

173 Duane Street, Suite 3A
New York, NY 10013-3334
Phone: 212.226.5525
Website: www.acor.org

Offers cancer-related information and support through online discussion
groups.

Cancer Care, Inc.

275 Seventh Avenue, 22nd floor
New York, NY 10001
Phone: 800.813.HOPE (4673), 212.712.8400
Website: www.cancercare.org

Provides free, professional support services for anyone affected by cancer.

Cancer Hope Network

2 North Road – Suite A
Chester, NJ 07930
Phone: 877.467.3638, 908.879.4039
Website: www.cancerhopenetwork.org

Offers free and confidential one-on-one support to cancer patients and their families
by matching cancer patients and/or family members with trained volunteers who
themselves have undergone and recovered from a similar cancer experience.

Cancer Survivors Network

Website: www.acscsn.org

An online community of cancer survivors, families, and friends, created and run
by the American Cancer Society. The website provides a private, secure way to
find and communicate with others who share your interests and experiences.

Fertile Hope

65 Broadway, Suite 603
New York, NY 10006
Phone: 888.994.HOPE (4673)
Website: www.fertilehope.org

Provides information and support for cancer patients faced with infertility.

Gilda's Club Worldwide

322 Eighth Avenue, Suite 1402
New York, NY 10001
Phone: 888.GILDA.4.U, 917.305.1200
Website: www.gildasclub.org

Offers nationwide support and networking groups, lectures, workshops and
social events where cancer patients, their family members, and friends can plan
and build life-changing emotional and social support networks.

Lance Armstrong Foundation

P.O. Box 161150
Austin, TX 78716-1150
Phone: 866.235.7205, 512.236.8820
Website: www.livestrong.org

Provides practical information, resources, and support for people living with a cancer diagnosis. Major areas of focus include education, advocacy, public health, and research.

National Cancer Institute

NCI Public Inquiries Office
6116 Executive Boulevard, Room 3036A
Bethesda, MD 20892-8322
Phone: 800.422.6237, TTY: 800.332.8615
Website: www.cancer.gov

The National Institute of Health's principal agency for cancer research. Offers consumer-oriented information on a wide range of topics as well as comprehensive descriptions of research programs and clinical trials.

National Coalition for Cancer Survivorship

1010 Wayne Avenue, Suite 770
Silver Spring, MD 20910
Phone. 301.650.9127
Website: www.canceradvocacy.org

Provides support and information to cancer survivors.

People Living With Cancer

American Society of Clinical Oncology
1900 Duke Street, Suite 200
Alexandria, VA 22314
Phone: 888.651.3038, 703.519.2927
Website: www.plwc.org

A patient information website, presented by The American Society of Clinical Oncology, that provides timely, oncologist-approved information to help patients and families make informed health care decisions.

The Wellness Community

919 18th Street, NW, Suite 54
Washington, DC 20006
Phone: 888.793.9355, 202.659.9709
Website: www.thewellnesscommunity.org

Provides free support and education to people with cancer and their loved ones. Offers professionally led support groups, educational workshops, nutrition and exercise programs, and mind/body classes to people affected by cancer in locations throughout the world.

Cancer Resources – Children and Adolescents

Candlelighters Childhood Cancer Foundation

P.O. Box 498
Kensington, MD 20895-0498
Phone: 800.366.2223, 301.962.3520
Website: www.candlelighters.org

Provides information and awareness for children and adolescents with cancer and their families, advocates for their needs, and supports medical research.

Children's Cancer Association

433 NW 4th Avenue, Suite 100
Portland, OR 97209
Phone: 503.244.3141
Website: www.childrenscancerassociation.org

Offers child-centered programs and provides information, advocacy, and support for families who have a child with cancer or other life-threatening illness. While many of their programs are based in the northwest United States, they serve as a resource link to other programs and organizations across the country. Distributes the *Kid's Cancer Pages*, a national resource guide relating to all aspects of pediatric cancer, free of charge to patients and families.

CureSearch

National Childhood Cancer Foundation
4600 East West Highway, Suite 600
Bethesda, MD 20814-3457
Children's Oncology Group
Research Operations Center
440 E. Huntington Drive, Suite 400
Arcadia, CA 91006-3776
Phone: 800.458.6223
Website: www.curesearch.org

Provides information on childhood cancer and treatments, including side effects and survivorship issues. Focuses on research, patient care, public awareness, and fund-raising. Made possible through the combined efforts of the National Childhood Cancer Foundation and the Children's Oncology Group.

Group Loop

The Wellness Community
National Office – ATTN: grouploop
919 18th Street, NW, Suite 54

Washington, DC 20006
Phone: 888.793.WELL (9355), 202.659.9709
Website: www.grouploop.org

Offered by The Wellness Community, this program provides online information and support for teens with cancer and their parents.

National Children's Cancer Society

1015 Locust, Suite 600
St. Louis, MO 63101
Phone: 800.5.FAMILY, 314.241.1600
Website: www.nationalchildrenscancersociety.com

Provides financial assistance, emotional support, advocacy, and educational
information to children with cancer and their families.

Related Conditions/Resources

ABLEDATA

8630 Fenton Street, Suite 930
Silver Spring, MD 20910
Phone: 800.227.0216, TT: 301.608.8912
Website: www.abledata.com

Provides objective information about assistive technology products and rehabilitation equipment available from domestic and international sources.

American Physical Therapy Association

1111 North Fairfax Street
Alexandria, VA 22314-1488
Phone: 800.999.APTA (2782), 703.684.APTA (2782), TDD: 703.683.6748
Website: www.apta.org

A national professional organization representing more than 66,000 members.
Its goal is to foster advancements in physical therapy practice, research, and
education.

American Speech-Language-Hearing Association

10801 Rockville Pike
Rockville, MD 20852
Phone: 800.498.2071 (Members), 800.638.8255 (Non-Members)
Website: www.asha.org

A professional, scientific, and credentialing association for audiologists,
speech-language pathologists, and speech, language, and hearing scientists.

Aphasia Hope Foundation

2436 West 137th St.
Leawood, KS 66224
Phone: 866.449.5804, 913.402.8306
Website: www.aphasiahope.org

Promotes research into the prevention and cure of aphasia, and works to ensure that all survivors of aphasia and their caregivers are aware of and have access to the best possible treatments available.

Brain Injury Association of America

8201 Greensboro Drive, Suite 611
McLean, VA 22102
Phone: 800.444.6443, 703.761.0750
Website: www.biausa.org

Provides information, education, and support to assist people with traumatic brain injury and their families.

Cushing's Support and Research Foundation

65 E. India Row, #22B
Boston, MA 02110
Phone: 617.723.3674
Website: www.csrf.net

Provides support to patients with Cushing's and their families. Offers information for patients on the medical aspects of Cushing's via newsletters and brochures and puts Cushing's patients in contact with other Cushing's patients.

Epilepsy Foundation

8301 Professional Place
Landover, MD 20785
Phone: 800.332.1000
Website: www.epilepsyfoundation.org

Works to ensure that people with seizures are able to participate in all life experiences. Seeks to prevent, control, and cure epilepsy through research, education, advocacy and services.

Hydrocephalus Association

870 Market Street, Suite 705
San Francisco, CA 94102
Phone: 888.598.3789, 415.732.7040
Website: www.hydroassoc.org

Provides support, education, and advocacy for anyone dealing with the complex issues of hydrocephalus. Works to ensure that families and individuals diagnosed with hydrocephalus receive personal support, educational materials, and ongoing quality health care.

National Aphasia Association

350 Seventh Avenue, Suite 902
New York, NY 10001
Phone: 800.922.4622
Website: www.aphasia.org

Promotes public education, research, rehabilitation, and support services to assist people with aphasia and their families.

National Ataxia Foundation

2600 Fernbrook Lane, Suite 119
Minneapolis, MN 55447
Phone: 763.553.0020
Website: www.ataxia.org

Improves the lives of people affected by ataxia through support, education, and research.

National Institute on Deafness and Other Communication Disorders

31 Center Drive, MSC 2320
Bethesda, MD 20892-2320
Phone: 800.241.1044, TTY: 800.241.1055
Website: www.nidcd.nih.gov

One of the Institutes that comprise the National Institutes of Health. Responsible for conducting and supporting biomedical and behavioral research, as well as research training in the normal and disordered processes of hearing, balance, smell, taste, voice, speech, and language. The Institute also conducts and supports research and research training related to disease prevention and health promotion; addresses special biomedical and behavioral problems associated with people who have communication impairments or disorders, and supports efforts to create devices which substitute for lost or impaired sensory and communication function.

Neurofibromatosis, Inc.

P.O. Box 18246
Minneapolis, MN 55418
Phone: 800.942.6825, 301.918.4600
Website: www.nfinc.org

Provides a community of support for those affected by NF through education, advocacy, coalitions, the raising of public awareness, and the support of research for treatments and a cure.

Other Resources

Caregiver.com

3005 Greene Street
Hollywood, FL 33020
Phone: 800.829.2734, 954.893.0550
Website: www.caregiver.com

Provides information, support, and guidance for family and progessional caregivers. Offers *Today's Caregiver* magazine, dedicated to caregivers, the "Sharing Wisdom Caregivers Conferences," and a website which includes topic-specific newsletters, online discussion lists, back issue articles of *Today's Caregiver* magazine, and chat rooms.

Centers for Medicare and Medicaid Services

7500 Security Boulevard
Baltimore, MD 21244
Phone: Medicare Service Center – 800.633.4227, TTY: 877.486.2048
Social Security, Disability Issues, or Supplemental Security Income – 800.772.1213
Website: www.cms.hhs.gov

The federal agency responsible for administering Medicare, Medicaid, SCHIP (State Children's Health Insurance), HIPAA (Health Insurance Portability and Accountability Act), CLIA (Clinical Laboratory Improvement Amendments), and several other health care-related programs.

Children's Hospice International

1101 King Street, Suite 360
Alexandria, VA 22314
Phone: 800.242.4453, 703.684.0330
Website: www.chionline.org

Provides education, training, and technical assistance to those who care for children with life-threatening conditions and the children's families.

DisabilityInfo.gov

Phone: 800.FED.INFO (800.333.46360), Voice and TTY
Website: www.disabilityinfo.gov

The federal government's one-stop website for people with disabilities, their families, employers, veterans, workforce professionals and many others.

Family Caregiver Alliance

180 Montgomery Street, Suite 1100
San Francisco, CA 94104
Phone: 800.445.8106, 415.434.3388
Website: www.caregiver.org

Provides education, services, research, and advocacy for families and friends caring for loved ones at home.

Hill-Burton Program

Phone: 800.638.0742, Maryland Residents: 800.492.0359
Website: www.hrsa.gov/hillburton/

A program administered by the Department of Health and Human Services. Provides federal funds to hospitals for construction or modernization. In return, these facilities provide a specific amount of free or below-cost health care services to people with low incomes. Eligibility standards vary between facilities and are based on income and family size.

National Center for Complementary and Alternative Medicine

NCCAM Clearinghouse
P.O. Box 7923
Gaithersburg, MD 20898
Phone: 888.644.6226, International: 301.519.3153, TTY: 866.464.3615
Website: nccam.nih.gov

The United States government's lead agency for scientific research on Complementary and Alternative Medicine (CAM).

National Hospice and Palliative Care Organization

1700 Diagonal Road, Suite 625
Alexandria, VA 22314
Phone: 800.658.8898, 703.837.1500
Website: www.nhpco.org

Advocates for the terminally ill and their families; develops public and professional educational programs and materials to enhance understanding and availability of hospice and palliative care; convenes frequent meetings and symposia on emerging issues; provides technical informational resources to its membership; conducts research; monitors Congressional and regulatory activities, and works closely with other organizations that share an interest in end-of-life care.

National Institute of Neurological Disorders and Stroke

NIH Neurological Institute
P.O. Box 5801
Bethesda, MD 20824
Phone: 800.352.9424, TTY: 301.496.5751
Website: www.ninds.nih.gov

A branch of the National Institutes of Health. Responsible for conducting and supporting research on brain and nervous system disorders. Provides information on neurological and neurodevelopment disorders.

National Library of Medicine

Reference and Web Services
8600 Rockville Pike
Bethesda, MD 20894
Phone: 888.346.3656, Local and International: 301.594.5983, TDD: 800.735.2258
Website: www.nlm.nih.gov

The world's largest medical library, containing materials in all areas of biomedicine and health care, as well as works on biomedical aspects of technology, the humanities, and the physical, life, and social sciences.

National Organization for Rare Disorders

55 Kenosia Avenue
PO Box 1968
Danbury, CT 06813-1968
Phone: 203.744.0100, 800.999.6673 (voicemail only), TDD: 203.797.9590
Website: www.rarediseases.org

A group of voluntary health organizations dedicated to helping people with rare "orphan" diseases and assisting the organizations that serve them. NORD is committed to the identification, treatment, and cure of rare disorders through education, advocacy, research, and service.

RadiologyInfo

Website: www.radiologyinfo.org

Public information website developed and funded by the American College of Radiology (ACR) and the Radiological Society of North America (RSNA). Established to inform and educate the public about radiologic procedures and the role of radiologists in health care, and to improve communications between physicians and their patients.

Index

Note: Page numbers for entries occurring in tables are suffixed with a "t".

Printed in the United States of America